Handbook of Neuroanesthesia

Third Edition

Handbook of Neuroanesthesia

Third Edition

Editors

Philippa Newfield, M.D.
California Pacific Medical Center;
Department of Anesthesiology
University of California San Francisco
San Francisco, California

James E. Cottrell, M.D.
Department of Anesthesiology
State University of New York
Health Science Center at Brooklyn
College of Medicine
Brooklyn, New York

Foreword by
Thomas Herrick Milhorat, M.D.
Professor and Chairman
Department of Neurosurgery
State University of New York
Health Science Center at Brooklyn
College of Medicine
Brooklyn, New York

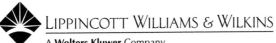
LIPPINCOTT WILLIAMS & WILKINS
A **Wolters Kluwer** Company
Philadelphia · Baltimore · New York · London
Buenos Aires · Hong Kong · Sydney · Tokyo

Acquisitions Editor: R. Craig Percy
Developmental Editor: Sonya L. Seigafuse
Production Editor: Emily Harkavy
Manufacturing Manager: Kevin Watt
Cover Illustrator: Kevin Kall
Compositor: The PRD Group, Inc.
Printer: R.R. Donnelley, Crawfordsville

© **1999, by LIPPINCOTT WILLIAMS & WILKINS**
227 East Washington Square
Philadelphia, PA 19106-3780 USA
LWW.com

Printed in the USA

Library of Congress Cataloging-in-Publication Data

Handbook of neuroanesthesia / edited by Philippa Newfield, James E. Cottrell ; foreword by Thomas Herrick Milhorat.—3rd ed.
    p. cm.
    Includes bibliographical references and index.
    ISBN 0-7817-1607-1
    1. Anesthesia in neurology Handbooks, manuals, etc. 2. Nervous system—Surgery—Complications Handbooks, manuals, etc.
I. Newfield, Philippa. II. Cottrell, James E.
III. Neuroanesthesia.
    [DNLM: 1. Anesthesia. 2. Nervous System—surgery. WO 200 H2358 1999]
RD87.3.N47H36 1999
617.9′6748—dc21
DNLM/DLC
for Library of Congress   99-22923
                                                                CIP

10 9 8 7 6 5 4 3 2 1

To my Neurological Anesthesia Residents and Fellows who have contributed to improving care for patients having neurosurgery and neurosurgical critical care.

Anthony Abadia, M.D.
Elisabeth Abramowicz, M.D.
David Acosta, M.D.
Edwarda Amadeu, M.D.
Pedro Amorim, M.D.
Audrée A. Bendo, M.D.
Jean Booning, M.D.
Jean G. Charchaflieh, M.D.
Elie Fried, M.D.
Bhagwandas Gupta, M.D.
Pavel Illner, M.D.
Michael Kittay, M.D.
Brad Litwak, M.D.
Michael Mendeszoon, M.D.
James K. Ohn, M.D.
Janet Pittman, M.D.
Lesly Pompy, M.D.
Andrew Robustelli, M.D.
Hector Torres, M.D.

And to our teachers and colleagues, who have led the way and supported us in our endeavors.

James E. Cottrell, M.D.
Philippa Newfield, M.D.

Contents

I. General Considerations

II. Anesthetic Management

III. Intensive Care

Contributing Authors

Steven J. Allen, M.D. *Medical Director, Neurointensive Care Unit, Hermann Hospital; Professor, Department of Anesthesiology, The University of Texas–Houston Medical School, Houston, Texas*

Audrée A. Bendo, M.D., M.P.H. *Associate Professor of Anesthesiology, Department of Anesthesiology, State University of New York Health Science Center at Brooklyn College of Medicine, Brooklyn, New York*

Paolo Bolognese, M.D. *Department of Neurosurgery, State University of New York Health Science Center at Brooklyn College of Medicine, Brooklyn, New York*

Jean G. Charchaflieh, M.D. *Assistant Professor of Anesthesiology and Critical Care, Department of Anesthesiology, State University of New York Health Science Center at Brooklyn College of Medicine, Brooklyn, New York*

Daniel J. Cole, M.D. *Professor of Anesthesiology, Department of Anesthesiology, Loma Linda University School of Medicine, Loma Linda, California*

James E. Cottrell, M.D. *Professor and Chairman, Department of Anesthesiology, State University of New York Health Science Center at Brooklyn College of Medicine, Brooklyn, New York*

Gregory Crosby, M.D. *Associate Professor, Department of Anesthesia, Harvard Medical School, Brigham and Women's Hospital, Boston, Massachusetts*

Deborah J. Culley, M.D. *Instructor, Department of Anesthesia, Harvard Medical School, Brigham and Women's Hospital, Boston, Massachusetts*

Timothy R. Deer, M.D. *Director of Pain Medicine, Center for Pain Relief, Charleston, West Virginia*

Karen B. Domino, M.D., M.P.H. *Professor of Anesthesiology, Adjunct Professor of Neurological Surgery, University of Washington School of Medicine, Seattle, Washington*

Elie Fried, M.D. *Clinical Associate Professor of Anesthesiology, State University of New York Health Science Center at Brooklyn College of Medicine, Brooklyn, New York*

Adrian W. Gelb, M.B., Ch.B., D.A., F.R.C.P.C. *Professor and Chair, Department of Anaesthesia, The University of Western Ontario; Chief of Anaesthesia, London Health Sciences Centre, London, Ontario, Canada*

Joseph P. Giffin, M.D.   *Professor of Clinical Anesthesiology, State University of New York Health Science Center at Brooklyn College of Medicine, Brooklyn, New York*

Wiebke Gogarten, M.D.   *Fellow, Klinik und Poliklinik für Anästhesiologie und Operative Intensivmedizin, West Fälische Wilhelms Universität, Münster, Germany*

Rukaiya K. A. Hamid, M.B.B.S., F.F.A.R.C.S., M.D.   *Attending Anesthesiologist, Children's Hospital of Los Angeles; Associate Professor of Anesthesiology, University of Southern California, Los Angeles, California*

Ian A. Herrick, B.S., M.D., F.R.C.P.C.   *Associate Professor, Department of Anaesthesia, London Health Sciences Centre, London, Ontario, Canada*

Rosemary Hickey, M.D.   *Professor of Anesthesiology, Department of Anesthesiology, The University of Texas Health Science Center at San Antonio, San Antonio, Texas*

Shailendra Joshi, M.D.   *Department of Anesthesiology, College of Physicians and Surgeons of Columbia University, The Presbyterian Hospital Medical Center, New York, New York*

Ira S. Kass, Ph.D.   *Professor of Anesthesiology, Departments of Anesthesiology, Physiology, and Pharmacology, State University of New York Health Science Center at Brooklyn College of Medicine, Brooklyn, New York*

Arthur M. Lam, M.D.   *Professor of Anesthesiology and Neurosurgery, Department of Anesthesiology, University of Washington School of Medicine; Harborview Medical Center, Seattle, Washington*

Linda L. Liu, M.D.   *Assistant Clinical Professor, Department of Anesthesia and Perioperative Care, University of California San Francisco, San Francisco, California*

Pirjo Helen Manninen, M.D., F.R.C.P.C.   *Associate Professor, University of Toronto; Department of Anesthesia, The Toronto Hospital, Western Division, Toronto, Ontario, Canada*

M. Jane Matjasko, M.D.   *Martin Helrich Professor and Chairman, Department of Anesthesiology, University of Maryland, Baltimore, Maryland*

Philippa Newfield, M.D.   *Attending Anesthesiologist, California Pacific Medical Center; Assistant Clinical Professor of Anesthesia and Neurosurgery, University of California, San Francisco, San Francisco, California*

C. Lee Parmley, M.D., J.D. *Associate Professor of Anesthesiology, Department of Anesthesiology, The University of Texas–Houston Medical School, Houston, Texas*

Patricia H. Petrozza, M.D. *Associate Professor of Anesthesiology, Department of Anesthesiology, Wake Forest University School of Medicine, Baptist Medical Center, Winston-Salem, North Carolina*

Janet Pittman, M.D. *Department of Anesthesiology, State University of New York Health Science Center at Brooklyn College of Medicine, Brooklyn, New York*

Patrick A. Ravussin, M.D. *Professor of Medicine, Departement D'Anesthesiologie et de Reanimation, Hôpital Regional, Sion, Switzerland*

Takefumi Sakabe, M.D. *Professor of Anesthesiology, Department of Anesthesiology–Resuscitology, Yamaguchi University Hospital, Ube, Yamaguchi, Japan*

Gary R. Stier, M.D. *Associate Professor of Anesthesiology; Head, Section of Critical Care, Department of Anesthesiology, Loma Linda University School of Medicine, Loma Linda, California*

Concezione Tommasino, M.D. *Assistant Professor of Anesthesiology, Department of Anesthesiology, University of Milano–San Raffaele Hospital, Milano, Italy*

Roger E. Traill, M.B., B.S., F.A.N.Z.C.A. *Doctor, Department of Anesthetics, Royal Prince Alfred Hospital, Camperdown, New South Wales, Australia*

Hugo Van Aken, M.D., Ph.D. *Professor and Chairman of Anesthesiology, Klinik und Poliklinik für Anästhesiologie und Operative Intensivmedizin, West Fälische Wilhelms Universität, Münster, Germany*

O. H. G. Wilder-Smith, M.D., M.B., Ch.B. *Director, Nociception Research Group, Bern University, Bern, Switzerland*

David J. Wlody, M.D. *Clinical Associate Professor of Anesthesiology, Department of Anesthesiology, State University of New York Health Science Center at Brooklyn College of Medicine, Brooklyn, New York*

William L. Young, A.B., M.D. *Professor of Anesthesiology, Neurological Surgery, and Radiology, Department of Anesthesiology, College of Physicians and Surgeons of Columbia University, The Presbyterian Hospital Medical Center, New York, New York*

Foreword

I confess to a certain fondness for small medical books, such as Zachary Cope's *The Early Diagnosis of the Acute Abdomen,* that are easy to read and authoritative and to which one returns repeatedly for information and guidance. The third edition of *Handbook of Neuroanesthesia* fulfills these criteria. It is a credit to the editors that a variety of specialists merged their expertise to author such a valuable handbook.

In recent years, the discipline of neuroanesthesia has evolved rapidly as advances in the basic sciences, coupled with improvements in neurosurgical technique and supportive management, have made it possible to treat increasingly complex disorders of the brain and spinal cord. More than a mere subspecialty of anesthesia, neuroanesthesia has become a core subject of the neurosciences with links extending from the laboratory to the bedside. As horizons expand, it is interesting to observe the increasing role of neuroanesthesiologists in pain management, neural monitoring, and intensive care. But it is in the operating room where neuroanesthesiologists and neurosurgeons are most at home. For nearly two decades, it has been my privilege and good fortune to work closely with one of the handbook's editors. I have learned much over the years, and have come to appreciate that continuing advances in neurosurgery would not be possible without excellence and parallel achievements in neuroanesthesia.

Readers of the second edition will welcome the third. While retaining the style that made the previous edition so popular, the text has been extensively revised and updated to include new chapters on preoperative evaluation, postoperative pain management, neuroendocrine procedures, epilepsy surgery, disruption of the blood–brain barrier, neurosurgery and the pregnant patient, induced hypotension, nutritional support, and head injury. These and other chapters represent the best efforts of a distinguished group of authors. *Handbook of Neuroanesthesia* has been skillfully edited to provide a comprehensive review of the art and science of neuroanesthesia that solidifies its place as a standard reference on the subject.

Thomas Herrick Milhorat, M.D.

Preface

In keeping with the editors' original goal of providing a current synopsis of clinical neuroanesthesia and its scientific foundations, the third edition of *Handbook of Neuroanesthesia* updates previous chapters and adds new chapters on epilepsy surgery, monitoring modalities, interventional neuroradiology, treatment of acute and chronic pain, and nutrition and energy balance—all presented in a more accessible and convenient format.

Several practices advocated in the first edition of this handbook have become routine aspects of neuroanesthetic management over the ensuing decade. For example, children are now more likely to be monitored for the effects of anesthetics on cerebral and spinal cord pathophysiology, and the same anesthetic judgments and precautions exercised in operating rooms are now observed in locations where neurodiagnostic and neurotherapeutic procedures are performed.

These kinds of advances would not have been possible without the intellectual curiosity and uncompromising resolve of physicians who have worked to improve the treatment of neurosurgical patients. We acknowledge all anesthesiologists who devote much of their careers to teaching and practicing safe and enlightened neuroanesthesiology, especially those who have so generously contributed to this volume.

We also express our appreciation for the cooperation and support of the neurosurgeons, neuroradiologists, neuropathologists, neurointensivists, and neurophysiologists with whom we enjoy a close working relationship. Consultation, collaboration, and communication among specialists is critically important to the excellent care that neurosurgical patients receive today.

James E. Cottrell, M.D.
Philippa Newfield, M.D.

General Considerations

1

Physiology and Metabolism of the Brain and Spinal Cord

Ira S. Kass

I. **Brain and spinal cord physiology.** In order to understand the effects of anesthesia and surgery on the nervous system, one needs to know basic cellular neurophysiology as well as organ level physiologic function. In this section we provide a brief description of the basic principles of neurophysiology.

   A. **Cellular neurophysiology.** The basic properties of neuronal excitability are due to a change in the membrane potential such that a threshold is reached and the neuron fires an action potential. This propagates to the axon terminal and releases a neurotransmitter that influences the membrane potential of a second neuron.

   1. Membrane potentials are voltages measured across the cell membrane due to an unequal distribution of ions across that membrane. A combination of the equilibrium potential for a particular ion and the membrane's conductance (permeability) for that ion determines that ion's contribution to the membrane potential.

      a. The equilibrium potential (E) for an ion can be calculated using the Nernst equation if the intra- (for potassium K_i) and extracellular (K_o) concentration of that ion is known. For an ion with a single positive charge the equation simplifies to $E_k = -61 \log[K_i/K_o]$ at 37°C. Under normal conditions in the nervous system the equilibrium potential for potassium is approximately -90 mV and for sodium it is $+45$ mV.

         (1) The relative conductance of the neuronal membrane to different ions determines the membrane potential. This conductance (g) for the different ions varies with conditions, input to that neuron, and time. The membrane potential of a neuron at any point in time can be described by a modification of the Goldman equation:

         $$E_m = \frac{g_k(E_k) + g_{Na}(E_{Na}) + g_x(E_x)}{g_k + g_{Na} + g_x}$$

         where g_x is the conductance for ion x and E_x is the equilibrium potential for that ion. The resting membrane potential for a neuron is approximately -70 mV, which is closer to the E_k (-90mV) than the E_{Na} ($+45$mV) because g_k is much greater than g_{Na} in resting (unexcited) neurons.

2. Action potentials are regenerative changes in a neuron's membrane potential due to excitation of the neuron such that its membrane potential depolarizes past a certain threshold. During an action potential there is a rapid initial increase in the g_{Na} followed by a return to baseline and a slower increase in the g_k. These conductance changes lead to a short and rapid depolarization followed by a repolarization. This is sometimes followed by a hyperpolarization after the action potential (Fig. 1-1).

   a. The sodium conductance changes are due to opening a lipoprotein channel in the membrane that is selectively permeable to Na ions. This channel has one activation and one inactivation gate, both of which have to be in the open configuration if the channel is to allow Na through it. The rapid opening and closing of this channel are in part responsible for the brief duration of the action potential.

   b. More potassium than sodium channels are open at rest. With the action potential more sodium channels open such that the g_{Na} is greater than the g_k and the neurons depolarize. The depolarization causes a slow opening of potassium channels, increasing g_k and leading to a repolarization ($g_k > g_{Na}$). In the period after the action potential, when the Na channels have become inactivated, the increased g_k can actually cause a hyperpolarization below the resting potential; this so-called after-hyperpolarization is frequently found in neurons.

3. Synaptic transmission is how one neuron (presynaptic neuron) influences the membrane potential and thereby the action potential generation in a second neuron (postsynaptic neuron). The axon terminals of a neuron contain vesicles with neurotransmitter molecules in them. When the terminal is depolarized, voltage-sensitive Ca channels open, increasing the calcium concentration in the terminal. This increase in calcium causes the vesicles to release neurotransmitter into the synaptic cleft. The transmitter diffuses across the synapse and binds to a specific receptor on the post-synaptic neuron. Its effect on the postsynaptic neuron depends on ion channels opened or biochemical processes altered by activation of that receptor.

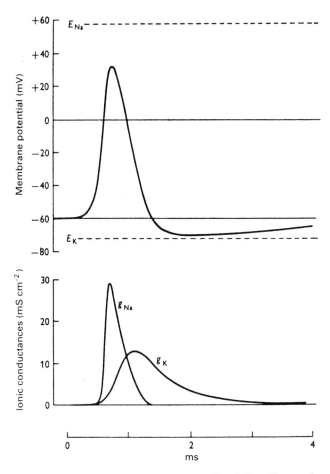

Fig. 1-1.   Changes in the membrane potential and the sodium and potassium conductances (g_{Na} and g_K) during an action potential. E_{Na} and E_k are the sodium and potassium equilibrium potentials. (From Aidley DJ. *The physiology of excitable cells.* Cambridge: Cambridge University Press, 1989:65, as redrawn from Hodgkin AI, Huxley AF. A quantitative description of membrane and excitation in nerve current and its application to conduction. *J Physiol* 1952;117:500–544)

a. Ionotropic receptor activation opens membrane channels for certain ions that can either hyperpolarize or depolarize the postsynaptic neuron, making it less or more likely to fire an action potential.

b. Metabotropic receptors can activate second messengers that alter neuronal biochemical parameters. This can effect long-term changes in a neuron's activity.

4. Glutamate is a major excitatory neurotransmitter in the central nervous system (CNS). Its activation depolarizes neurons, increasing the number of action potentials generated.

   a. There are three major ionotropic glutamate receptors: α-amino-3-hydroxy-5-methyl-4-isoxazole propionic acid (AMPA), kainate, and n-methyl-d-aspartic acid (NMDA). The AMPA and kainate receptors are attached to ion channels that allow Na and K to pass through them; a small number of AMPA receptors are permeable to calcium also. The NMDA channels are activated when neurons are already depolarized and are permeable to Na, K, and Ca. Activation of NMDA channels has been associated with long-term changes in neuronal activity that may be cellular correlates of learning and memory. Over activation of glutamate receptors has been associated with neuronal injury from epilepsy, trauma, and ischemia.

   b. Metabotropic receptors are also activated by glutamate. These receptors act via guanosine 5′-triphosphate (GTP)–binding proteins (G proteins) to affect ion channels or second-messenger pathways [e.g., cyclic AMP, inositol 1,4,5-trisphosphate (IP_3) IP_3], which in turn can alter ionic conductance, cell calcium levels, and a host of other biochemical changes. The effect of metabotropic receptor activation is of longer duration than that of inotropic receptor activation.

5. γ-Aminobutyric acid (GABA) and glycine are major inhibitory neurotransmitters in the CNS. Their activation hyperpolarizes neurons, decreasing the number of action potentials generated. Inhibition is important for the brain and spinal cord to function. When inhibition is substantially reduced, seizures may lead to complete loss of function and permanent brain damage.

   a. GABA is a major inhibitory transmitter in the brain and spinal cord. The $GABA_A$ receptor contains a chloride channel that is opened when GABA binds. This activity is augmented by benzodiazepines and barbiturates. The $GABA_B$ receptor acts via a second messenger to open K or Ca channels.

   b. Glycine is a major inhibitory transmitter in the spinal cord. Strychnine blocks the action of glycine.

6. Active transport maintains the ionic concentrations required for neuronal function. There is a constant leak of ions down their concentration

and electrical gradients. If not corrected this leak leads to a loss of these gradients. Ion pumps use energy to maintain the ion concentrations necessary for neuronal viability. During ischemia there is a decrease in energy production and a loss of ion gradients (Fig. 1-2).

a. ATP is a source of energy for many ion pumps. The Na-K-ATPase pump maintains high intracellular K concentrations and low intracellular Na concentrations. It compensates for the leak of these ions in inactive neurons and the large changes in these ions during the action potential. If this pump is blocked neurons quickly lose their ability to function. Low cytosolic Ca concentrations are

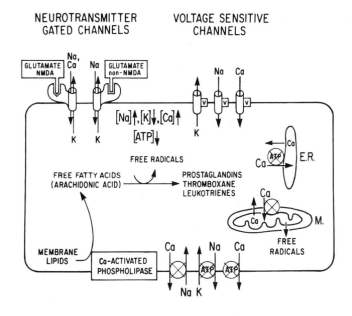

EVENTS DURING ISCHEMIA

Fig. 1-2. Effect of ischemia on ion and metabolite levels in neurons. For clarity, ion channels are shown on the top membrane and ion pumps on the bottom membrane; their actual location can be on any membrane surface. Circles indicate energy-driven pumps; an "x" through the circle indicates that this pump is blocked or has reduced activity during ischemia. "V" indicates a voltage-dependent channel. (From Bendo AA, Kass IS, Hartung J, Cottrell JE. Anesthesia for neurosurgery. In: Barash PG, Cullen BF, Stoelting RK, eds. *Clinical anesthesia*, 3rd ed. Philadelphia: Lippincott–Raven Publishers, 1997:699–746.)

maintained in neurons by ATPase pumps in the plasma membrane and the endoplasmic reticulum.
    b. The Na gradient is a source of energy for ion pumps and amino acid transporters. These active transporters couple the energy of Na going down its gradient to the pumping of other ions and metabolites against their gradients. Na–Ca exchange and Na–H exchange are important transporters maintaining appropriate cellular levels of Ca and H. The transport of glutamate and other amino acids from the extracellular to the intracellular compartment uses the energy of the Na gradient.
B. **Regional neurophysiology.** Different regions of the brain subserve different and distinct functions. We can provide only a very brief summary; for details, see the book *Principles of Neural Science* by Kandel et al.
    1. The primary somatosensory cortex located on the postcentral gyrus is the cortical locus where somatic sensations converge. Association areas that aid in the interpretation of these sensations are located posterior to this gyrus.
    2. The primary motor cortex is located on the precentral gyrus and has output to motor neurons in the spinal cord. Premotor association areas are located anterior to this gyrus and receive input from other important motor centers of the brain including the cerebellum, the basal ganglia, and the red nucleus. The reticular formation also has important motor functions.
    3. The primary visual and visual association areas are located on the occipital lobe.
    4. The primary auditory and auditory association areas are located on the temporal lobe.
    5. Wernicke's area is located on the angular gyrus in the dominant hemisphere. It is a multimodal association area. Lesions of this area are devastating and can lead to the loss of comprehension of written and spoken words.
    6. The prefrontal association areas are important for controlling personality and directing intellectual activity through sequential steps toward a goal.
    7. The limbic areas of the brain include the hypothalamus, the amygdala, the hippocampus, and the limbic cortex. These areas are associated with feelings of reward and punishment, emotional behavior, learning, and memory. The hippocampus is essential for the transformation of short-term to long-term memory. The hypothalamus controls many vegetative functions of the body such as cardiovascular function, temperature, and water regulation.
    8. The brain stem contains the reticular activat-

ing system, which is responsible for maintaining alertness. Lesions in this area can lead to coma. The vasomotor areas located in the brain stem are important for circulatory control.

9. The spinal cord is important as a pathway for information between the body and the brain as well as for the generation of certain reflexes. Input to the spinal cord comes via the dorsal root to the dorsal horn; output from motor neurons, which are located in the ventral horn, is via the ventral root. Input to the brain via the spinal cord can be modified before transmission to the brain via ascending tracts. Indeed pain input can be reduced at the spinal level via descending pathways. These pathways are activated by periaqueductal and periventricular gray regions of the brain.

II. Brain and spinal cord metabolism

A. **Energy utilization by neurons in the brain and spinal cord.** Neurons have a high metabolic rate and use more energy than their mass would account for. The brain accounts for 2% of total body weight yet uses 20% of total body oxygen consumption. Most energy-requiring processes in cells use either ATP directly or energy stores indirectly derived from ATP such as ion gradients.

1. Ion pumping accounts for a large part of a neuron's energy requirement. The Na-K pump alone accounts for 25% to 40% of a neuron's ATP utilization. Calcium and the transport of other cations (e.g., H) or anions (Cl or HCO_3) account for significant energy utilization. Some pumping of Ca and H is coupled to Na for an energy source and depletes the Na gradient; thus Ca and H are indirectly coupled to ATP utilization via the Na-K pump. In addition to pumping molecules across the plasmalemma, energy is required to pump ions from the cytosol to intracellular organelles.

2. Transport of amino acids and other essential small molecules across the cell membrane might also require energy. Glutamate and many other neurotransmitters are removed from the extracellular space by active pumps that require energy. Reduced activity of the glutamate pump can lead to excessive excitability and neuronal damage.

3. Neuronal structure and function require the synthesis of proteins, lipids, and carbohydrates. These substances are continually being formed, modified, and degraded, and ATP is required for their synthesis.

4. The transport of substances within cells also requires energy. Most synthesis takes place in the cell body and an energy-dependent transport system is used to distribute these substances to the

parts of the neuron that require them. The enormity of the task is apparent when one considers the length of the axons and dendrites of a typical neuron; diffusion is not sufficient, and active transport is required.

B. Energy synthesis by neurons in the brain and spinal cord

1. Efficient ATP production from glucose requires oxygen (Fig. 1-3).

    a. The vast majority of energy is generated by glycolysis (breakdown of glucose), the citric acid cycle [a pathway that generates nicotinamide adenine dinucleotide, reduced form (NADH) from nicotinamide adenine dinucleotide (NAD)], and oxidative phosphorylation (coupling of the regeneration of NAD from NADH to the production of ATP). The mitochondria and oxygen are critical for the efficient production of ATP from glucose. Glucose $+ 6O_2 + 38ADP + 38P_i \rightarrow 6CO_2 + 44H_2O + 38ATP$.

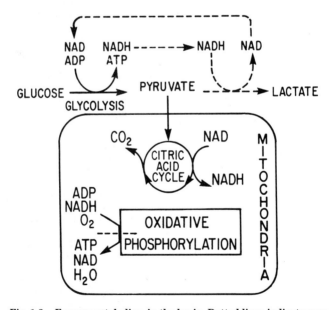

Fig. 1-3. Energy metabolism in the brain. Dotted lines indicate reactions that occur during ischemia. The dotted line across the oxidative phosphorylation reaction indicates that this reaction is blocked during ischemia. (From Bendo AA, Kass IS, Hartung J, Cottrell JE. Anesthesia for neurosurgery. In: Barash PG, Cullen BF, Stoelting RK, eds. *Clinical anesthesia*, 3rd ed. Philadelphia: Lippincott–Raven Publishers, 1997:699–746.)

b. In the absence of oxygen, the mitochondria cannot convert NADH to NAD and much of the energy of glucose oxidation is lost. Each molecule of glucose yields only 2 ATP molecules. This is insufficient to meet the energy demands of the brain. Glucose + 2ADP + $2P_i$ + 2NAD → pyruvate + 2ATP + 2NADH → lactate + 2H + 2NAD. The last step, called anaerobic glycolysis, is required to regenerate the NAD from NADH; no energy is obtained from this step in the absence of oxygen.

C. Emergency sources of energy during metabolic stress

1. There are two immediate sources of ATP when energy production does not meet the cell's demand for energy.

   a. The enzyme adenylate kinase can convert ADP to ATP. When energy production recovers, this process is reversed. ADP + ADP ⇆ ATP + AMP.

   b. Phosphocreatine (PCr) acts as a store of high-energy phosphate that can be rapidly converted to ATP. Normally there is 2 to 3 times more phosphocreatine than ATP. Nevertheless, phosphocreatine levels fall rapidly during ischemia.

   PCr + ADP + H ⇄ ATP + Cr

2. **Energy production and saving during ischemia**

   a. In addition to the formation of ATP from 2ADP or PCr, anaerobic glycolysis contributes to ATP maintenance. The latter, however, also leads to acidosis, which may be damaging to neurons. With ischemia that lasts for more than a couple of minutes, the first two processes are exhausted and the latter continues only so long as glucose is available. Some glucose is produced from the breakdown of glycogen.

   b. Shortly after the onset of ischemia (in about 30 seconds) spontaneous neuronal activity stops and the EEG becomes quiet. This reduces the neurons' metabolic rate and ATP utilization.

D. The overall metabolic rate for the brain of awake young adults is 3.5 mL O_2 per 100 g/minute or 5.5 mg glucose per 100 g/minute. This rate is virtually identical in healthy elderly persons. Children have a higher metabolic rate, i.e., 5.2 mL O_2 per 100 g/minute. The reason for the higher metabolic rate in children is unknown, but it may represent continuing growth and development of the nervous system.

III. Cerebral and spinal cord blood flow

A. Cerebral blood flow (CBF) rates are largely determined by the cerebral metabolic rate; there is exquisite coupling of blood flow and metabolism on a regional basis. The global blood flow to the brain remains fairly stable for a given physiologic state (e.g., awake adult). Anesthetics and hypothermia tend to decrease metabolism throughout the brain and thereby reduce global CBF.

1. The global CBF in adults is approximately 50 mL per 100 g/minute. This global measure is composed of flow from two very different regions: the gray matter, which is where neuronal cell bodies and synapses are located, has a blood flow of 75 mL per 100 g/minute whereas the white matter, which consists mainly of fiber tracts, has a blood flow of 20 mL per 100 g/minute. The higher blood flow to gray matter is primarily due to its greater metabolic rate.

2. The global CBF of children is approximately 95 mL per 100 g/minute and is greater than that of adults. In contrast, infants have a slightly lower CBF than adults (40 mL per 100 g/minute).

3. Spinal cord blood flow has been less extensively studied; the gray matter has a rate of 60 mL per 100 g/minute and the white matter a rate of 20 mL per 100 g/minute.

B. Regulation of cerebral blood flow

1. Regional flow–metabolism coupling is dependent on the buildup of metabolites that cause local dilatation of the microvessels.

a. The precise mechanism of this coupling is unknown. It might be due to the buildup of K or H in the extracellular fluid surrounding the arterioles. Other agents that may mediate flow–metabolism coupling include calcium, adenosine, and eicosanoids such as thromboxane and prostaglandin. A combination of the factors listed above is likely to contribute to coupling.

2. Nitric oxide (NO) is a vasodilator that is released locally by the vascular endothelial cells. It is important for vascular regulation throughout the body, but its precise role in the control of CBF remains to be determined. It is likely to be an important regulator of local CBF perhaps by affecting arterioles upstream of the microvessels dilated by metabolic factors.

3. Carbon dioxide (CO_2) enhances vasodilatation and increases CBF. It is hydrated with the help of carbonic anhydrase leading to an acidification. This reduction in pH is thought to cause the vasodilatation. When CO_2 is halved from 40 to 20 mm Hg, the CBF is reduced by approximately half (Fig. 1-4).

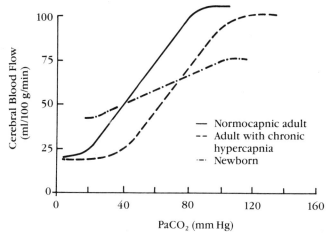

Fig. 1-4.   Relationship between cerebral blood flow and arterial carbon dioxide tension ($PaCO_2$) in the normocapnic adult, the hypercapnic adult, and the newborn.

    a. Hyperventilation leads to a reduction in CO_2, an increase in pH, and thereby a reduction in CBF. If hyperventilation is maintained over a period of 6 to 8 hours, the pH returns to normal due to bicarbonate transport and CBF returns to its pre-hyperventilation levels.

    (1) If hyperventilation is discontinued abruptly, the increase in CO_2 back to normal in the presence of reduced HCO_3 leads to acidosis and an increase in CBF above normal. This can be a critical problem when hyperventilation is used to reduce intracranial pressure (ICP) (see below).

    (2) It is possible that extreme hyperventilation to levels below 20 mm Hg can lead to relative ischemia due to vasoconstriction; the physiologic importance of this has yet to be demonstrated.

  4. Autoregulation allows CBF to remain constant if the cerebral perfusion pressure varies between 50 and 150 mm Hg. Below 50 mm Hg signs of cerebral ischemia are seen; above 150 mm Hg disruption of the blood–brain barrier (BBB) and cerebral edema might occur. The adjustment of flow to abrupt changes in pressure requires 30 to 180 seconds (Fig. 1-5).

    a. The mechanism of autoregulation is not completely understood but is likely to be a combination of effects including myogenic and metabolic factors.

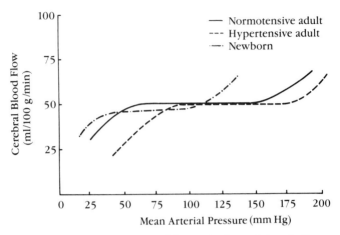

Fig. 1-5. Autoregulatory curve of the cerebral vasculature in the normotensive adult, the hypertensive adult, and the newborn.

(1) Myogenic activity of the vessel wall musculature occurs in response to increased distending pressure. In isolated vessels, when the vessel wall is stretched, as it would be by increased blood pressure, the smooth muscle contracts causing a vasoconstriction that reduces flow. This balances out the increase in blood flow due to the increased pressure and there is little net change in blood flow.

(2) The metabolic theory states that reduced pressure leads to reduced flow and the buildup of metabolites. This buildup in metabolites and the decrease in local pH lead to a local vasodilatation and thereby an increase in blood flow back to normal.

(3) Autoregulation can be impaired by hypoxia, ischemia, hypercapnia, trauma, and certain anesthetic agents.

(4) Patients who are chronically hypertensive or have high sympathetic tone have a shift in the autoregulatory curve to the right. They may demonstrate signs of ischemia due to reduced blood flow at pressures above the lower limit for normotensive individuals.

5. The partial pressure of oxygen has little effect on global CBF until it falls below 50 mm Hg. At this point there is a dramatic increase in blood flow

with further reductions in PaO_2. Since the oxygen-carrying capacity of blood is high, there may not be a critical reduction in oxygen content of the blood until the PaO_2 falls below a threshold of 50 mm Hg (Fig. 1-6).

6. Neurogenic factors also influence CBF. They have their greatest influence on the larger blood vessels. Adrenergic, cholinergic, and serotonergic systems influence blood flow.

7. The hematocrit alters blood viscosity and thereby can affect blood flow. A low hematocrit can increase blood flow by decreasing blood viscosity.

8. Hypothermia decreases neuronal metabolism and thereby reduces CBF; hyperthermia has the opposite effect.

9. Regional blood flow is regulated by the metabolic rate of neurons surrounding the microvasculature. If the activity of these neurons increases, their metabolic rate increases, and the blood flow to that region increases to meet the demand for oxygen and glucose. This property has been exploited using positron emission tomography to functionally map brain activity.

IV. **Cerebrospinal fluid and the blood–brain barrier**
    A. Cerebrospinal fluid (CSF) is formed in the choroid plexus of the cerebral ventricles (70%) and across the pial and ependymal surfaces (30%) at a rate of 0.4 mL/minute. The total volume of CSF is between 100 and 150 mL.
        1. Cerebrospinal fluid is an ultrafiltrate of plasma whose final composition is modified by active (mainly Na) and passive (most importantly glu-

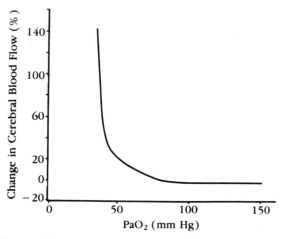

Fig. 1-6. **Relationship between cerebral blood flow and PaO_2.**

cose) transport of ions and other metabolites (Table 1-1). Proteins and other hydrophilic molecules are poorly permeable and excluded from the CSF. The capillary endothelium in the choroid plexus is freely permeable to substances. The epithelial cells of the choroid plexus contain tight junctions and are the site of the blood–CSF barrier.

   a. CSF formation is reduced by (a) decreased choroidal blood flow and capillary hydrostatic pressure, (b) hypothermia, (c) increased serum osmolarity, and (d) increased ICP.

  2. Cerebrospinal fluid flows through the ventricles and out to the subarachnoid space of the brain and the spinal cord. It is reabsorbed into venous blood via the arachnoid villi. If reabsorption is impeded, then CSF builds up and the ICP increases.

B. The blood-brain barrier (BBB) isolates the brain from substances in the plasma and is important for normal brain function.

  1. The site of the BBB is the capillary endothelial cells. They are connected to each other via tight junctions that exclude the passage of substances between them. Any substance that crosses into the brain from the blood must cross the capillary epithelial cell. The tight junctions and therefore the BBB are not present in the choroid plexus and certain other small areas of the brain (e.g., restricted areas of the hypothalamus).

  2. Water, gases, and lipophilic substances are freely permeable to the BBB. Proteins and polar (hydro-

Table 1-1. Composition of cerebrospinal fluid and serum in humans

Component	CSF	Serum
Sodium (mEq/L)	141	140
Potassium (mEq/L)	2.9	4.6
Calcium (mEq/L)	2.5	5.0
Magnesium (mEq/L)	2.4	1.7
Chloride (mEq/L)	124	101
Bicarbonate (mEq/L)	21	23
Glucose (mg/100 mL)	61	92
Protein (mg/100 mL)	28	7000
pH	7.31	7.41
Osmolality (mosmol/kg H_2O)	289	289

Adapted with permission from Artru AA. Cerebrospinal fluid. In: Cottrell JE, Smith DS, eds. *Anesthesia and neurosurgery.* St. Louis: Mosby, 1994:95.

philic) substances are poorly permeable to the BBB and only cross this barrier if there is a specific transport system for them. Glucose, ions, and certain amino acids are transported across the BBB. Since glucose is passively transported to and metabolized in the CNS, its concentration in the brain is usually 60% of its plasma level. This transport is saturable, so that large changes in glucose concentrations require time to equilibrate (Table 1-1).

V. Intracranial pressure

A. Normal ICP is approximately 10 mm Hg. Intracranial pressure is determined by the volume of the various intracranial components. Since the cranium has a fixed volume, an increase in the volume of any intracranial component must be compensated for by a decrease in the volume of another component. Otherwise the pressure in the cranium will increase.

1. There are three major intracranial components:

   a. Brain tissue represents 80% to 85% of the intracranial volume and is composed of a cellular component that includes the neurons and glia and an extracellular component consisting of the interstitial fluid.

   b. The CSF volume accounts for 7% to 10% of the intracranial volume.

   c. The cerebral blood volume accounts for 5% to 8% of the intracranial volume and includes the blood in the vascular space.

2. There is an elastance or compliance to the components in the cranium such that a small increase in the volume of one component does not cause an increase in pressure. Once this compliance is exhausted, small increases in volume lead to large increases in ICP (Fig. 1-7).

3. Increases in cranial volume can be caused by:

   a. Increases in CSF volume due to blockage of circulation or absorption of CSF.

   b. Increased cerebral blood volume due to vasodilatation (intravascular) or hematoma (extravascular).

   c. Increased brain tissue volume due to a tumor or edema.

B. Brain edema is classified as cytotoxic or vasogenic and can increase ICP.

1. Cytotoxic edema is due to swelling of the neuronal and/or glial cellular component and is frequently the result of cerebral ischemia.

2. Vasogenic edema is caused by a breakdown of the BBB. The resultant extra vascularization of protein increases interstitial water due to an increase in osmotic equivalents in the extravascular space.

C. An increase in ICP can have severe pathophysiologic consequences.

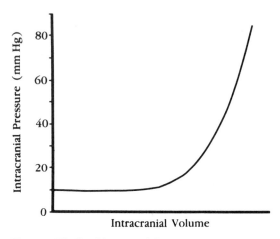

Fig. 1-7. Idealized intracranial pressure–volume curve.

1. Cerebral perfusion pressure (CPP) can be calculated by subtracting ICP from mean arterial blood pressure (MAP), i.e., CPP = MAP − ICP.

   a. As ICP increases, CPP decreases. This leads to cerebral ischemia. Normally cerebral ischemia leads to the Cushing reflex, which will increase the MAP. However, this can compensate only up to a certain point beyond which CPP will fall further, leading to severe ischemia, coma, and death if ICP is uncontrolled.

   b. Increased ICP can also cause herniation of the brain, which can lead to rapid neurologic deterioration and death (Fig. 1-7).

SUGGESTED READING

Aidley DJ. *The Physiology of Excitable Cells*. Cambridge: Cambridge University Press, 1989:65.

Albers RW, Siegel GJ, Stahl WL. Membrane transport. In: Siegel GJ, Agranoff BW, Albers RW, Molinoff PB, eds. *Basic neurochemistry*, 5th ed. New York: Raven Press, 1994:4–74.

Artru AA. Cerebrospinal fluid. In: Cottrell JE, Smith DS, eds. *Anesthesia and neurosurgery*, 3rd ed. St. Louis: Mosby, 1994:93–116.

Bendo AA, Kass IS, Hartung J, Cottrell JE. Anesthesia for neurosurgery. In: Barash PG, Cullen BF, Stoelting RK, ed s. *Clinical anesthesia*, 3rd ed. Philadelphia: Lippincott–Raven Publishers, 1997:699–746.

Dingledine R, McBain CJ. Excitatory amino acid transmitters. In: Siegel GJ, Agranoff BW, Albers RW, Molinoff PB, eds. *Basic neurochemistry*, 5th ed. New York: Raven Press, 1994:367–387.

Drummond JC, Shapiro HM. Cerebral physiology. In: Miller RD, ed.

Anesthesia, 4th ed. New York: Churchill Livingstone, 1994:689–729.

Fitch W. Brain metabolism. In: Cottrell JE, Smith DS, eds. *Anesthesia and neurosurgery*, 3rd ed. St. Louis: Mosby, 1994:1–16.

Ganong WF. Excitable tissue nerve. In: *Review of medical physiology*, 18th ed. Norwalk: Appleton & Lange, 1997:47–59.

Hodgkin AI, Huxley AF. A quantitative description of membrane and excitation in nerve current and its application to conduction. *J Physiol* 1952;117:500–544.

Kandel ER, Schwartz JH, Jessell TM, eds. *Principles of neural science*, 3rd ed. Norwalk: Appleton & Lange, 1991:81–94.

Young WL, Ornstein E. Cerebral and spinal cord blood flow. In: Cottrell JE, Smith DS, eds. *Anesthesia and neurosurgery*, 3rd ed. St. Louis: Mosby, 1994:17–58.

Effects of Anesthesia on Cerebral and Spinal Cord Physiology

Rosemary Hickey

Anesthetic treatment of neurosurgical patients must be based on knowledge of how the selected agents influence central nervous system physiology. The specific anesthetic regimen is a combination of agents that favorably affects cerebral hemodynamics, cerebral metabolism, and intracranial pressure (ICP) to provide good operating conditions and enhance the probability of a quality outcome. Most anesthetic agents have been studied in this regard and, as new anesthetic agents are developed, their effects on cerebral physiology should be elucidated. The varying effects of anesthetic agents on cerebrospinal fluid (CSF) volume (as determined by the rate of formation and resistance to reabsorption of CSF) have also been recently recognized.

Few studies, however, have addressed the effects of anesthetic agents on spinal cord physiology. This may be in part due to the fact that noninvasive methods of measuring various aspects of spinal cord physiology in the human are not available, so that most data are derived from animal studies. Although it has been assumed that the effects of anesthetic agents on the spinal cord mimic their effects in the brain (and this is likely to be qualitatively correct), in order to make true comparisons investigators must examine both brain and spinal cord parameters simultaneously. This chapter will also outline the effects of anesthetic agents on spinal cord physiology where known.

I. **Intravenous agents**
   A. **Barbiturates**
      1. **Effect on cerebral blood flow and cerebral oxygen consumption (Table 2-1).** Barbiturates were the first anesthetics to be examined for their cerebral vascular effects. Thiopental decreases cerebral blood flow (CBF) and cerebral oxygen consumption ($CMRO_2$) in a parallel fashion up to the point of an isoelectric electroencephalogram (EEG). The changes in CBF are thought to be secondary to the changes in $CMRO_2$ (a coupled decrease in flow and metabolism). At the point at which an isoelectric EEG occurs with thiopental, there is an approximately 50% decrease in $CMRO_2$ and no cerebral metabolic evidence of toxicity. If barbiturates are used clinically for the purpose of brain protection, an endpoint of EEG burst suppression is often used to provide near-maximal brain metabolic suppression. Reductions

Table 2-1. Effects of anesthetic agents on cerebral blood flow, cerebral metabolic oxygen consumption, and intracranial pressure

Anesthetic	CBF	CMRO$_2$	ICP
Thiopental	Decrease	Decrease	Decrease
Etomidate	Decrease	Decrease	Decrease
Propofol	Decrease	Decrease	Decrease
Fentanyl	0/Decrease	0/Decrease	0/Decrease
Alfentanil	0/Decrease/ increase	0/Decrease	0/Decrease/ increase
Sufentanil	0/Decrease/ increase	0/Decrease	0/Decrease/ increase
Ketamine	Increase	0/Increase	Increase
Midazolam	Decrease	Decrease	0/Decrease
Nitrous oxide	Increase	0/Increase	Increase
Halothane	Increase	Decrease	Increase
Enflurane	Increase	Decrease	Increase
Isoflurane	Increase	Decrease	Increase
Desflurane	Increase	Decrease	Increase
Sevoflurane	Increase	Decrease	Increase

CBF, cerebral blood flow; CMRO$_2$, cerebral metabolic oxygen consumption; ICP, intracranial pressure.

in mean arterial pressure (MAP) with high doses of thiopental needed to provide EEG burst suppression may require concomitant use of a vasopressor to maintain cerebral perfusion pressure (CPP). Methohexital is an exception to other barbiturates in regard to epileptiform activity in that it may activate seizure activity in patients with epilepsy.

2. **Effect on autoregulation and CO$_2$ reactivity.** Thiopental, even in high doses, does not appear to abolish cerebral autoregulation or CO$_2$ reactivity.

3. **Effect on CSF dynamics (Table 2-2).** Low doses of thiopental cause no change in V_f (rate of CSF formation) and no change or an increase in R_a (resistance to reabsorption of CSF). This would predict no change or an increase in ICP. High doses of thiopental cause a decrease in V_f and no change or a decrease in R_a (with a predicted decrease in ICP).

4. **Effect on ICP.** As a result of a reduction in both CBF and cerebral blood volume (CBV), barbiturates lower ICP. Barbiturates are used clinically for this purpose and may even be effective when other methods for lowering ICP have failed.

Table 2-2. Effects of intravenous drugs on rate of cerebrospinal fluid formation, resistance to reabsorption of cerebrospinal fluid, and the predicted effect on intracranial pressure

Intravenous drug	V_f	R_a	Predicted ICP effect
Thiopental			
Low dose	0	+, 0*	+, 0*
High dose	—	0, −*	—
Etomidate			
Low dose	0	0	0
High dose	—	0, −*	—
Propofol	0	0	0
Ketamine	0	+	+
Midazolam			
Low dose	0	+, 0*	+, 0*
High dose	−	0, +*	—, ?*

V_f, rate of CSF formation; R_a, resistance to CSF reabsorption; ICP, intracranial pressure.
0, no change; —, decrease; *, effect dependent on dose; ?, uncertain.
Adapted from Artru AA. CSF dynamics, cerebral edema, and intracranial pressure. In: Albin MS, ed. *Textbook of neuroanesthesia with neurosurgical and neuroscience perspectives.* New York: McGraw-Hill, 1997:61.

     5. Effect on spinal cord blood flow and metabolism. Barbiturates produce a significant reduction in spinal cord blood flow (SCBF). Autoregulation of SCBF is intact under barbiturate anesthesia (demonstrated with thiopental), with an autoregulatory range of approximately 60 to 120 mm Hg. Pentobarbital has been shown to produce a decrease in local spinal cord glucose utilization, although the magnitude of this effect is lower than that seen in the brain.

B. Etomidate

     1. Effect on CBF and $CMRO_2$. Etomidate, like the barbiturates, reduces CBF and $CMRO_2$. An isoelectric EEG can be induced with etomidate, and, as with thiopental, there is no evidence of cerebral toxicity as reflected by normal brain metabolites. Myoclonus produced by the drug has the disadvantage in neurosurgical patients of being misinterpreted as seizure activity. Prolonged use of etomidate may suppress the adrenocortical response to stress. However, this is not an issue in patients with intracranial tumors because they frequently are already receiving steroids. Less cardiovascular depression with etomidate compared to thiopental makes this drug advantageous for induction in the trauma patient or the older neurosurgical patient who has multiple medical problems.

2. **Effect on CSF dynamics.** Low-dose etomidate causes no change in V_f and R_a (no predicted effect on ICP). High-dose etomidate causes a decrease in V_f and no change or a decrease in R_a (predicted decrease in ICP).

3. **Effect on ICP.** Although there are no data on CBV and etomidate, the drug has been shown to reduce ICP and is clinically useful in neurosurgical patients for this purpose.

C. **Propofol**

1. **Effect on CBF and CMRO$_2$.** Propofol produces dose-related reductions in both CBF and CMRO$_2$. Mean arterial pressure reductions might be substantial in patients receiving large doses of propofol for induction. Therefore, this drug is often reserved for induction in the younger neurosurgical patient with a stable hemodynamic status. A continuous infusion of propofol may be used intraoperatively as part of a total intravenous technique, in combination with an inhalational agent, or as a substitute for an inhalational agent at the end of the case to shorten wake-up time.

2. **Effect on autoregulation and CO$_2$ response.** Propofol does not interfere with autoregulation or CO$_2$ reactivity.

3. **Effect on CSF dynamics.** Propofol causes no change in V_f or R_a (no predicted effect on ICP).

4. **Effect on ICP.** Propofol reduces ICP. Because it also reduces MAP, its effect on CPP must be carefully monitored (CPP = MAP − ICP). Continuous infusions of propofol are also useful postoperatively in the intensive care unit to provide sedation in patients with elevated ICP. The antinausea effect of propofol is advantageous in neurosurgical patients, many of whom receive moderate to large doses of narcotics which are associated with a high incidence of nausea and vomiting (retching, nausea, and vomiting might increase ICP). Careful attention must be given to sterile technique when using propofol infusions, as the solubilizing agent in which propofol is prepared provides an excellent medium for bacterial growth.

5. **Effect on spinal cord metabolism.** Propofol decreases local spinal cord metabolism in both the gray and white matter, as expressed by decreases in glucose utilization.

D. **Narcotics**

1. **Effect on CBF and cerebral CMRO$_2$.** The effects of narcotics on CBF are difficult to characterize accurately because of conflicting experimental reports. It appears, however, that low doses of narcotics have little effect on CBF and

$CMRO_2$, whereas higher doses progressively decrease both CBF and $CMRO_2$. It is also possible that the baseline anesthetic state plays a role. If a cerebral vasodilator is used as the control state to which a narcotic is added, a decrease in CBF and $CMRO_2$ occurs. If a vasoconstricting or no anesthetic is used as the control, little effect of narcotics on CBF is seen. Observed reductions in CBF and $CMRO_2$ are paralleled by progressive EEG slowing. However, burst suppression and an isoelectric EEG are never achieved. High doses of narcotics have been shown to produce seizures in laboratory animals and, rarely, in humans. Seizures have been reported from high-dose fentanyl and meperidine has the known convulsant metabolite normeperidine.

2. **Effect on autoregulation and CO_2 reactivity.** Cerebral autoregulation and CO_2 reactivity are maintained with narcotics.

3. **Effect on CSF dynamics (Table 2-3).** At low doses, fentanyl, alfentanil, and sufentanil cause no change of V_f and a decrease in R_a (predicted decrease in ICP). At high doses, fentanyl decreases V_f and causes no change or an increase in R_a (predicted decrease or uncertain effect on ICP). At high doses, alfentanil causes no change in V_f or R_a (no predicted effect on ICP), and sufentanil causes no change of V_f and no change or an increase in R_a (no predicted change or an increase in ICP).

4. **Effect on ICP.** Under most conditions, narcotics produce no change or a slight decrease in ICP.

Table 2-3. Effects of narcotics on rate of cerebrospinal fluid formation, resistance to reabsorption of cerebrospinal fluid, and the predicted effect on intracranial pressure

Narcotic	V_f	R_a	Predicted ICP effect
Fentanyl, alfentanil, and sufentanil (low dose)	0	−	−
Fentanyl (high dose)	−	0, +*	−, ?*
Alfentanil (high dose)	0	0	0
Sufentanil (high dose)	0	+, 0*	+, 0*

V_f, rate of CSF formation; R_a, resistance to CSF reabsorption; ICP, intracranial pressure.
0, no change; −, decrease; +, increase; *, effect dependent on dose; ?, uncertain.
Adapted from Artru AA. CSF dynamics, cerebral edema, and intracranial pressure. In: Albin MS, ed. *Textbook of neuroanesthesia with neurosurgical and neuroscience perspectives.* New York: McGraw-Hill, 1997:61.

However, narcotics have been shown to increase ICP under certain study conditions. For example, bolus administration of sufentanil has been shown to produce transient but pronounced increases in ICP in patients with severe head injury. Likewise, bolus administration of sufentanil and alfentanil has been shown to produce increases in cerebrospinal fluid pressure (CSFP) in patients with supratentorial tumors. Autoregulatory vasodilatation of cerebral vessels from decreases in MAP may explain the changes in CSFP. The new short-acting narcotic remifentanil may find a particularly useful place in neuroanesthesia because of its beneficial effects on ICP (no change) and its lack of accumulation, which allows prompt evaluation of neurologic function at the end of the case. The narcotic antagonist naloxone, when carefully titrated, has little effect on CBF and ICP. However, when used in large doses for reversal of narcotic effects, it may be associated with hypertension, cardiac arrhythmias, and intracranial hemorrhage.

E. **Ketamine**
1. **Effect on CBF and CMRO$_2$.** Ketamine produces an increase in CBF with no change or a slight increase in CMRO$_2$. The mechanism of the increase in CBF may be several fold: respiratory depression with mild hypercapnia in spontaneously ventilating subjects; regional neuroexcitation with a concomitant increase in cerebral metabolism; and direct cerebral vasodilatation as demonstrated by an increase in CBF during normocapnia and in the absence of changes in cerebral metabolism. Although seizures have been reported in epilepsy patients receiving ketamine, generally no epileptiform activity is seen on EEG analysis.
2. **Effect on CSF dynamics.** Ketamine increases R_a and causes no change in V_f (predicted increase in ICP).
3. **Effect on ICP.** During spontaneous ventilation, ketamine produces an increase in PaCO$_2$ and ICP (both in the presence or absence of preexisting intracranial hypertension). Increases in ICP might also occur in the presence of normoventilation. Interestingly, ketamine is a no•competitive N-methyl-D-aspartate antagonist, and in one animal model of incomplete cerebral ischemia, ketamine was shown to reduce cerebral infarct size. However, the results of this one laboratory study should not be extrapolated to the clinical arena, and ketamine is still avoided in most neurosurgical patients, particularly those with mass lesions and the potential for increased ICP.

F. Benzodiazepines

1. **Effect on CBF and CMRO$_2$.** Benzodiazepines, including diazepam, midazolam, and lorazepam, produce small decreases in CBF and CMRO$_2$, in both small and large doses. A ceiling effect on these parameters is seen, which may represent saturation of receptor-specific binding sites. As with the barbiturates, some of the CBF lowering effect of benzodiazepines is thought to be secondary to a reduction in CMRO$_2$. Electroencephalographic effects include a shift from alpha to low-voltage beta and then theta waves, although an isoelectric EEG is not produced. These agents are known anticonvulsants and are used clinically for this purpose.

2. **Effect on cerebral autoregulation and CO$_2$ reactivity.** Cerebral blood flow autoregulation and CO$_2$ reactivity are maintained with benzodiazepines.

3. **Effect on CSF dynamics.** Midazolam causes no change in V_f at low doses and a decrease in V_f at high doses. R_a is not changed or increased. The predicted effect on ICP from a change in CSF dynamics is uncertain.

4. **Effect on ICP.** Intracranial pressure effects are small with benzodiazepines, causing either no change or a slight reduction in ICP. Midazolam is commonly used as a premedication in neuroanesthesia, with small intravenous doses titrated to patient response. It may also be used as an anesthetic adjuvant, but large doses are generally avoided because of the potential for prolonged sedation. Flumazenil is a receptor-specific benzodiazepine antagonist that can increase CBF and ICP when used in large doses to reverse midazolam sedation. Seizures can also be precipitated by large doses of flumazenil.

II. Inhalational agents

A. Nitrous oxide

1. **Effect on CBF and CMRO$_2$.** Although once thought by many clinicians to be devoid of cerebrovascular effects, it is now known that nitrous oxide (N$_2$O) can cause large increases in CBF. When the effects of a 1 MAC (minimum alveolar concentration) anesthetic produced by a volatile agent alone are compared to the effects of a 1 MAC anesthetic provided by the combination of 0.5 MAC volatile agent and 0.5 MAC N$_2$O, CBF is greater in the presence of N$_2$O. CMRO$_2$ is unchanged or increased with N$_2$O. Although EEG brain activity might be increased with N$_2$O, it does not cause seizures.

2. **Effect on CSF dynamics (Table 2-4).** Addition or withdrawal of N$_2$O to the inhalational agents halothane or enflurane causes no change of V_f or R_a (no predicted effect on ICP).

Table 2-4.   Effects of inhaled agents on rate of cerebrospinal fluid formation, resistance to reabsorption of cerebrospinal fluid, and the predicted effect on intracranial pressure

Inhaled agent	V_f	R_a	Predicted ICP effect
Nitrous oxide	0	0	0
Halothane	—	+	+
Enflurane			
Low dose	0	+	+
High dose	+	0	+
Isoflurane			
Low dose	0	0, +*	0, +*
High dose	0	—	—
Desflurane	0, +[a]	0	0, +[a]
Sevoflurane	—	+	?

V_f, rate of CSF formation; R_a, resistance to CSF reabsorption; ICP, intracranial pressure.

0, no change; −, decrease; +, increase; *, effect dependent on dose; ?, uncertain.

[a] Effect occurs only during hypocapnia combined with increased CSF pressure.

Adapted from Artru AA. CSF dynamics, cerebral edema, and intracranial pressure. In: Albin MS, ed. *Textbook of neuroanesthesia with neurosurgical and neuroscience perspectives.* New York: McGraw-Hill, 1997:61.

3. **Effect on ICP.** Nitrous oxide can increase CBV and ICP in patients with mass lesions. The ICP response can be attenuated if intracranial compliance is improved or if agents that decrease CBV, e.g., barbiturates, are administered. Nitrous oxide is known to diffuse rapidly into and expand closed air-filled spaces. Pneumocephalus produced by a recent craniotomy contraindicates the use of N_2O for the repeat procedure. If a venous air embolism (VAE) occurs, N_2O increases the size of the air bubble and worsens the consequences of the air embolism. N_2O should be discontinued if a VAE occurs, and some clinicians would avoid its use altogether in procedures in which the likelihood of VAE is high, such as a sitting position posterior fossa craniectomy.

4. **Effect on spinal cord metabolism.** N_2O increases spinal cord glucose utilization, which is quantitatively similar to that produced in the brain (approximately 25%).

B. **Halothane**

1. **Effect on CBF and $CMRO_2$.** Halothane has direct vasodilatory effects that increase CBF. Regionally specific changes in CBF are seen with

halothane, with an increase in flow to the cerebral cortex and a decrease in subcortical flow. Halothane lowers $CMRO_2$, but to a lesser extent than with other volatile agents. A concentration of 4.5% is required to produce an isoelectric EEG. Significant cardiac depression is seen at concentrations greater than 2%; however, induction of an isoelectric EEG is not clinically feasible with halothane. High concentrations of halothane are also associated with a deterioration in the brain energy state, with increased levels of lactate. Unlike thiopental and isoflurane, $CMRO_2$ does not plateau at the point where an isoelectric EEG is reached with halothane but continues to decrease with increasing concentrations.

2. **Effect on cerebral autoregulation and CO_2 reactivity.** Cerebral autoregulation is attenuated with halothane and at high concentrations is abolished. The CO_2 reactivity is preserved with halothane.

3. **Effect on CSF dynamics.** Halothane increases R_a to a greater extent than it decreases V_f (predicted increase in ICP).

4. **Effect on ICP.** Halothane causes an increase in ICP when given during normocapnia or when introduced simultaneously with hyperventilation. The increase in ICP might be prevented when hypocarbia is induced prior to the introduction of halothane.

5. **Effect of spinal cord metabolism.** Halothane reduces local spinal cord glucose utilization, although the magnitude of the effect is less than that in the brain.

C. **Enflurane**

1. **Effect on CBF and $CMRO_2$.** Enflurane increases CBF and decreases $CMRO_2$. The increase in CBF with enflurane is less than that seen with halothane but more than that with isoflurane. The decrease in $CMRO_2$ is greater than that of halothane but less than that of isoflurane. One disadvantage of enflurane is its potential to cause seizure activity at high concentrations (greater than 1.5 MAC) in the presence of hypocapnia (less than 30 mm Hg).

2. **Effect on cerebral autoregulation and CO_2 reactivity.** Like other volatile anesthetics, enflurane interferes with cerebral autoregulation but CO_2 reactivity remains intact.

3. **Effect on CSF dynamics.** At low doses, enflurane causes no change in V_f and an increase in R_a (predicted increase in ICP). At high doses, enflurane causes an increase in V_f and no change in R_a (predicted increase in ICP).

4. **Effect on ICP.** An increase in ICP can occur with enflurane, as with other volatile agents. The use

of hyperventilation to attenuate this response might be limited because of the possibility of increasing the likelihood of seizure activity with low CO_2 levels.

D. Isoflurane

1. **Effect on CBF and CMRO$_2$.** Isoflurane is a cerebrovasodilator that increases CBF. Compared to halothane and enflurane, it is the least potent cerebrovasodilator and the most potent depressant of CMRO$_2$. The techniques of CBF measurement may influence the interpretation of CBF studies with the different inhalational agents. As noted above, halothane selectively increases flow to the cerebral cortex. By contrast, isoflurane causes more uniform flow patterns. Therefore, if a technique of CBF measurement is used that selectively looks at cortical flow, halothane might demonstrate a greater influence than isoflurane on CBF. If whole-brain blood flow is measured, the effects might appear more similar.

   Isoflurane is unique among the inhalational agents in that it has the capacity to induce an isoelectric EEG at a concentration that is clinically relevant because it is tolerated hemodynamically (approximately 2 MAC). At the point at which an isoelectric EEG is reached, the reduction in CMRO$_2$ plateaus. Also at this point a normal cerebral energy state is present (in contrast to halothane).

2. **Effect on cerebral autoregulation and CO$_2$ reactivity.** Cerebral autoregulation is maintained with 1 MAC isoflurane but is impaired at higher concentrations. The CO_2 reactivity is generally maintained with isoflurane, except at high concentrations (more than 2 MAC) where preexisting cerebral vasodilatation might impair the response to hypocapnia.

3. **Effect on CSF dynamics.** At low concentrations, isoflurane causes no change in V_f and no change or increased R_a (predicted no change or an increase in ICP). At high concentrations, isoflurane causes no change in V_f and a decrease in R_a (predicted decrease in ICP).

4. **Effect on ICP.** Like halothane and enflurane, isoflurane has the potential to increase ICP. Unlike halothane, however, it may not be necessary to induce hypocapnia prior to introducing the anesthetic. The simultaneous introduction of hyperventilation and isoflurane is said to prevent ICP increases.

5. **Effect on spinal cord blood flow and metabolism.** At both 1.0 and 2.0 MAC concentrations, isoflurane produces an increase in SCBF and an attenuation of autoregulation. The changes seen

at 2.0 MAC are greater for the spinal cord than for the cortex or subcortex.

E. **Desflurane**

1. **Effect on CBF and CMRO$_2$.** The effects of desflurane on CBF and CMRO$_2$ appear to be very similar to those of isoflurane. It is associated with a dose-related decrease in CMRO$_2$ and, if blood pressure is maintained, an increase in CBF. At 2.0 MAC, EEG burst suppression is seen, but it may revert with the passage of time. Desflurane has a low blood gas partition coefficient (0.4) which provides rapid titration of anesthetic depth and emergence. The pungency of desflurane is a disadvantage in neurosurgical patients if it results in coughing on emergence from anesthesia.

2. **Effect on cerebral autoregulation and CO$_2$ reactivity.** Cerebral autoregulation is impaired with concentrations of desflurane greater than 1 MAC. The CO$_2$ reactivity is maintained at desflurane concentrations between 0.5 and 1.5 MAC.

3. **Effect on CSF dynamics.** Desflurane causes no change in V_f or R_a under several conditions (normocapnia and normal or increased CSF pressure, hypocapnia, and normal CSF pressure). This would predict no effect on ICP. However, at hypocapnia and increased CSF pressure, desflurane increases V_f (predicted increase in ICP).

4. **Effect on ICP.** Desflurane produces an increase in ICP due to general cerebrovascular dilatation. Altered CSF dynamics (an increase in V_f as noted above) might also play a role in decreasing intracranial compliance with desflurane.

F. **Sevoflurane**

1. **Effect on CBF and CMRO$_2$.** Sevoflurane's effects on CBF and CMRO$_2$ are similar to those of isoflurane and desflurane. Cerebral blood flow is increased with sevoflurane secondary to cerebral vasodilatation. CMRO$_2$ is decreased and EEG burst suppression can be reached with a clinically relevant concentration of approximately 2 MAC (similar to isoflurane). There is also no evidence of cerebral toxicity with high concentrations of sevoflurane. Its relatively low blood gas partition coefficient (0.6) provides fast induction and emergence. Unlike desflurane, it is not irritating to the airway and can be used for inhalational induction (although inhalational inductions are avoided in most neurosurgical procedures because of the potential for producing hypercapnia and subsequent increases in ICP). Approximately 2% of the sevoflurane that is absorbed is metabolized, with inorganic fluoride produced as one of the metabolites. The clinical significance of the levels of fluoride that are produced is not agreed on, but

because of their potential to adversely affect renal function, low gas flow rates are avoided with sevoflurane.

2. **Effect on cerebral autoregulation and CO_2 reactivity.** Cerebral autoregulation and CO_2 reactivity are preserved with low concentrations of sevoflurane.

3. **Effect on CSF dynamics.** Sevoflurane decreases V_f and increases R_a (predicted effect on ICP uncertain).

4. **Effect on ICP.** The effect of sevoflurane on ICP is similar to isoflurane. Little or no increase in ICP has been seen at concentrations up to 1.5 MAC, both in normocapnic and hypocapnic models.

III. **Muscle relaxants**

Muscle relaxants do not cross the blood–brain barrier and thus any cerebral effects are due to secondary effects such as histamine release, systemic hemodynamic effects, effects of metabolites, or altered cerebral afferent input.

A. **Nondepolarizing muscle relaxants**

1. **Short-acting agents.** Mivacurium is a short-acting agent that is metabolized in vitro by plasma cholinesterase (at about 88% the rate of succinylcholine) and undergoes ester hydrolysis in the liver. It is commonly given by infusion because of its rapid metabolism. If large doses of mivacurium are given rapidly, some histamine release can occur. Therefore, if bolus doses are given, they should be given slowly, over a period of 30 to 60 seconds, to avoid histamine release and the potential for an increase in CBF and ICP.

2. **Intermediate-acting agents.** Atracurium causes histamine release when given in large bolus doses but has less of an effect than d-tubocurarine. It is metabolized by ester hydrolysis and Hoffmann elimination, and has the advantage that its metabolism is not altered by renal or liver dysfunction. One metabolite of Hoffmann elimination of atracurium is laudanosine, which has been shown to cause seizures in laboratory animals (although this has not been noted at the levels obtained clinically). cis-Atracurium, the newer analog of atracurium, has the advantage of not causing histamine release and is not associated with the formation of toxic metabolites.

   Vecuronium has the advantage of maintaining stable hemodynamics even when given in large doses. One possible exception is that bradycardia may be noted when vecuronium is combined with large doses of narcotics for induction, leaving the vagotonic effect of the narcotic unopposed. Vecuronium does not alter ICP or CSF dynamics (no change in V_f or R_a). Its lack of cerebral effects and its stable hemodynamics have made vecuronium a popular choice in neuroanesthesia.

Rocuronium is a new nondepolarizing muscle relaxant that has a relatively stable hemodynamic profile (weakly vagolytic) and is excreted unchanged by the biliary system and the kidneys. Unlike vecuronium, it is not associated with any active metabolites. The rapid onset of rocururonium makes it an excellent choice for intubation in the neurosurgical patient who is at risk for succinylcholine side effects but in whom rapid onset of action is desirable.

3. **Long-acting agents.** d-Tubocurarine is known to release histamine, and, when given in large doses as a bolus, decreases blood pressure and increases heart rate. This may be accompanied by an increase in CBF and ICP. Although d-tubocurarine is rarely used now for neurosurgical patients (except possibly in a defasciculating dose prior to succinylcholine), if chosen for induction or maintenance it should be given slowly, in incremental doses.

Pancuronium decreases the MAC of halothane by 25%, secondary to decreased cerebral input from paralyzed muscle spindles. Large doses of pancuronium may cause hypertension and tachycardia, which could increase CBF and ICP. These effects may not be seen when pancuronium is combined with narcotics for induction or when it is given in smaller maintenance doses.

Doxacurium, a long-acting muscle relaxant, is devoid of significant cardiovascular side effects and has not been shown to have any adverse cerebral effects. It is eliminated unchanged in the kidney and bile. Its lack of side effects and long duration of action make this agent desirable for very lengthy neurosurgical procedures.

B. **Depolarizing muscle relaxants.** Succinylcholine can cause an increase in CBF that is associated with an increase in ICP. This is secondary to increases in muscle spindle activity which increase cerebral afferent input. These effects can be blocked by prior paralysis or precurarization with pancuronium or metocurine. The changes in ICP are modest and transient, however, and may be outweighed by the benefit of rapid and reliable onset in instances when rapid control of the airway is necessary. Succinylcholine produces no change in V_f or R_a (no predicted effect on ICP). Of more concern with succinylcholine than its ICP effects in the neurosurgical patient is the exaggerated release of potassium seen with certain neurologic injuries such as closed head trauma, cerebrovascular accidents, hemiparesis, spinal cord trauma, and neuromuscular disorders.

SUGGESTED READING

Artru AA. CSF dynamics, cerebral edema, and intracranial pressure. In: Albin MS, ed. *Textbook of neuroanesthesia with neuro-*

surgical and neuroscience perspectives. New York: McGraw-Hill, 1997:61.

Marx W, Shah N, Long C, et al. Sufentanil, alfentanil, and fentanyl: impact on cerebrospinal fluid pressure in patients with brain tumors. *J Neurosurg Anesthesiol* 1989;1:3.

Pinaud M, Lelausque J-N, Chetanneau A, et al. Effects of propofol on cerebral hemodynamics and metabolism in patients with brain trauma. *Anesthesiology* 1990;73:404.

Warner DS, Hindman BJ, Todd MM, et al. Intracranial pressure and hemodynamic effects of remifentanil versus alfentanil in patients undergoing supratentorial craniotomy. *Anesth Analg* 1996; 83:348.

Young WL. Effects of desflurane on the central nervous system. *Anesth Analg* 1992:75:S32.

Neurophysiologic Monitoring

Arthur M. Lam

Patients with neurologic disease undergoing surgical procedures have an increased risk of ischemic/hypoxic damage to the central nervous system (CNS). This risk may be related to hemodynamic/embolic events associated with a nonneurosurgical operation, e.g., patients with significant carotid stenosis undergoing cardiopulmonary bypass procedures. The risk may also be inherent in the neurosurgical procedure, e.g., temporary clipping of feeding artery during cerebral aneurysm surgery.

Intraoperative neurophysiologic monitoring may improve patient outcome by (a) allowing early diagnosis of ischemia/hypoxia before irreversible damage occurs and (b) enabling surgeons to provide optimal operative treatment as indicated by the monitoring parameter. Although not universally adopted, in many centers neurophysiologic monitoring has become routine for certain surgical procedures. Broadly speaking, the brain can be monitored in terms of (a) function, (b) blood flow, and (c) metabolism (Tables 3-1 to 3-3).

I. **Monitoring of function**

   A. **Electroencephalography.** Summation of the excitatory postsynaptic potential generated by the pyramidal cells of the cerebral cortex gives rise to the electrical activity of the brain, which can be recorded as the electroencephalogram (EEG). The EEG is composed of many underlying components with different frequencies and harmonics. The component waves are typically classified according to the respective frequencies (Table 3-4). This electrical activity is volume-conducted and can be recorded from the scalp and forehead using surface or needle electrodes.

   1. **Recording techniques.** Since there is no electrically neutral area, EEG is typically recorded using a montage (electrode arrangement) with bipolar recording. Thus both electrodes are active and the polarity of the signal recorded is dependent on the arbitrary designation of the recording versus the referential electrode. Other electrical activities generated in the body such as electromyographic and electrocardiographic are minimized but not eliminated using common mode rejection, i.e., rejecting the electrical signals that are measured (common) in both recording sites in comparison to a third "ground electrode."

   The number of channels used and the placement of electrodes determine the specificity of the EEG as a monitor of the occurrence of regional ischemia. The gold standard for raw EEG re-

Table 3-1. Monitoring of function

Electroencephalogram
  Raw EEG
  Computerized processed
    Compressed spectral array
    Density spectral array
    Aperiodic analysis
  Bispectral analysis
Evoked potentials
  Sensory evoked potentials
    Somatosensory EP
    Brainstem auditory EP
    Visual EP
  Motor evoked potentials
    Transcranial magnetic MEP
    Transcranial electric MEP
    Direct spinal cord stimulation
Elecromyography
  Cranial nerve functions (V, VII, IX, X, XI, XII)

EEG, electroencephalogram; EP, evoked potential; MEP, motor evoked potential.

Table 3-2. Monitoring of flow/pressure

Cerebral blood flow
  Nitrous oxide washin
  Radioactive xenon clearance
  Laser Doppler blood flow
  Transcranial Doppler
Intracranial pressure
  Intraventricular catheter
  Fiberoptic intraparenchymal catheter
  Subarachnoid bolt
  Epidural catheter

Table 3-3. Monitoring of metabolism

Invasive monitor
  Intracerebral PO_2 electrode
Noninvasive monitor
  Transcranial cerebral oximetry (near-infrared spectroscopy)
  Jugular venous oximetry

Table 3-4. Electroencephalogram

beta	13–30 Hz: high frequency, low amplitude, dominant during awake state
alpha	9–12 Hz: medium frequency, higher amplitude, seen in occipital cortex with eyes closed while awake
theta	4–8 Hz: low frequency, not predominant in any condition
delta	0–4 Hz: very low frequency, low to high amplitude, signifies depressed functions, consistent with deep coma (cause can be anesthesia, metabolic factor, or hypoxia)

cording is 16-channel recording (8 channels for each hemisphere) with electrodes placed according to the International 10–20 system (Fig. 3-1). With the exception of monitoring in carotid endarterectomy in some centers, 16-channel EEG recording is seldom performed intraoperatively because of the relative complexity and the inaccessibility of recording sites in intracranial surgical procedures.

To simplify recording and interpretation of EEG, most EEG machines designed for intraoperative monitoring use 2- to 4-channel recording, with computer processing to simplify the output. Although different algorithms are used by different vendors, the basic premise is to filter out the high-frequency activity (likely to be artifacts or interference), typically at 30 Hz, separate the raw EEG into the component waves using fast Fourier transform, and then group them together according to their frequency spectrum. Thus raw EEG recorded in a time domain is now displayed in a frequency domain. The resultant power (square of the amplitude of the EEG wave) spectrum can be displayed in a number of ways, the most common being compressed spectral array and density spectral array, with either the peaks and valleys or the density of the gray scale representing the power of the spectrum. Aperiodic analysis is another method of EEG processing whereby each wave is tracked and plotted as a "telephone pole" with its height representing the amplitude or power of the wave.

2. **Interpretation of EEG**
   a. The EEG is random activity reflecting the state of "wakefulness" and metabolic activity. The generation of electrical activity is an energy-requiring process that is dependent on an adequate supply of substrates, i.e., oxygen and glucose. Thus significant reductions of

blood flow, oxygen, or glucose all lead to depression of EEG activity. Gradual reduction of cerebral blood flow (CBF) can be correlated with characteristic changes in EEG, and constitutes the most frequent underlying indication for EEG monitoring.

b. Awake EEG is dominated by beta activity with high-frequency and low-amplitude waves. With the onset of ischemia/hypoxia there is initially a transient increase in beta activity, followed by development of slow waves (theta and delta waves) with large amplitude, disappearance of beta activity, and, eventually, the occurrence of delta waves with low amplitude. This can progress to suppression of electrical activity with an occasional burst of activity (burst suppression), and finally to complete electrical silence with flat EEG, signaling the onset of irreversible damage.

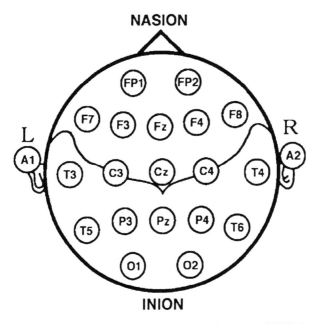

Fig. 3-1. The international 10–20 system for placement of EEG electrodes. It is based on dividing each head circumference (anteroposterior from nasion to inion over the vertex, coronal from tragus of one ear to the other) into two halves and then subdividing each half (50%) into 10%, 20%, 20% sectors. Fp, frontal pole; F, frontal; C, central; P, parietal; T, temporal; A, ear lobe; M, mastoid (not shown). Odd number subscripts denote the left hemisphere, and even numbers denote the right hemisphere.

Table 3-5.   Influence of inhalation anesthetics on electroencephalogram

Dose (MAC)	Anesthetic agents	Dominant EEG pattern
1.0	Isoflurane/enflurane/ desflurane/sevoflurane/ halothane	Beta activity at 12–15 Hz
1.5	Isoflurane	Burst suppression
	Halothane/enflurane/ desflurane/sevoflurane	Alpha/beta activity
2.0	Isoflurane	Electrical silence
	Desflurane	Burst suppression/silence
	Enflurane	Delta/theta with spike activity
	Sevoflurane	Delta/burst suppression/ silence
	Halothane	Delta/theta activity

MAC, minimum alveolar concentration.

Thus the sudden development of delta waves coincident with a surgical maneuver, e.g., cross-clamp of the common carotid artery, would provide warning to the anesthesiologist and the surgeon that the patient is now placed at risk. Because of the existence of the ischemic penumbra, where blood flow is inadequate to generate electrical activity but sufficient to maintain neuronal viability for a period of time, EEG has poor predictive power for brain damage. EEG is therefore sensitive to the occurrence of ischemia but lacks specificity as a diagnostic test for irreversible damage. In general, the quicker the onset of the ischemic EEG changes, the higher is the probability for irreversible damage.

3. **Confounding factors.** The changes in EEG seen with ischemia/hypoxia are not unique, and similar changes are seen with anesthetic-induced metabolic depression, albeit in a reversible manner. Most intravenous (with the exception of ketamine) and inhalation anesthetics cause a dose-dependent depression of EEG, and virtually all can produce a burst suppression pattern on EEG (Table 3-5). Similarly, hypothermia decreases cerebral metabolism and causes slowing of the EEG. Therefore the EEG changes should always be interpreted in concert with other physiologic variables, and not in isolation.

4. Indications for EEG monitoring

    a. All surgical procedures that potentially place the brain at risk are theoretically amenable to EEG monitoring. In practice, EEG monitoring is often difficult to perform during intracranial procedures because of lack of access to scalp recording. To a certain extent, the use of needle electrodes obviates this problem. Carotid endarterectomy, which places the ipsilateral hemisphere at risk during cross-clamp of the common carotid artery, is the most common indication for EEG monitoring. When EEG changes indicate that CBF is inadequate, the placement of an intraluminal shunt will restore blood flow.

    b. Anesthesia-induced metabolic suppression is utilized by some anesthesiologists/surgeons to provide cerebral protection during risky procedures. Electroencephalographic monitoring in these circumstances allows optimal metabolic suppression with anesthesia administered by titration to achieve burst suppression. The main indications for EEG monitoring are listed in Table 3-6.

5. Bispectral analysis.

The bispectral index is a derived EEG parameter designed not to detect ischemia but to monitor the degree of hypnosis. Based on both power spectrum analysis and phase change or coherence of the different frequencies, the value is normalized to a range of 0 to 100. A value between 40 and 60 is considered adequate hypnosis to prevent possible recall, whereas a value above 80 is consistent with impending emergence from anesthesia. Strictly speaking, this is not a parameter used to monitor integrity of the CNS. But it is derived from the raw EEG and as such is potentially influenced by the occurrence of ischemia that results in changes in the EEG. The frontal location of electrode placement, however, renders the bispectral index less sensitive to development of regional ischemia.

Table 3-6. Indications for electroencephalographic monitoring

1. Carotid endarterectomy
2. Cerebral aneurysm surgery when temporary clipping is used
3. Cardiopulmonary bypass procedures
4. Extracranial-intracranial bypass procedures
5. Deliberate metabolic suppression for cerebral protection

B. Evoked potential monitoring

1. **Sensory evoked potentials.** Sensory evoked potential (SEP) is a time-locked, event-related, pathway-specific electroencephalographic activity generated in response to a specific stimulus, e.g., electrical stimuli applied to the median nerve. The typical peaks and troughs are described by their polarity and the latency. For example, the cortical negative peak that typically occurs 20 milliseconds after stimulation of the median nerve is called N_{20}. Alternatively, it is numbered according to the sequence in which it is generated; thus, the first positive wave that occurs after posterior tibial nerve stimulation is called P1. The amplitude of evoked potential waves is small relative to conventional EEG and is not easily visualized without computer averaging of repetitive stimuli. Sensory evoked potentials are anatomically pathway-specific and theoretically only assess the integrity of the pathway monitored. The contrast between conventional EEG and SEP is summarized in Table 3-7.

   a. Sensory evoked potential can be recorded in response to stimulation of any sensory nerve, cranial or peripheral. The common modalities of evoked potentials used in clinical practice are (a) somatosensory evoked potentials (SSEPs), (b) visual evoked potentials (VEPs), and (c) brain stem auditory evoked potentials (BAEPs) (Fig. 3-2). Of these three, VEP is profoundly influenced by inhalation anesthesia, difficult to perform, and is seldom utilized as an intraoperative monitor. The SSEPs recorded in response to stimulation of

Table 3-7.   Difference between sensory evoked potential and electroencephalogram

SEP	EEG
Event-related	Random
Anatomically pathway-specific	Primarily cortical activity
Monitors integrity of the pathway	Monitors cortex only
Small amplitude	Large amplitude
Requires computer averaging	No averaging required
Resistant to intravenous anesthetics, recordable during inhaled anesthetics	Abolished by high-dose intravenous or inhalation anesthetics

SEP, sensory evoked potential; EEG, electroencephalogram.

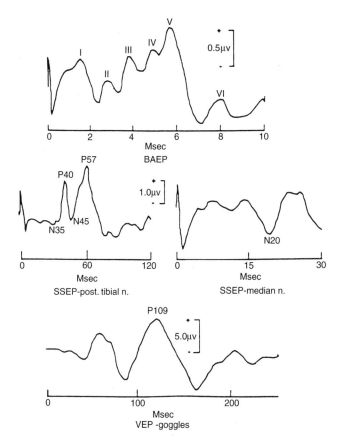

Fig. 3-2. Common modalities of sensory evoked responses. BAEP,
brain stem auditory evoked potentials; SSEP-median n, somatosensory evoked potential with median nerve stimulation; SSEP-post tibial n, somatosensory evoked potential with posterior tibial nerve
stimulation; VEP-goggles, visual evoked potential in response to
stimulation with light-emitted diode goggles. (Reproduced from Lam
AM. Monitoring neurologic evoked potentials. *ASA Refresher Course*
1989;17(13):175–192, with permission.)

the median nerve, ulnar nerve, and posterior
tibial nerve monitor the integrity of the respective pathway from the periphery to the
cortex. They are a routine monitor for surgical procedures on the spinal column with potential risk to the spinal cord, e.g., scoliosis
surgery, in a number of centers.

Somatosensory evoked potentials are also
used during carotid endarterectomy, with the

theoretical advantage over EEG that even subcortical ischemia can be detected. Indications for different SEP monitoring modalities are summarized in Table 3-8.

    b. Brain stem auditory evoked potentials are a series of seven short-latency peaks generated in response to stimulation of the auditory nerve, typically with repetitive clicks delivered to the ears by a head phone or by ear-insert transducers. Each peak, numbered with Roman numerals, is produced by a specific neurogenerator; by examining the change in latency interval between various peaks, the specific site of the injury can be localized. Monitoring of BAEP during acoustic neuroma surgery, when feasible, has been shown to help preserve the integrity of the auditory nerve. Although the neurogenerators are specific to the VIIIth nerve, BAEP monitoring has also been used to reflect the general well-being of the brain stem in posterior fossa procedures.

  2. **Interpretation of evoked potentials.** In a manner similar to EEG, ischemia/hypoxia leads to depression of conduction of evoked potentials with resultant decrease in amplitude and increase in latency of the specific peaks. For SSEPs, it is generally accepted that a 50% reduction in amplitude from baseline in response to a specific surgical maneuver is considered to be a significant change warranting alteration of surgical strategy to avert potential damage. For BAEP, an increase in latency of more than 1 millisecond is considered to be clinically significant.

  3. **Confounding factors.** As with EEG, cortical evoked potentials are influenced by anesthetic agents. Unlike EEG, SSEPs are resistant to the influence of intravenous agents. Although the amplitude may be slightly reduced and the latency increased, cortical SSEPs can be recorded

Table 3-8.   Indications for sensory evoked potential monitoring

SSEP monitoring
    Spinal column surgery
    Carotid endarterectomy
    Cerebral aneurysm surgery

BAEP monitoring
    Acoustic neuroma
    Vertebral-basilar aneurysms
    Other posterior fossa procedures

SSEP, somatosensory evoked potential; BAEP, brain stem auditory evoked potential.

even during deep barbiturate-induced coma with isoelectric EEG. In contrast, inhalation anesthetics cause a dose-related decrease in amplitude and increase in latency. With high doses, SSEP can become unrecordable. Nitrous oxide also has a profound depressant effect on the amplitude of SSEP, particularly when used in combination with an inhalation anesthetic. Therefore, the combination of inhalation anesthetic and nitrous oxide is to be avoided. Intraoperative recording of SSEP is best accomplished using an intravenous anesthetic technique or low-dose inhalation anesthetic (less than 1 MAC). Opioids have a negligible effect on SSEP. Ketamine and etomidate have a paradoxical effect of augmenting the amplitude of SSEP and have been utilized to make monitoring possible in patients with otherwise unrecordable SSEP.

Brain stem auditory evoked potential, unlike cortical SSEP, is resistant to the influence of anesthetic agents and can be recorded even during high-dose inhalation anesthetics. For surgical procedures on the spinal column, evoked potentials can also be recorded directly from the epidural space, and these potentials are robust and can be recorded regardless of anesthetic agents used. As with EEG, hypothermia will also decrease amplitude and increase latency.

4. **Motor evoked potentials.** Because SSEP only monitors the integrity of the sensory pathway, it is theoretically possible to miss injury specifically affecting the motor pathway but sparing the sensory tracts. Thus motor evoked potential (MEP) recording was introduced into clinical practice to complement SSEP recording. The motor evoked potential is basically an electromyographic potential recorded over muscles in the hand or foot in response to depolarization of the motor cortex. Depolarization can be achieved using transcranial magnetic or electrical stimulation.

Unfortunately, both modalities are profoundly influenced by anesthetic agents, rendering the former essentially unrecordable during anesthesia, and the latter recordable only during intravenous anesthesia. Motor evoked potentials cannot be recorded in the presence of complete neuromuscular blockade.

C. **Monitoring of cranial nerve functions.** Operations in the posterior fossa and the lower brain stem are associated with potential injury to the cranial nerves. By monitoring the electromyographic potential of the cranial nerves with motor components (V, VII, IX, X, XI, XII), the integrity of these cranial nerves can be preserved. Two types of potentials can be recorded: spontaneous and evoked activity. By measuring spontaneous activity, injury potential can be detected, signifying accidental surgical trespass. Evoking the nerve with electrical stimulation facilitates identification and thus preservation of the cranial nerve. Although theoretically EMG can be recorded during partial neuromuscular blockade, it is best not to administer any muscle relaxants during cranial nerve monitoring.

II. Monitoring of cerebral blood flow/intracranial pressure

A. Absolute cerebral blood flow.
Most methods of CBF measurement are not applicable to intraoperative monitoring. Nitrous oxide wash-in is the classic method of measuring global hemispheric CBF, but it necessitates cannulation of the jugular bulb and clinically is cumbersome to use. Radioactive xenon clearance is a method that allows noninvasive measurement of regional CBF. Although some centers use it clinically to determine adequacy of hemispheric CBF during carotid endarterectomy, it is primarily a research tool.

B. Relative cerebral blood flow.
Recent advances for measurement of regional flow include the introduction of laser Doppler flowmetry (LDF) and transcranial Doppler sonography (TCD).

1. **Laser Doppler flowmetry.** This is a parenchymal or surface Doppler probe that measures tissue local CBF in a quantitative manner. However, the flow can only be expressed in a relative manner in arbitrary units. Because the volume of tissue monitored is limited to 1 mm, its clinical use, both in the operating room and in the intensive care unit, remains limited. A burr hole is also required for its insertion. Its incorporation into the intracranial pressure (ICP) monitor might increase its functionality.

2. **Transcranial Doppler sonography.** This allows measurement of CBF velocity in the major vessels of the circle of Wills noninvasively and continuously. For intraoperative purposes, velocity in the middle cerebral artery (V_{mca}) is measured transtemporally over the zygomatic arch. Although the absolute CBF cannot be derived, relative changes in CBF are measured in a quantitative manner. The waveform profile also provides a qualitative assessment of intracranial pressure/cerebral perfusion pressure and the occurrence of air or particulate emboli can be detected. It can also be used to determine cerebral autoregulation and CO_2 reactivity.

   a. **Physiological principles of transcranial Doppler**
      (1) **The diameter of the basal cerebral arteries is constant.** Flow velocity is proportional to CBF only when the diam-

eter of the insonated vessel and the angle of insonation remain constant. There is considerable evidence to suggest that the basal cerebral arteries, as conductance vessels, do not dilate or constrict as the vascular resistance changes. Angiographic and CO_2 reactivity studies confirm that changes in carbon dioxide tension and blood pressure have negligible influence on the diameter of the proximal basal arteries. Intravenous and inhaled anesthetic agents do not constrict or dilate the MCA appreciably.

Probably the only clinically important situation in which the basal cerebral vessels vasoconstrict is when vasospasm occurs as a complication of subarachnoid hemorrhage. Vasospasm renders the relationship between CBF velocity and CBF invalid; as the vessel constricts, the flow velocity increases but the CBF actually decreases. This increase in flow velocity with constriction of the basal cerebral artery represents one of the most important and established uses of TCD. Once the diagnosis of vasospasm is confirmed by angiography, TCD can be used to track the patient's response to therapy and the time course of resolution of the vasospasm.

(2) **Changes in CBF velocity reflect relative changes in CBF.** Although correlation between absolute flow velocity and CBF in any given population is poor, there is good correlation between relative changes in flow velocity and CBF.

b. **Clinical applications of intraoperative TCD monitoring**

(1) **Carotid endarterectomy**

Detection of ischemia: TCD monitoring during carotid endarterectomy (CEA) can detect cerebral ischemia during cross-clamping of the carotid artery and allows selective shunting. The correlation between flow–velocity changes and EEG changes appears to be excellent in many studies. A decrease in V_{mca} of more than 60% compared to preclamped baseline suggests inadequate CBF and the need for an intraluminal shunt. Transcranial Doppler can also detect malfunctioning shunts due to kinking or thrombosis.

Detection of microemboli: Microemboli occur frequently during carotid endarterectomy and embolic events may outweigh hemodynamic events as an etiology of perioperative stroke. Both air and particulate emboli can be detected with TCD.

Diagnosis and treatment of postoperative hyperperfusion syndrome: Approximately 1% of patients develop hyperperfusion syndrome following carotid endarterectomy resulting in cerebral hemorrhage. Transcranial Doppler monitoring allows this diagnosis to be made and treatment to be implemented. Patients who develop the hyperperfusion syndrome show sustained elevation of flow velocities after release of carotid occlusion and often develop headaches. Prompt reduction of blood pressure is effective in normalizing the ipsilateral flow velocity and alleviating symptoms.

Diagnosis and treatment of postoperative intimal flap or thrombosis: Occlusion of the carotid artery postoperatively can occur due to clot formation or the presence of an intimal flap. Clinically, sudden development of symptoms in the recovery room should prompt an immediate TCD examination. A prompt exploration may prevent an impending stroke.

(2) Cardiac surgery. Stroke as a complication of cardiac surgical procedures occurs in up to 10% of patients. More subtle neurologic and cognitive dysfunction has been reported in 30% to 70% of patients. Adverse cerebral outcomes are due either to embolic events or hypoperfusion, or both.

Cerebral emboli during cardiopulmonary bypass (CPB): There is considerable evidence to suggest that the delivery of microemboli (air, platelet aggregate, and thrombus) into the cerebral circulation is responsible for the neuropsychologic deterioration seen after bypass procedures. It has been observed that patients with the highest emboli counts had greater neurologic deterioration. Other studies have shown that the presence of arterial line filters reduces the incidence of emboli detected by TCD. Despite these published findings, TCD monitoring of emboli is still in evolution and a number of technical challenges remain.

Cerebral perfusion during CPB: Brain injury during CPB may also occur as a result of hypoperfusion. Transcranial Doppler sonography has been used as a noninvasive tool for the examination of CBF in patients having cardiac surgical procedures performed under CPB. However, the validity of TCD as an estimate of CBF during CPB is unclear at present.

(3) **Closed head injury.** TCD monitoring can be used to assess autoregulation and diagnose hyperemia and vasospasm as well as intracranial circulatory arrest. Although less widely used intraoperatively, TCD may be useful in monitoring head-injured patients undergoing nonneurosurgical procedures.

c. **Limitations of TCD as a routine intraoperative monitor**

(1) Most TCD monitors are designed for diagnostic and not for monitoring purposes. There is a need for a fixation device that allows continuous, reliable recording and does not interfere with the surgical procedure.

(2) Although most TCD equipment is fairly easy to operate, skill and training are nevertheless required.

(3) The successful transmission of ultrasound through the skull is dependent on the thickness of the skull, and the temporal bone thickness varies with gender, race, and age. The failure rate can be anywhere from 5% to 20%, depending on the patient population.

C. **Intracranial pressure.** Cerebral perfusion pressure (CPP) is determined by the difference between mean arterial pressure (MAP) and ICP. The monitoring of ICP (a) allows optimization of CPP and (b) prevents brain herniation by prompt institution of treatment for elevated ICP. Since the components of the intracranial contents (brain, blood, and cerebrospinal fluid) are essentially incompressible and there is limited buffering capacity (dislocation of CSF to the lumbosacral axis, compression of venous sinuses), any significant increase in intracranial volume will lead to an inordinately steep rise in ICP. This is often referred to as the intracranial compliance curve, although it is more appropriately labeled the elastance curve (Fig. 3-3).

Current monitoring methods include ventriculostomy, subarachnoid bolt, epidural sensor, and fiberoptic intraparenchymal monitor, with the latter

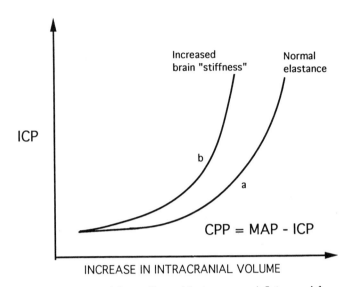

Fig. 3-3. Intracranial compliance (elastance curve). Intracranial pressure increases as the apparent intracranial volume increases. The steepness of the slope is dependent on the preexisting elastance of the system. The stiff brain has a steeper rise in ICP (curve B) than the normal curve (curve A). CPP, cerebral perfusion pressure; MAP, mean arterial pressure; ICP, intracranial pressure.

being the most commonly in use (Fig. 3-4). The ventricular catheter allows drainage of CSF for treatment but is associated with increased risk of infection compared to the fiberoptic catheter, which can be inserted at the bedside. New generations of fiberoptic ICP monitors may allow simultaneous measurement of LDF, PaO_2, $PaCO_2$, and pH, as well as temperature. Although the use of ICP monitors is fairly common in the management of patients with head injury in the intensive care unit, they are seldom available as intraoperative monitors.

III. **Monitoring of cerebral oxygenation/metabolism**
   A. **Invasive monitoring**
      1. **Brain tissue PO_2.** Using a miniature Clarke-type polarographic electrode originally designed for continuous intra-arterial monitoring, it is now possible to measure brain tissue PaO_2, $PaCO_2$, and pH. Coupled with a dialysis catheter, other metabolic markers including lactate, glucose, and excitotoxic amino acids can be measured. Although theoretically attractive, it is invasive and the measurement is limited to the parenchyma where the electrode is inserted. For now it remains an investigative tool.

2. **Jugular bulb venous oximetry.** This allows continuous or intermittent estimation of the global balance between cerebral oxygen demand and supply. Provided cerebral metabolic rate for oxygen ($CMRO_2$) stays constant, calculation of the arteriovenous oxygen content ($CAVDO_2$) would allow estimation of the relative CBF. Even if $CMRO_2$ does not stay constant, the arteriovenous oxygen content difference always reflects the balance between oxygen demand and supply of the brain. Since arterial oxygenation is usually 100%,

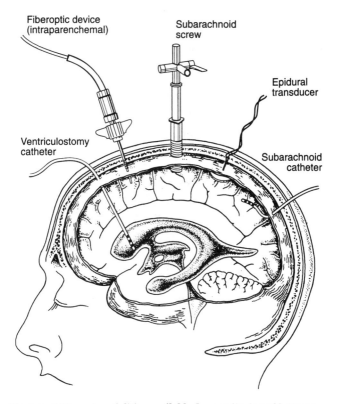

Fig. 3-4. **Different modalities available for monitoring of intracranial pressure. One of the most commonly used fiberoptic devices (Camino Catheter, Camino Laboratories, San Diego, CA) can be placed epidurally, subarachnoidally, or intraparenchymally. Other modalities include ventriculostomy catheter, subarachnoid screw, epidural transducer, and subarachnoid catheter. (Reproduced with permission from Lam AM, Mayberg TS. Anesthetic management of patients with traumatic head injury. In: Lam AM, ed. *Anesthetic management of acute head injury.* New York: McGraw-Hill, 1995:181–221.)**

provided hematocrit stays constant, the jugular venous oxygen saturation ($SjvO_2$) will equally reflect this balance. The physiologic principles behind jugular venous oximetry are shown in Table 3-9.

Intraoperative cerebral ischemia from inadequate perfusion pressure or excessive hyperventilation can be diagnosed readily. The influence of jugular venous desaturation on prognosis in head-injured patients has been documented, and continuous jugular venous oximetry has become a routine monitor in many neurointensive care units. The thermistor-tipped catheter also measures temperature approximating that of the brain. Its major limitations include its global nature and therefore inability to detect focal cerebral ischemia, as well as its invasive nature. Its reliability during cardiopulmonary bypass is also controversial.

a. **Interpretation of $SjvO_2$.** The normal $AVDO_2$ is 2.8 μmol/mL or 6.3 vol% of oxygen (range 2.2 to 3.3 μmol/mL, or 5 to 7.5 vol%), and $SjvO_2$ is between 60% and 70%. When oxygen delivery is greater than oxygen demand, as in hyperemia, $AVDO_2$ will decrease and $SjvO_2$ will increase. During periods of global cerebral ischemia, $AVDO_2$ will widen and $SjvO_2$ will decrease.

   (1) *Increased values:* An $SjvO_2$ of greater then 90% is indicative of absolute or relative hyperemia. This can occur as a result of a reduced metabolic need (e.g., a comatose or brain-dead patient) or from excessive flow (e.g., severe hypercapnia).

Table 3-9.   Physiologic principles of jugular venous oximetry

$CMRO_2 = CBF \times AVDO_2$

$CMRO_2 \div CBF = AVDO_2$

$AVDO_2$ = arterial O_2 content (CaO_2) − jugular venous O_2 content ($CjvO_2$)

$\qquad = (Hgb \times 1.39 \times SaO_2 + 0.003 \times PaO_2) − (Hgb \times 1.39 \times SjvO_2 + 0.003 \times PjvO_2)$

$\qquad = Hgb \times 1.39 (SaO_2 − SjvO_2) + 0.003 (PaO_2 − PjvO_2)$

$\qquad = Hgb \times 1.39 (SaO_2 − SjvO_2)$ (ignoring the amount of dissolved O_2)

Since under most circumstances $SaO_2 = 1$, $AVDO_2 \propto 1 − SjvO_2$ where $AVDO_2$ is arteriovenous O_2 content, $SjvO_2$ is jugular venous O_2 saturation, $PjvO_2$ is jugular venous O_2 tension; and "a" refers to arterial. Therefore, a change in $SjvO_2$ will reflect a corresponding change in $AVDO_2$ provided hemoglobin saturation remains constant.

Patients with cerebral arteriovenous malformations have a direct arterial shunt into the venous circulation and thus have abnormally increased $SjvO_2$ values. Extracranial contamination, either from the facial vein or from rapid withdrawal in blood sampling (intermittent measurement), will also result in an elevated value.

(2) *Normal values:* Although a normal balance between flow and metabolism will result in a normal $SjvO_2$, this does not exclude the presence of focal ischemia. Since the blood in the jugular veins drains from all areas of the brain, a discrete area of ischemia or infarction might not influence the overall level of saturation.

(3) *Decreased values:* On the other hand, $SjvO_2$ is sensitive to global cerebral ischemia. A value of less than 50% reflects increased oxygen extraction and is indicative of a potential risk of ischemic injury. This may be due to increased metabolic demand not matched by an equivalent increase in flow, as in fever or seizure, or it may be due to an absolute reduction in flow. A significant decrease in oxygen carrying capacity due to a decrease in hematocrit will also lead to desaturation. Ischemia may also alter $CMRO_2$ and affect the interpretation of $SjvO_2$. As ischemia progresses to infarction, oxygen consumption will decrease and $SjvO_2$ will normalize.

B. **Noninvasive monitoring.** Near-infrared spectroscopy or transcranial oximetry measures cerebral regional oxygen saturation by measuring near-infrared light reflected off the chromophobes in the brain, the most important of which are oxyhemoglobin, deoxyhemoglobin, and cytochrome AA3. It has been studied in a variety of clinical settings including carotid endarterectomy and hypothermic circulatory arrest. Its major limitations include the intersubject variability, the variable optical pathlength, the potential contamination from extracranial blood, and, most importantly, the lack of a definable threshold. Because of the thin scalp and skull in the neonate and infant, it holds promise in this patient population. It remains an investigative tool in its present form.

SUGGESTED READING

Lam AM. Do evoked potentials have any value in anesthesia? *Anesthesiol Clin North Am* 1992;10:657–682.

Lam AM, Mayberg TS. Jugular venous oximetry. *Anesthesiol Clin North Am* 1997;15:533–549.

MacLennan N, Lam AM. Intraoperative transcranial Doppler monitoring. *Semin Anesthesiol* 1997;16:56–68.

Rampil I. What every neuroanesthesiologist should know about electroencephalograms and computerized monitors. *Anesthesiol Clin North Am* 1992;10:683–718.

Rosow C, Manberg PJ. Bispectral index monitoring. *Anesthesiol Clin North Am (Annu Anesthetic Pharmacol)* 1998;2:89–107.

4

Cerebral Protection and Resuscitation

Janet Pittman and James E. Cottrell

I. **Cerebral protection and resuscitation**
   A. **Cerebral protection** is the preemptive use of therapeutic interventions to improve neurologic outcome in patients who will be at risk for cerebral ischemia. The primary objective is **prevention** of the deleterious effects of ischemia.
   B. **Resuscitation** refers to therapeutic interventions initiated after an ischemic event. The goal is treatment of ischemia and attenuation of neuronal injury.

II. **The normal brain**
   A. **Cerebral metabolic rate for oxygen consumption (CMRO$_2$).** Normal CMRO$_2$ is 3.5 mL/100 g (brain tissue)/minute for an adult. Although the brain accounts for only 2% of body weight, it consumes 20% of total body oxygen supply and receives 15% of total cardiac output. CMRO$_2$ is 25% higher in children and 10% lower in elderly individuals.
   B. **Cerebral blood flow (CBF)** is normally 50 mL/100 g/minute (15% of cardiac output).
      1. **Flow–metabolism coupling.** In the normal brain the ratio of CBF to CMRO$_2$ is stable at 14:18 (Fig. 4-1A). This phenomenon of flow–metabolism coupling explains the difference in CBF between gray matter (75 to 80 mL/100 g/minute) and white matter (20 to 30 mL/100 g/minute). Gray matter consists of cell bodies that have greater metabolic requirements than white matter, which consists primarily of nerve fibers.
      2. **Autoregulation.** In the normal brain, CBF remains constant between a mean arterial pressure (MAP) of 60 and 160 mm Hg [cerebral perfusion pressure (CPP) = 50 to 150 mm Hg] through a mechanism of rapid (30 to 120 seconds) vascular response to changes in MAP (Fig. 4-1B). Above and below these values, the relationship between CBF and MAP is linear, i.e., flow is directly proportional to pressure. Ischemia quickly leads to loss of autoregulation because of vasomotor paralysis. The autoregulation curve is shifted to the right in untreated chronic hypertensive patients. With effective blood pressure control, the curve returns to near normal.
      3. **Carbon dioxide reactivity.** In the normal individual, CBF varies from 3% to 4% per mm Hg change in PaCO$_2$ between 20 and 80 mm Hg (Fig. 4-1C). The CBF response to changes in PaCO$_2$ oc-

curs within 20 to 30 seconds. CO_2 reactivity is more resistant to ischemia than autoregulation but may also be lost under ischemic conditions.

4. **Hypoxemia** refers to deficient oxygenation of arterial blood. Hypoxia is a reduction of oxygen supply to a tissue below that required for aerobic metabolism. Cerebral blood flow is not affected by PaO_2 values within the normal physiologic range. However, hypoxemia is a powerful stimulus for cerebrovasodilatation, thereby increasing CBF (Fig 4-1D). Cerebral blood flow begins to increase at PaO_2 levels below 50 mm Hg and is doubled at a PaO_2 of 30 mm Hg. Hyperoxemia has a slight vasoconstrictor effect, leading to a 10% to 15% decrease in CBF at one atmosphere (i.e., $F_IO_2 = 1.0$). Further decrease in CBF may occur with hyperbaric oxygenation.

C. **Cerebral perfusion pressure,** the perfusion force of blood to the brain, is defined as the difference between MAP and intracranial pressure (ICP):

CPP = MAP − ICP.

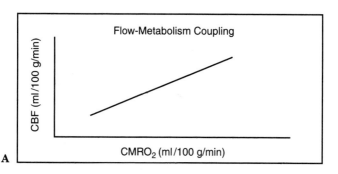

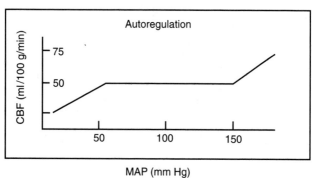

Fig. 4-1. Mechanisms of cerebral blood flow regulation in the normal brain. A: Flow-metabolism coupling. B: Autoregulation.

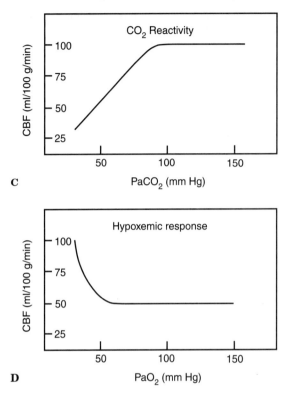

Fig. 4-1. (*continued*) C: CO_2 reactivity. D: The hypoxemic response. (Adapted from Lam AM. Anesthetic management of patients with traumatic head injury. In: Lam Am, ed. *Anesthetic management of acute head injury.* New York: McGraw-Hill, 1995:183.)

Normal CPP is 100 mm Hg. The generally accepted lower limit of CPP in a normal patient is 50 mm Hg. An isolated increase in ICP causes a decrease in CPP, which can result in ischemia.

D. Oxygen delivery (DO_2) is the amount of oxygen delivered to the brain per minute:

$$DO_2 = CaO_2 \times CBF$$

where **CaO_2** is arterial oxygen content, a function of hemoglobin and PaO_2. Normal CaO_2 is 16 to 20 mL O_2/100 mL arterial blood. Normal DO_2 is 8 to 10 mL O_2/100 g/minute, which when compared to $CMRO_2$ indicates a physiologic safety factor of 2. Oxygen delivery can be compromised by insufficient CaO_2 from severe anemia or hypoxemia and by hypoxia from inadequate blood flow to the brain despite adequate arterial oxygen content.

E. **Intracranial pressure** is determined by total intra-cranial volume, consisting of brain parenchyma (80% to 85% by volume), blood (4% to 8%), and cerebrospinal fluid (CSF) (10% to 12%). Normal ICP is 5 to 13 mm Hg. A sustained ICP greater than 20 mm Hg should be treated (see V.A.5).

F. **Intracranial elastance** describes change in ICP as a function of volume ($\delta P/\delta V$) (Fig. 4-2). Intracranial compliance ($\delta V/\delta P$) or a change in volume as a function of pressure is a misnomer that is frequently used interchangeably with elastance. Increased intracranial volume is initially compensated by shifts in CSF and blood volume until this mechanism is overwhelmed. Subsequently small volume increases lead to a pronounced increase in ICP and clinical deterioration.

G. **Cerebral metabolic rate for glucose (CMRgl)** is normally 5 mg/100 g of brain/minute. Under normal conditions, more than 90% of glucose is metabolized aerobically through oxidative phosphorylation; the remainder is converted anaerobically to lactic acid. The former process is extremely efficient: each molecule of glucose yields 38 molecules of adenosine triphosphate (ATP). In contrast, anaerobic glycolysis yields only two ATP molecules for each molecule of glucose.

H. **Electroencephalogram (EEG).** The electrical activity of the brain, shown on the EEG, is usually measured via scalp electrodes. Different EEG waveforms have characteristic frequencies and amplitudes.

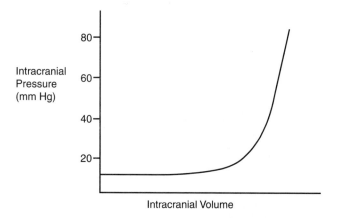

Fig. 4-2. **Pressure–volume curve of intracranial elastance.** Increased intracranial pressure (ICP) is initially compensated by cerebrospinal fluid and blood volume redistribution until this mechanism is overwhelmed. Subsequently, small volume increases lead to pronounced ICP increases. (Adapted from Langfitt TW, Weinstein JD, Kassell NF. Cerebral vasomotor paralysis produced by intracranial hypertension. *Neurology* 1965; 15:622–641 (Fig. 1, p. 625).)

1. **Beta** (13 to 30 Hz) waves are fast (cycles/second), low-voltage waves. Beta activity is seen in awake, alert individuals with open eyes or in patients receiving low-dose barbiturates or 50% N_2O.

2. **Alpha** (8 to 13 Hz) waves are seen in alert, awake patients with closed eyes and during light anesthesia.

3. **Theta** (4 to 8 Hz) waves are slow, high-amplitude waves seen with drowsiness or moderate to deep anesthesia.

4. **Delta** (1 to 4 Hz) waves are very low-frequency, high-amplitude waves seen normally during deep sleep or deep anesthesia. They indicate ischemia or other neuropathology when seen during wakefulness.

5. **Burst suppression** is characterized by an EEG tracing that is predominantly isoelectric but interspersed with bursts of electrical activity occurring every 3 to 10 seconds. Burst suppression is seen with high-dose barbiturates, other intravenous medications (etomidate and propofol), potent inhaled volatile agents (particularly isoflurane), and ischemia.

III. **The ischemic brain**
   A. **Cerebral ischemia** is defined as perfusion insufficient to provide the supply of oxygen and nutrients needed for maintenance of **neuronal metabolic integrity (40% to 45% of total $CMRO_2$)** and **function (55% to 60% of $CMRO_2$)**. It is assumed that a hierarchy of ischemic damage exists in which neuronal function is lost before cellular integrity.
      1. **Integrity.** The brain utilizes **glucose** as its primary substrate for energy production. In the nonfasting state, glucose is metabolized via oxidative phosphorylation to ATP, which is needed for cellular activities such as homeostasis, protein synthesis, maintenance of ionic gradients, cell membrane stability, mitochondrial activity, and CO_2 removal.
      2. **Function.** Normal neuronal functional activity consists of the generation and transmission of nerve impulses and is reflected by the presence of normal EEG activity.
   B. **Ischemia** may be **global or focal**, as well as **complete or incomplete.** Complete global ischemia is seen with **cardiac arrest**; incomplete global ischemia occurs with hypotension or shock. Focal ischemia involves the occlusion of a single vessel and is thus incomplete.
   C. **The ischemic cascade.** Inadequate cerebral perfusion leads rapidly to a cascade of pathophysiologic changes (Fig. 4-3) involving a multitude of chemical mediators of neuronal damage.
      1. Decreased availability of oxygen and glucose leads to immediate depletion of ATP required for

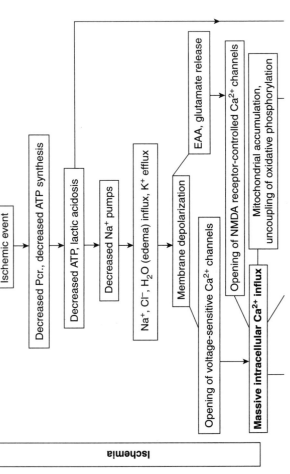

Fig. 4-3. The ischemic cascade of immediate and delayed neuronal damage. (Adapted from Milde LN, Weglinski MR. Pathophysiology of metabolic brain injury. In: Cottrell JE, Smith DS, eds. *Anesthesia and neurosurgery.* St. Louis: Mosby, 1994:61.)

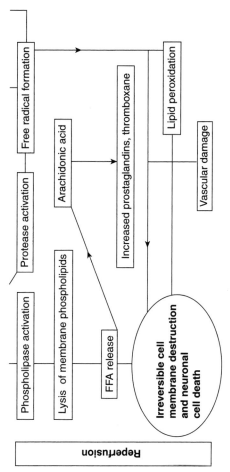

Fig. 4-3. (*continued*)

all active cellular processes. This occurs within 2 to 4 minutes. Phosphocreatine (Pcr), a high-energy compound, is both a precursor of ATP and a byproduct of ATP resynthesis from adenosine diphosphate (ADP). Brain Pcr levels are normally 3 times those of ATP. A decrease in Pcr is one of the earliest harbingers of ischemia.

2. **Lactate** levels increase due to anaerobic metabolism of glucose. Lactic acidosis aggravates ischemic damage. Lactate reduces ferric to ferrous iron, which in turn promotes free radical formation followed by lipid peroxidation of cell membranes. With incomplete ischemia, the persistence of residual perfusion leads to increased lactate production in the presence of ongoing anaerobic metabolism and is thought to be the mechanism for increased damage with this type of ischemia. In contrast, complete ischemia results in complete cessation of metabolism.

3. Increased plasma **glucose** is an independent risk factor for aggravation of ischemia. The primary mechanism appears to be the increased production of lactate. Hyperglycemia also prevents the increase in brain adenosine occurring with ischemia. Adenosine, a purine nucleotide, inhibits excitatory amino acid (EAA) release and promotes cerebrovasodilatation, thus theoretically attenuating ischemic damage. In addition, there is some evidence that insulin has neuroprotective effects independent of its glucose-lowering properties.

4. Cerebral ischemia increases release of the **EAA neurotransmitters glutamate** and **aspartate.**
   a. Three receptors for the excitatory neurotransmitters are currently identified:
      (1) **N-methyl-D-aspartate (NMDA)** receptors are located in layers three, five, and six of the cerebral cortex, thalamus, striatum, Purkinje, and granule cell layers of the cerebellum, and the CA_1 region of the hippocampus, which is particularly susceptible to ischemia. The NMDA receptors mediate the influx of Na^+ and Ca^{2+} through membrane channels. Magnesium and the experimental drug dizocilipine maleate (MK-801) block the NMDA receptor site in a noncompetitive fashion.
      (2) **Quisqualate [α-amino-3-hydroxy-5-methyl-4-isoxazole-propionic   acid (AMPA)]** receptors occur in the deep cortical layers, thalamus, striatum, molecular layer of the cerebellum, and pyramidal cell layer and striatum lucidum of the hippocampus. The AMPA receptors mediate the influx of Na^+.

(3) **Kainate** receptors, located in the striatum lucidum of the hippocampus, mediate the influx of Na^+.

Glutamate stimulates all three receptors, but aspartate affects only the NMDA receptor. The presence of glycine is necessary for activation of the NMDA receptor by glutamate.

b. Glutamate causes neuronal cell death by two mechanisms: **immediate** and **delayed.** In immediate neurotoxicity, glutamate activates the NMDA receptor, leading to Na^+, Cl^-, and H_2O influx, which results in cellular edema, membrane lysis, and cell death. In delayed neurotoxicity (24 to 72 hours), the activated NMDA receptor promotes a cycle of ischemia initiated by Ca^{2+} influx. This leads to activation of phospholipases, proteases, and eventually free fatty acids (FFAs), formation of arachidonic acid and free radicals, lipid peroxidation, and, ultimately, cell death.

5. Increased **calcium** influx is an early, pivotal event in the ischemic cascade and is due to several mechanisms.

a. Depletion of ATP results in failure of energy-requiring Na^+/K^+ ATPase-dependent ion pumps. Na^+ and Cl^- influx and K^+ efflux ensue. Influx of H_2O and edema occur secondarily. The resulting membrane depolarization leads to opening of voltage-sensitive Ca^{2+} channels and calcium influx.

b. Decreased ATP leads to calcium release from the endoplasmic reticulum.

c. The EAA levels increase during ischemia, leading to stimulation of glutamate receptors and the opening of NMDA-mediated Ca^{2+} channels.

d. Calcium extrusion from the cell is an active process that is halted when ATP stores are exhausted.

6. The numerous ischemic effects of calcium form a common pathway leading to neuronal cell destruction. Increased intracellular calcium activates **phospholipase A_1, A_2,** and **C,** which lead to the hydrolysis of membrane phospholipids and the release of FFAs. Loss of membrane phospholipids also results in mitochondrial and cell membrane destruction.

a. **Arachidonic acid,** the major **FFA,** is metabolized to **prostaglandins, leukotrienes,** and **free radicals.** Both prostaglandins (via the cyclooxygenase pathway) and leukotrienes (via lipoxygenase) cause cerebral edema. **Thromboxane A_2,** a prostaglandin derived from arachidonic acid with potent vasoconstrictor and platelet aggregation properties, potentiates ischemia and has been implicated in reperfusion injury (see III.E below).

   b.   **Free radical formation. Superoxide, peroxide,** and **hydroxyl radicals** cause lipid peroxidation within neuronal cell membranes. This alters membrane function and releases toxic byproducts (aldehydes, hydrocarbon gases). These byproducts cause edema, blood–brain barrier (BBB) disruption, and inflammation. The superoxide radical itself can create an inflammatory response with vascular plugging.

D.   Clinical ischemia

   1.   Of all of the body organs the brain is the most vulnerable to ischemia. Loss of consciousness occurs within 15 seconds of cardiac arrest. Brain Pcr becomes negligible within one minute. Glucose and ATP stores are exhausted within 4 to 5 minutes.

      a.   Critical levels for CBF, CPP, and PaO_2 have been determined below which cerebral ischemia occurs (see Fig. 4-4) with characteristic EEG changes.

   2.   **Critical CBF** is 18 to 20 mL/100 g/minute. The **penumbra** is a hypoperfused region that may remain viable depending on timely reperfusion. The EEG becomes isoelectric at a CBF of 15 mL/100

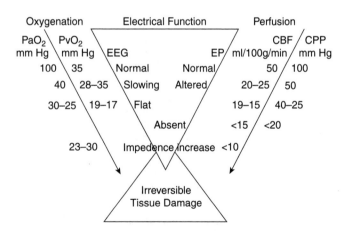

Fig. 4-4. Critical levels for PaO_2, cerebral blood flow, and cerebral perfusion pressure below which ischemic electroencephalographic changes are seen. (Adapted from Shapiro HM. Anesthesia effects upon cerebral blood flow, cerebral metabolism, electroencephalogram, and evoked potentials. In: Miller RD, ed. *Anesthesia*, 2nd ed. New York: Churchill Livingstone, 1986:1276.)

g/minute. Metabolic failure occurs at a CBF of 10 mL/100 g/minute.

3. **Critical CPP** is 50 mm Hg in the normal individual.

4. **Critical PaO$_2$** is 30 to 35 mm Hg in healthy awake patients.

E. **Reperfusion injury** refers to ischemic damage that occurs after the restoration of cerebral perfusion. An initial phase of hyperperfusion occurs, followed by a gradual decline in CBF to a negligible level referred to as the **"no-reflow phenomenon."** Hypoperfusion results from thromboxane-induced vasoconstriction and platelet aggregation, impaired red cell deformability, tissue edema, and the persistence of abnormal calcium levels. In addition, intracellular acidosis, continued EAA neurotransmitter and catecholamine release, and free radical formation contribute to delayed neuronal damage. This no-reflow phenomenon can last for 24 hours.

IV. **Clinical cerebral protection**

A. **Rationale for treatment.** The goal is to maximize the available oxygen by **increasing oxygen supply (delivery)** and **decreasing oxygen demand.** Preservation of CBF and avoidance of hypoxia and hypoxemia are critical.

B. Patients who are candidates for **cerebral protection** include the following:

1. Patients with space-occupying lesions such as tumor, abscess, hematoma, hydrocephalus, and chronic cystic fluid collections with or without increased ICP who are scheduled for neurosurgical procedures.

2. Patients scheduled for intracranial vascular procedures, such as cerebral aneurysm clipping or excision of arteriovenous malformation (AVM) or cavernous angioma, and extracranial vascular procedures including carotid endarterectomy (CEA) or superficial temporal artery to middle cerebral artery (STA-MCA) bypass, which involve temporary vessel occlusion and the possibility of focal ischemia.

3. Patients with giant or complex basilar artery aneurysms for aneurysm clipping, which may be facilitated by **deep hypothermic circulatory arrest (DHCA).**

4. Cardiac bypass patients typically at risk from global ischemia due to low-flow states or focal ischemia from multiple small emboli.

V. **Clinical therapies**

A. **Nonpharmacologic treatment**

1. **Hypothermia** decreases both metabolic and functional activities of the brain. Although hypothermia reduces CMRO$_2$ by 7% for each degree Celsius, the mechanism is not uniformly linear. The temperature coefficient (Q_{10}), used to de-

scribe the relationship between temperature and $CMRO_2$, is the ratio of two $CMRO_2$ values separated by 10°C. For most biological reactions, the Q_{10} is approximately 2.0 (a 50% decrease in $CMRO_2$ for every 10°C decrease). Thus, if the normothermic brain (37°C) can tolerate 5 minutes of complete ischemia, then at 27°C the brain should tolerate 10 minutes of ischemia. The actual Q_{10} is 2.2 to 2.4 between 37°C and 27°C, resulting in a greater than 50% reduction in $CMRO_2$ at 27°C. Between 27°C and 17°C, the Q_{10} is approximately 5.0. This correlates with the gradual loss of neuronal function demonstrated by an isoelectric EEG (which occurs between 18°C and 21°C) and the ability of the brain to tolerate more prolonged ischemia than would be predicted based on a linear model. Below 17°C, the Q_{10} is 2.2 to 2.4 again.

However, small decreases in temperature have also resulted in significant reductions in the effects of cerebral ischemia. Possible mechanisms of auxiliary hypothermic protection include decreased calcium influx, decreased EAA release, BBB preservation, and prevention of lipid peroxidation.

The current therapeutic recommendation is mild hypothermia (brain temperature of 32°C to 35°C). Correlation of esophageal and brain temperatures should not be assumed. Tympanic membrane or nasopharyngeal temperature should therefore be measured as a more accurate estimate of brain temperature. Avoidance of hyperthermia is paramount since above-normal temperatures markedly increase $CMRO_2$ and exacerbate ischemic damage.

a. **Deep hypothermic respiratory arrest** to core temperatures of 13°C to 21°C might be indicated for clipping of giant or complex basilar artery aneurysms. Peripheral arterial and large-bore intravenous catheters are inserted before induction. After induction, either a central venous or a pulmonary artery catheter, a second arterial line for phlebotomy, and a lumbar subarachnoid drain are placed. Electrophysiologic monitoring of EEG, somatosensory evoked potentials (SSEPs), and brain stem auditory evoked potentials (BAEPs) is begun. The SSEPs persist to 15°C to 18°C, and a CBF of 10 to 15 mL/100 g/minute, which is beyond hypothermic EEG isoelectricity (18°C to 20°C).

Cooling at a rate of 0.2°C/minute is performed by the use of a cooling blanket, infusion of cold saline, and decreased ambient temperature. Barbiturate-induced burst suppression is initiated and maintained intraoperatively. Hemodilution to a hematocrit of 28% to 30% is accomplished by phlebotomy; this blood is reserved in an anticoagulant solution to be reinfused after termination of bypass for replacement of essential clotting factors.

The aneurysm is dissected with meticulous attention to hemostasis before beginning femoral artery–femoral vein bypass. Heparin 300 to 400 IU/kg is administered; and the activated clotting time (ACT) is kept between 450 and 480 seconds. Cardiopulmonary bypass is begun when the patient's temperature is 34°C and continued until the desired core temperature is reached. Spontaneous atrial fibrillation may occur below 30°C and continuous ventricular fibrillation frequently occurs below 28°C. In order to prevent myocardial ischemic injury, persistent ventricular fibrillation should be terminated by potassium chloride (KCl) 20 to 60 mEq. Cardioversion with 100 to 250 joules may be used to induce asystole in patients resistant to KCl or in anephric patients in whom KCl is contraindicated. Mean arterial pressure should be maintained between 40 to 80 mm Hg during bypass.

Circulatory arrest occurs between 22°C and 18°C. The bypass pump is stopped. The duration of circulatory arrest is limited to aneurysm clip application time. Bypass is resumed and rewarming proceeds at 0.2 to 0.5°C/minute. Spontaneous ventricular fibrillation occurs with rewarming. Cardioversion (200 to 400 joules) is required to restore sinus rhythm. Extracorporeal bypass is terminated when the patient's temperature reaches 34°C, and normal sinus rhythm and cardiac output are present. Inotropic support may be required. The previously removed whole blood is reinfused to promote normal coagulation. Heparin is reversed with protamine to achieve an ACT of 100 to 150 seconds. Complications of this technique include coagulopathy, postoperative hemorrhage, metabolic acidosis, hyperglycemia, myocardial depression, and dysrhythmias.

2. **Avoidance of hyperglycemia.** The current recommendation is to keep the serum glucose below 150 mg/dL. Serum glucose is monitored frequently; hypoglycemia (serum glucose below 60 mg/dL) is scrupulously avoided.

3. **Avoidance of hypotension, hypoxia,** and **hypercapnia.** Induced hypertension may be requested by the surgeon to improve CPP during

temporary proximal occlusion of the parent vessel prior to definitive aneurysm clip placement. Induced hypotension can also be detrimental in patients at risk for vasospasm.

4. **Hemodilution** to a hematocrit of 32% to 34% will increase CBF by decreasing viscosity, thereby improving oxygen delivery.

5. **Normalization of increased ICP** is achieved through moderate hyperventilation (PaCO$_2$ 25 to 30 mm Hg), head elevation to 30° in the neutral position, mannitol and/or furosemide diuresis, CSF drainage via ventriculostomy, limited fluid restriction, and barbiturate coma in patients unresponsive to the above techniques. Subtemporal decompressive craniotomy with anterior temporal lobectomy may be performed as a last resort.

6. **Correction of acidosis** and **electrolyte imbalance** including Na$^+$ and K$^+$ abnormalities should be prompt.

B. **Pharmacologic treatment**

1. **Barbiturates** remain the only drugs proven to be effective for pharmacologic cerebral protection against focal ischemic damage.

   a. **Thiopental sodium,** a potent cerebrovasoconstrictor, decreases CBF, CBV, and ICP. Carbon dioxide reactivity is preserved.

      (1) The primary mechanism of protection involves a reduction in CMRO$_2$ of up to 55% to 60% at which point the EEG becomes isoelectric. Further reduction in CMRO$_2$ confers no further protection. Thiopental's beneficial effects are thus limited to preservation of neuronal function.

      (2) Thiopental may cause an **inverse steal** phenomenon whereby vasoconstriction in normal tissue improves perfusion of ischemic areas that are unable to vasoconstrict.

      (3) Thiopental is an effective **anticonvulsant.**

      (4) Other possible mechanisms include γ-aminobutyric acid (GABA) agonism, free radical scavenging, membrane stabilization, NMDA antagonism, and calcium channel blockade.

      (5) Thiopental does not improve outcome in global or complete ischemia as after cardiac arrest.

      (6) The thiopental dose in focal ischemia is 3 to 5 mg/kg every 5 to 10 minutes titrated to EEG burst suppression up to a total of 15 to 20 mg/kg. Maintenance of cardiovascular stability may determine the rate of administration.

b. **Pentobarbital's** cerebral effects are similar to those of thiopental. Pentobarbital is longer acting ($t\frac{1}{2}$ = 30 hours). Current clinical use of pentobarbital is limited to barbiturate coma in patients with increased ICP resistant to standard therapy. A loading dose of 3 to 10 mg/kg over 0.5 to 3 hours is given, followed by a maintenance infusion of 0.5 to 3.0 mg/kg/hour titrated to EEG burst suppression. The currently accepted therapeutic range for plasma concentration of pentobarbital is 2.5 to 4.0 mg/dL.

c. **Methohexital,** a very short-acting barbiturate, may precipitate seizures in individuals with epilepsy. Methohexital is useful for induction of anesthesia for brief procedures where seizure activity is desired: e.g., electroconvulsive therapy (ECT) or epilepsy surgery.

2. **Other intravenous anesthetics.** Anesthetic drugs that maintain ATP levels by decreasing cerebral metabolism while simultaneously preserving CBF and cardiovascular stability have theoretical potential for cerebral protection.

a. **Etomidate** is a short-acting imidazole compound which, like the barbiturates, causes cerebral vasoconstriction. Electroencephalogram burst suppression occurs with higher doses.

(1) Etomidate reduces $CMRO_2$ (by as much as 50%), CBF, and ICP while maintaining cardiovascular stability and CPP. Carbon dioxide reactivity is preserved.

(2) Etomidate can cause **adrenocortical suppression** for up to 24 hours after a single induction dose (inhibition of 11β-hydroxylase). This may be of clinical concern when etomidate is used as an infusion, especially in patients who are not concomitantly receiving steroids.

(3) Myoclonic activity has been reported with etomidate and seizures may occur.

(4) Side effects of etomidate include nausea and vomiting as well as pain on injection.

b. **Propofol** (2,6-diisopropylphenol), a short-acting induction agent also used for maintenance of anesthesia, has a cerebrovascular profile similar to that of the barbiturates:

(1) Propofol decreases $CMRO_2$, ICP, and CBF (via cerebrovasoconstriction). Hemodynamic depression, greater than with barbiturates, decreases CPP.

(2) An EEG burst suppression occurs with larger doses of propofol.

   (3) Propofol may decrease nausea and vomiting postoperatively.

c. **Benzodiazepines,** which are sedative-hypnotic drugs most commonly used as anesthetic adjuncts, stimulate the inhibitory neurotransmitter GABA and decrease $CMRO_2$ and CBF while preserving CO_2 reactivity. Intracranial pressure may be decreased slightly. Benzodiazepines are potent anticonvulsants; in addition they produce amnesia and anxiolysis.

   (1) **Diazepam** is most commonly used for oral premedication in a dose of 0.1 to 0.25 mg/kg. Its prolonged $t\frac{1}{2}$ of 21 to 37 hours limits its use in neurosurgical patients in whom prompt emergence and postoperative neurologic assessment are critical. Diazepam remains an effective treatment for status epilepticus.

   (2) **Midazolam** has a $t\frac{1}{2}$ of 1 to 4 hours. The intravenous dose of midazolam for premedication is 0.5 to 2.5 mg up to 0.1 mg/kg. Excessive sedation and the possibility of hypoventilation-induced hypercapnia should be avoided in patients at risk for increased ICP.

   (3) **Lorazepam** is also an effective premedicant in doses of 0.5 to 4 mg p.o. or 2 to 4 mg i.v. or i.m. Like diazepam, its use is limited in neurosurgery by a $t\frac{1}{2}$ of 10 to 20 hours.

d. **Opioids** produce sedation and analgesia and cause a reduction in neurotransmitter release while preserving autoregulation, CO_2 reactivity, and cardiovascular stability. Values of CBF, $CMRO_2$, and ICP are unchanged or slightly decreased. Delta waves are seen on EEG; burst suppression does not occur.

   (1) **Morphine** is a potent analgesic with relatively poor central nervous system (CNS) penetration. Commonly used for postoperative analgesia in neurosurgical patients, morphine can cause hypotension secondary to histamine release.

   (2) **Meperidine** may increase heart rate due to its atropine-like structure and effect. Normeperidine is a metabolite of meperidine that can cause CNS excitation and seizures.

   (3) **Fentanyl** is 100 times more potent than morphine. Fentanyl does not cause histamine release; is shorter acting than morphine; and decreases ICP and CBV slightly while maintaining CPP.

   (4) **Sufentanil** is more potent than fentanyl and may increase ICP (via vasodilatation) in patients with severe head trauma; use of another opioid should be considered in such instances.

(5) **Remifentanil** is a very short-acting ($t\frac{1}{2}$ = 3 to 10 minutes) esterase-metabolized opioid that compared favorably to fentanyl in a recent clinical trial.

e. **Calcium channel blockers** provide cerebral protection by vasodilatation and diminution of the consequences of Ca^{2+} influx.

(1) **Nimodipine** improves neurologic outcome in patients at risk for vasospasm due to aneurysmal subarachnoid hemorrhage (SAH) and after ischemic stroke but not after cardiac arrest. Nimodipine may increase CBF to underperfused areas by redistribution through an inverse steal effect. The dosage of nimodipine, available only in oral form at present, is 60 mg every 4 hours for 21 days after SAH. Hypotension may occur with administration of nimodipine.

(2) **Nicardipine,** available for intravenous administration, has decreased ischemic damage in animal studies, but clinical trials have not shown improved neurologic outcome after ischemia.

f. **Ketamine,** a phencyclidine derivative, produces dissociative anesthesia.

(1) Ketamine markedly increases ICP and CBF (60%) via cerebrovasodilatation. The $CMRO_2$ is unchanged or slightly increased. Autoregulation is abolished.

(2) **Seizures** might occur.

(3) Although ketamine is a noncompetitive NMDA antagonist, ketamine is not recommended for patients with intracranial pathology.

g. **Local anesthetics** are commonly used as adjuvants in neuroanesthesia.

(1) Lidocaine's clinical effects are determined by the dosage. When administered after EEG isoelectricity induced by pentobarbital, lidocaine may decrease $CMRO_2$ by an additional 15% to 20%. At clinically recommended doses (1.5 mg/kg), lidocaine has not consistently been shown to reduce ischemic damage. However, lidocaine may be useful in blunting the hemodynamic response to intubation and increasing anesthetic depth. At lower doses, lidocaine possesses anticonvulsant activity and can be used as ancillary therapy for status epilepticus. At toxic doses, lidocaine causes seizures.

C. Potent inhaled anesthetics

1. **Potent inhaled volatile agents.** All potent inhaled volatile anesthetics are cerebrovasodilators and thereby increase CBF and ICP to different degrees. This effect is attenuated by hyperventilation. They also decrease $CMRO_2$ while uncoupling CBF and $CMRO_2$. Autoregulation is impaired but CO_2 reactivity is preserved.

   a. **Halothane,** the most potent cerebrovasodilator of all the volatile agents, causes the greatest increase in CBF. Halothane decreases CSF production and decreases CSF resorption by the arachnoid villi. The critical CBF (minimum CBF below which EEG changes are seen with unilateral carotid artery occlusion) for halothane is 18 to 20 mL/100 g/minute.

   b. **Isoflurane** causes the greatest decrease in $CMRO_2$ (40% to 50%), with isoelectric EEG at 2.0 minimum alveolar concentration (MAC) or 2.4%, and is the least potent cerebral vasodilator. Isoflurane has no effect on CSF production but increases its resorption. The critical CBF for isoflurane, the lowest of all the volatile agents, is 10 mL/100 g/minute. Thus, isoflurane use in patients undergoing CEA may have advantages.

   c. **Enflurane** causes seizure activity at doses above 1.5 MAC, an effect that is exacerbated by hypocapnia. Enflurane increases production and decreases resorption of CSF. The critical CBF for enflurane is 15 mL/100 g/minute.

   d. **Sevoflurane** is similar to isoflurane in its cerebral effects; both cause a slight increase in CBF and ICP and a decrease in $CMRO_2$. Nephrotoxic inorganic fluoride may accumulate in prolonged operations. Induction and emergence are rapid.

   e. **Desflurane** is similar to isoflurane in its cerebrovascular profile, but ICP might increase despite normocapnia with desflurane compared to isoflurane. Induction and emergence with desflurane are rapid.

2. **Nitrous oxide,** a cerebrovasodilator, increases CBF and ICP. $CMRO_2$ is slightly increased. The increase in CBF is attenuated by barbiturates, opioids, and hypocapnia. Nitrous oxide is 32 times more soluble in blood than nitrogen and is thus capable of diffusing into air-containing body cavities with extreme rapidity. Therefore, it is avoided in cases of pneumocephalus and any surgical procedure within 2 weeks of a craniotomy in which N_2O was used. The N_2O is discontinued immediately if air embolism is suspected.

   D. Anticonvulsant drugs are indicated in patients at risk for seizure activity including individuals with epilepsy, head trauma, or craniotomy, and are continued into the postoperative period. Seizure activity worsens the effects of ischemia through activation of anaerobic metabolic pathways; CBF, $CMRO_2$, and intracellular Ca^{2+} increase during seizures and EAA neurotransmitters, including glutamate, are released.
   1. Once seizure activity occurs, the patient's airway is immediately secured and adequate ventilation ensured to prevent hypoxemia and hypercapnia.
   2. Avoidance of hypotension is essential.
   3. Anticonvulsant therapy is administered promptly:
      - **Thiopental sodium,** 25 to 100 mg IV
      - **Diazepam,** 2 to 20 mg IV
      - **Midazolam,** 1 to 5 mg IV.
      a. **Fosphenytoin sodium** [15 to 20 mg phenytoin equivalents (PE)/kg] or **phenytoin sodium** (15 mg/kg) may be administered to prevent further seizure activity once the acute episode has been stopped. (Fosphenytoin 75 mg is equivalent to phenytoin 50 mg.) Fosphenytoin has the advantage of increased speed of administration (up to 150 mg PE/minute); phenytoin is limited to 50 mg/minute due to hypotension. The loading dose of fosphenytoin can be given in 5 to 7 minutes, whereas the equivalent dose of phenytoin would require 15 to 20 minutes.
VI. Cerebral resuscitation. Patients requiring resuscitation from preexisting cerebral ischemia include the following:
   A. Intensive care unit (ICU) patients with traumatic but nonoperative brain injury such as **diffuse axonal injury (DAI)** with increased ICP and cerebral edema who may be candidates for barbiturate coma. These patients may require anesthesia for emergent subtemporal decompressive craniotomy and anterior temporal lobectomy.
   B. Patients with **Reye's syndrome** and cerebral edema with increased ICP.
   C. Near-drowning victims with **anoxic encephalopathy,** cerebral edema, and intracranial hypertension who are treated like patients with Reye's syndrome.
   D. Patients with **nonhemorrhagic stroke** who may be candidates for fibrinolytic therapy with tissue plasminogen activator (TPA).
      Anesthesiologists may encounter these patients in the ICU when they are consulted for assistance with management of cerebral edema and increased ICP or induction and maintenance of barbiturate coma. These patients may also require sedation, analgesia, and neuromuscular blockade.
VII. Experimental modalities
   A. NMDA receptor antagonists. This category of drugs was developed to prevent neuronal damage due to ex-

cessive accumulation of the excitatory neurotransmitter glutamate. The NMDA receptor antagonists have not conferred consistently reproducible neuroprotection in experimental studies. One of the difficulties has been the development of drugs that effectively penetrate the BBB.

1. **Dizocilpine maleate (MK-801)** is a noncompetitive NMDA receptor antagonist whose beneficial effects may be partially attributable to drug-induced hypothermia.

2. **Magnesium,** a noncompetitive NMDA antagonist, binds within the ion channel, preventing ion flux.

3. **Glycine binding site antagonism (HA-966** and **7-chlorokynurenic acid)** is still in the investigational stage but shows promise.

4. **AMPA receptor antagonism** with 2,3-dihydroxy-6-nitro-7-sulfamoylbenzo(F)quinazoline **(NBQX)** has proven beneficial when given after the ischemic insult.

B. **Sodium channel blockers** such as **riluzole** may reduce glutamate release during ischemia. **Lamotrigine,** an anticonvulsant with Na^+ channel blocking activity, is known to reduce glutamate release and ischemic damage. Further studies are warranted.

C. **Tirilazad, a lipid-soluble 21-aminosteroid,** crosses the BBB and acts as a lipid antioxidant, inhibiting free radical formation and lipid peroxidation. Studies indicate protection only when tirilazad is administered before an ischemic insult.

D. **Free radical scavengers. Superoxide dismutase** (SOD) **deferoxamine, vitamin E, mannitol,** and **glucocorticoids** all possess free radical scavenging activity. The utility of SOD has been limited by its short $t\frac{1}{2}$ (8 minute) and poor BBB penetration. While glucocorticoids have membrane stabilizing properties and decrease cerebral edema from brain tumors, they have not been shown to improve outcome in cerebral ischemia. Clinical usefulness of free radical scavengers is still under investigation.

E. **Modification of arachidonic acid synthesis.** Ischemia-induced excess of the vasoconstrictor thromboxane relative to the vasodilator prostacyclin (PGI_2) has led to the development of **thromboxane synthetase inhibitors** and **PGI_2 synthetase stimulation** to prevent the formation of excessive thromboxane.

F. **The α_2 agonist dexmedetomidine** decreases central sympathetic activity by decreasing plasma norepinephrine release. Dexmedetomidine has been found to be neuroprotective in a model of focal ischemia, perhaps because excess catecholamine levels correlate with increased neuronal ischemic damage. Dexmedetomidine also decreases the MAC for halothane and isoflurane and decreases CBF without significantly altering $CMRO_2$.

G. Nitric oxide (NO) is a free radical with complex neuronal activity. Nitric oxide synthase (NOS) catalyzes the formation of NO from the amino acid L-arginine, which itself decreases neuronal damage in experimental focal ischemia. Three forms of NOS have been discovered:

1. **Neuronal NOS (nNOS)** enhances glutamate release and NMDA-mediated neurotoxicity. Selective nNOS inhibition has been shown to be neuroprotective.
2. **Immunologic NOS (iNOS)** is not detectable in healthy tissue. Induction of iNOS causes delayed neuronal cell death and can also exacerbate glutamate excitotoxicity. Inhibition of iNOS by **aminoguanidine** reduces ischemic damage in experimental models.
3. **Endothelial NOS (eNOS).** Stimulation of eNOS by increased intracellular Ca^{2+} due to ischemia improves CBF by dilatation of cerebral blood vessels and has been shown to reduce ischemic damage in a rodent model.

ACKNOWLEDGMENTS

The authors gratefully acknowledge the expert editorial assistance of James B. Eisenkraft, M.D., and the invaluable neurosurgical contribution of Hal W. Pittman, M.D. in the preparation of this manuscript.

SUGGESTED READINGS

Busto R, Dietrich WD, Globus MY, et al. Small differences in intraischemic brain temperature critically determine the extent of ischemic neuronal injury. *J Cereb Blood Flow Metab* 1987;7:729.

Farnsworth ST, Sperry RJ. Neurophysiology. In: Stone DJ, Sperry RJ, Johnson JO, et al., eds. *The neuroanesthesia handbook.* St. Louis: Mosby, 1996.

Guy J, Hindman BJ, Baker KZ, et al. Comparison of remifentanil and fentanyl in patients undergoing craniotomy for supratentorial space-occupying lesions. *Anesthesiology* 1997;86:514–524.

Lam AM. Anesthetic management of patients with traumatic head injury. In: Lam AM, ed. *Anesthetic management of acute head injury.* New York: McGraw-Hill, 1995:183.

Milde LN, Weglinski MR. Pathophysiology of metabolic brain injury. In: Cottrell JE, Smith DS, eds. *Anesthesia and neurosurgery.* St. Louis: Mosby, 1994:61.

The National Institute of Neurological Disorders and Stroke rt-PA Stroke Study Group. Tissue plasminogen activator for acute ischemic stroke. *N Engl J Med* 1995;333(24):1581–1587.

Shapiro HM. Anesthesia effects upon cerebral blood flow, cerebral metabolism, electroencephalogram, and evoked potentials. In: Miller RD, ed. *Anesthesia,* 2nd ed. New York: Churchill Livingstone, 1986:1276.

Spetzler RF, Hadley MN, Rigamonti D, et al. Aneurysms of the basilar artery treated with circulatory arrest, hypothermia, and barbiturate cerebral protection. *J Neurosurg* 1988;68:868–879.

Preoperative Evaluation

Roger E. Traill

I. **The patient**
   A. **General considerations.** Detailed preoperative knowledge of a patient's neurologic disease and its pathophysiologic effects as well as the usual assessment of his or her general medical state are essential to the proper planning of a neurosurgical anesthetic. The purpose of the preoperative evaluation is to allow this assessment to occur, to inform the patient of the risks and options for anesthetic management, and to formulate in conjunction with the surgeon an appropriate anesthetic management plan.
   B. **Neurologic history.** The neurologic history gives us valuable information about the patient's disease process and current neurologic state. The history is usually taken in a narrative fashion. If not volunteered, one needs to ask specifically about:
      1. **Symptoms and duration**
         a. **When patient can't give a history.** In these circumstances the patient is often unable to provide information and it is important to gather what information one can from witnesses to the injury/collapse or the paramedics who were involved in the resuscitation and transport. In many hospitals the anesthesia staff are not part of the trauma team and if this is the case then one should try and get information from the emergency room staff involved in the initial resuscitation. The key pieces of information that must be obtained are:
            (1) **Nature of the trauma, e.g., motor vehicle accident, gun shot, etc.** This gives valuable information about the likelihood of other injuries and the probable progression of their state.
            (2) **Level of consciousness.** Immediately after the injury and whether this has changed since then.
            (3) **Gross movement of limbs.** A history of all limbs moving indicates no gross spinal cord injury. Failure of leg movement raises the issue of paraplegia, and no movement in one arm raises the possibility of brachial plexus injury (and possible first-rib fracture and thoracic aortic damage).

(4) **Cardiorespiratory state since injury.**
Presence of hypo- or hypertension, hypoventilation, hypoxemia.

b. **When the patient can give a history.**

(1) **Seizures.** This is often the mode of presentation for tumors. One needs to find out whether these are generalized or focal, whether anticonvulsant treatment has been started, and whether or not it has been effective in controlling the seizures.

(2) **Focal signs.** A history of neurologic changes related to the location of the tumor is the other most common mode of presentation for tumors. The specific presentation depends on the location of the tumor. Supratentorial tumors involving the motor cortex may present with arm, face, or leg weakness. Brain stem lesions may present with cranial nerve palsies.

Chronic subdural hematomas may present with hemiparesis or arm weakness due to local pressure effects in addition to headaches and decreased mentation. Rarely, aneurysms, e.g., basilar aneurysms, may present with cranial nerve palsies when they become large enough to produce local pressure effects. The specific history will give clues as to the location of the lesion.

(3) **Symptoms/signs of raised intracranial pressure (ICP).** These are relatively nonspecific and depend greatly on the cause and rapidity of onset of the underlying pathology. The symptoms are either the result of compromised cerebral perfusion pressure (CPP) or from the effects of brain shift. If the effect is solely due to compromised CPP, e.g., as in benign intracranial hypertension, then the ICP will need to be as high as 40 to 50 mm Hg before marked symptoms occur. If the pressure rise is nonuniform, e.g., trauma or tumor, then brain shift will occur producing symptoms and signs related to herniation of brain tissue (see later). In these cases symptoms and signs may occur when the ICP is only 20 to 30 mm Hg.

General symptoms of raised ICP include headache (classically worse in the morning and made worse by coughing and straining), nausea, vomiting, altered mentation, and visual problems (IIIrd and VIth nerve palsies).

(4) **Signs of meningeal irritation.** Headache, photophobia, and stiff neck are the classical symptoms and signs of this. Meningitis and subarachnoid hemorrhage (SAH) are the two most important causes. Patients with SAH will often give a history of episodes of transient symptoms for 2 to 3 weeks preceding their final presentation. These are thought to represent minor hemorrhages (sentinel bleeding). Recognition of the importance of these symptoms prior to the final SAH can lead to timely diagnosis and treatment of the aneurysm with excellent outcome.

(5) **Peripheral nervous system.** A history of weakness of arms and/or legs and loss of sensation should be sought. The exact level of the motor or sensory change helps to determine the location of the lesion. Bladder dysfunction indicates sacral nerve root dysfunction.

(6) **Transient ischemic attack (TIA)/reversible ischemic neurologic deficits (RIND).** A TIA lasts from several minutes to up to 24 hours. If the deficit lasts longer than that but resolves within 72 hours, then it is called a RIND. If the deficit lasts longer than 72 hours, it is called a stroke.

Carotid artery disease produces symptoms by embolic phenomena (most common) or by hemodynamic insufficiency. In the latter case, the symptoms will occur when the blood pressure (BP) falls below some critical level. Symptoms that occur on rising from a supine or sitting position are suggestive of this. If the patient has been admitted to the hospital with TIAs and heparinized, the BP at the time of subsequent TIAs (if lower than usual) is helpful in determining the lower limit for BP during the anesthetic.

Knowing the type of TIAs helps to determine the vascular area most at risk. Amaurosis fugax (transient monocular blindness) is caused by platelet emboli to the ophthalmic arteries and is indicative of ipsilateral carotid disease. Transient weakness of the face and arm (often associated with difficulty in speaking) indicates ischemia of the contralateral middle cerebral artery. Leg weakness (less common) indicates ischemia of the contralateral anterior cerebral artery. Posterior circulation (basilar/vertebral arteries) TIAs cause more nebulous symptoms of dizziness and vertigo, numbness of the contralateral face/limbs, diplopia, hoarseness, dysarthria, and dysphagia. Hemiparesis is rare.

(7) **Stroke.** Past cerebrovascular accidents must be fully elucidated including when they occurred, their management, and how they have revolved.

2. **Interventions to date**
   a. **Surgery/anesthesia.** The patient's history of surgery and anesthesia gives vital information about management in this case. If at all possible, one should review the patient's past operative and anesthetic records. Specific problems raised by the patient need to be discussed in full. If necessary, one should contact prior anesthesiologists and surgeons to elucidate the nature of previous problems.

      Patients who have hydrocephalus, especially one presenting during the neonatal period, e.g., spina bifida or meningitis, usually have a long and detailed surgical history of repeated shunt revisions and associated operations, e.g., Arnold-Chiari malformation repairs, spinal surgery, temporal decompressions. These patients often have a very clear idea of what problems they have had with anesthetics and how they wish their anesthetic treatment to be conducted.

   b. **Radiation.** Local irradiation has little anesthetic importance. However, if the patient is presenting with metastases and has had radiation to the primary site, then the effects there need to be considered. Occasionally a patient who has had irradiation for spinal metastases may develop acute cord compression and need an urgent decompressive laminectomy.

   c. **Chemotherapy.** Patients with primary tumors do not commonly receive chemotherapy prior to presenting for surgery. Patients with metastases may well have had chemotherapy for their primary lesion. These drugs have important effects on the cardiac, respiratory, and hematologic systems. It is important to find out which drugs have been used and to assess the systems commonly affected by those drugs.

   d. **Aspirin, heparin, warfarin for TIAs.** Many patients with carotid disease will be taking aspirin. Those in whom aspirin does not control the TIAs will be given anticoagulants: warfarin in the chronic situation and heparin acutely. Whether this has controlled their TIAs is important.

   3. **Neurobehavioral evaluation.** This is often performed pre- and postoperatively to assess the effects of surgery. This tests memory, attention span, spatial perception, and higher cognition. Changes in areas of higher function might mean that someone who at first glance seems neurologically intact is in fact completely unable to function in normal society. These tests are usually carried out by a neuropsychologist.

C. **Medical history**
   1. **Cardiovascular.** The older patients get, the more likely they are to have cardiovascular disease. In addition, patients presenting for cerebrovascular surgery, e.g., carotid endarterectomies or clip ligation of cerebral aneurysms, have a higher incidence of cardiovascular disease. Patients with acromegaly or Cushing's disease (pituitary tumors) are also more likely to have cardiovascular disease.

      The patient needs to be specifically asked about prior myocardial infarction, the presence of angina (relationship with exercise, recent frequency, treatment), exercise capacity (often most easily quantified in terms of the number of flights of stairs climbed without a rest), nocturnal shortness of breath, and ankle edema. Those with a clear history of ischemic heart disease (IHD) or congestive heart failure (CHF) should be asked about investigation, e.g., stress tests, angiograms, echocardiograms, and interventions to date, such as medications, angioplasties, and coronary bypass. A determination of whether these interventions/treatments have had any beneficial effects is also important.

      Ischemic heart disease is a relative contraindication to induced hypotension. Those with compromised cardiac function may also be less able to tolerate the postural effects of the sitting position. A history of an atrial or ventricular septal defect or probe patent foramen ovale is an absolute contraindication to the sitting position (due to the risk of paradoxical air embolus).

      Myocardial infarction (MI) within the last 6 months is a relative contraindication to surgery. However, most neurosurgical procedures are not elective and postponement for this period of time is usually not prudent. In determining the best balance between cardiac risks and the risks of delaying surgery, one needs to assess the cardiac risk associated with the particular operation and anesthetic, obtain a cardiologic review, and do specific tests of cardiac function (echocardiogram) and ischemic potential (stress tests, thallium scans, coronary angiography). Clearly, the greater the risks of delay, e.g., grade 1 SAH, the more beneficial it is to proceed. The critical question to ask is whether the patient will be in a better state if surgery is delayed and, if so, how long it will take. Someone in florid cardiogenic shock in the setting of SAH will probably benefit from stabilization over a day or two, whereas someone with electrocardiogram (ECG) changes and no other evidence of cardiac disease probably would not.

2. **Respiratory.** Many of these patients are smokers and information about the extent and duration of cigarette exposure must be sought. A patient's exercise capacity must be assessed (as above) and its limiting factors determined, e.g., shortness of breath, angina, claudication, etc. The presence of reversible airways disease (asthma) is important as are treatments and current state. One needs to state specifically whether the assessment is by using airflow meters (reliable) or clinical symptoms (unreliable). Adult onset asthma is often more difficult to control. Information about the need for oral steroids, hospital admission, and intubation/ventilation is important in determining the severity of the disease.

3. **Endocrine**
   a. **Diabetes insipidus (DI).** This is associated with pituitary disease (posterior pituitary dysfunction). The patient will give a history of polyuria and polydypsia. Nocturia is also a useful clue in a young person. If patients are being treated, it is necessary to clarify what the treatment is, how often it is taken, and how effective it is. A patient with DI who becomes obtunded may rapidly become dehydrated and develop electrolyte abnormalities if fluid replacement is inappropriate.
   b. **Diabetes mellitus (DM).** Patients having intracranial surgery are often given steroids. It is not uncommon for this to induce or worsen DM. A history of high blood sugars, e.g., during pregnancy, makes this more likely. Assessment of a patient's DM includes the nature of the control, e.g., diet, oral hypoglycemic, or insulin (insulin requiring), and whether the patient has had any episodes of ketoacidosis (insulin-dependent). The patient should also be able to tell you how good the control has been recently and what complications have ensued. Diabetics have increased risk of vascular disease (cerebral, cardiac,

and peripheral especially), renal disease, and autonomic dysfunction. The perioperative management of DM is outlined in Roizen's contribution to Miller's book *Anesthesia,* 4th edition.

c. **Panhypopituitarism.** This is not uncommon after pituitary surgery or with large pituitary tumors. Clinical symptoms are often minimal. Pituitary adenomas may be associated with multiple endocrine neoplasia type 1 (parathyroid hyperplasia/adenoma, pancreatic islet cell hyperplasia/adenoma, pheochromocytoma, and carcinoid syndrome).

d. **Acromegaly.** The patients complain that their shoes and gloves no longer fit and their voice is deeper. They may also complain of polyuria and polydypsia from DM.

e. **Cushing's disease.** Patients complain of weakness, especially in getting out of a chair (proximal myopathy), central obesity, striae, easy bruising. They may also complain of polyuria and polydypsia from DM.

4. **Hematologic.** Most neurosurgical operations do not allow the placement of drains and the compartments operated are not distensible (intracranial and spinal operations). Postoperative hemorrhage therefore produces severe complications. A history of easy bruising, cuts that take a long time to stop bleeding, or problems with bleeding after previous operations or dental procedures should alert one to the possibility of a bleeding problem. This should be investigated further before surgery proceeds.

5. **Renal disease.** Renal impairment is associated with vascular disease. Symptoms are slight until the condition is very advanced. Renal impairment is associated with platelet abnormalities and is also a relative contraindication to the use of mannitol and furosemide due to the risk of hypovolemia or osmotic-induced renal failure. The use of contrast in computed tomographic (CT) scans must be restricted in the presence of renal impairment because of renal toxicity.

D. **Fasting status.** The time of the patient's last oral intake should be noted. It is important to remember that for a trauma patient it is the time from last oral intake to trauma that represents the duration of fasting regardless of when the operation occurs.

E. **Medications.** Neurosurgical patients often take numerous medications. There are some specific concerns related to some of these:
- Steroids can lead to DM.
- Aspirin, nonsteroidal anti-inflammatory drugs (NSAIDs), and valproate can cause platelet dysfunc-

tion. Aspirin must be stopped for 7 to 10 days before its effect will pass. The NSAIDs need to be stopped for 5 times their half-life. Valproate causes platelet dysfunction in about 30% of patients. However, some centers still perform craniotomies without stopping the drug.

- Anticonvulsants, especially phenytoin, carbamazepine, and barbiturates, increase metabolism of steroidal muscle relaxants (pancuronium, vecuronium, rocuronium).
- Angiotensin-converting enzyme inhibitors may be associated with intraoperative instability, so that some anesthesiologists recommend their discontinuation prior to surgery. This is not this author's practice.

F. Allergies. Patients who have spina bifida have a much higher incidence of latex allergy. Symptoms of latex allergy should be specifically sought in this group. Symptoms include previous allergies to latex products during surgery, facial edema or asthma with balloons, reactions to latex gloves or catheters. If symptoms suggestive of latex allergy are found, then the patient should be assumed to be allergic until testing proves otherwise.

G. Social. The patient's intake of alcohol, tobacco, and other nonprescription drugs (legal and illegal) must be quantified.

H. Physical examination.

1. **Trauma** (Table 5-1). Assessment of trauma patients should consist of an initial look at the patient for obvious injuries, followed by primary and secondary surveys. One needs to consider other injuries such as thoracic and abdominal and long bone fractures.

2. **Neurologic**

   a. **General**

      (1) **Glasgow Coma Scale (GCS)** (Table 5-2). This is the standard means of assessing the neurologic state of a patient and is useful in management and prognosis. An unconscious patient is unable to protect the airway. In an acute situation, this would necessitate intubation. A GCS score of ≤9 is usually an indication for intubation and ventilation.

      (2) **Signs of raised ICP.** Papilledema and IIIrd and VIth nerve palsies occur because of brain shift. Lesions, e.g., posterior fossa tumors and basilar aneurysms, that obstruct the CSF pathways may raise the ICP to a greater extent than would be expected on their size alone. Coma is a severe manifestation of raised ICP.

Table 5-1. Trauma patient examination

1) Look for obvious injuries
2) Primary survey:
   A Airway
   - Look for chest wall movement, retraction, and nasal flaring
   - Listen for breath sounds, stridor, and obstructed breathing
   - Feel for air movement

   B Breathing
   - Look to see if ventilation is adequate
   - Look for open pneumothorax, open chest wound, or flail segments
   - Listen for bilateral chest sounds

   C Circulation
   - Feel peripheral pulses, measure blood pressure and capillary refill
   - Perform an electrocardiogram

   D Disability (neurologic state)
   - Check level of consciousness

A	Alert
V	responds to **V**ocal command
P	responds to **P**ainful stimulus
D	unresponsive

   - Check pupillary response to light

   E Expose patient fully for complete examination
3) Secondary survey

Table 5-2. Glasgow coma score

Eye opening	
Spontaneous	4
To speech	3
To pain	2
None	1
Verbal response	
Oriented	5
Confused conversation	4
Incomprehensible words	3
Incomprehensible sounds	2
None	1
Best motor response	
Obeys	6
Localizes	5
Withdraws	4
Abnormal flexion	3
Extensor response	2
None	1
Total	15

b. Specific
   (1) Cranial nerves. The following cranial nerves may need assessment in neurosurgical patients:

   (a) I—Olfactory nerve. The loss of the sense of smell (anosmia) in the absence of nasal problems or inflammation is associated with frontal lobe and pituitary lesions, meningitis, or an anterior cranial fossa fracture. Unilateral anosmia is much more likely to be significant.

   (b) II—Optic nerve. Lesions distal to the optic chiasm produce monocular blindness (with no pupillary response to light in that eye but preserved response to light in the other eye). Lesions pressing on the center of the chiasm produce bitemporal hemianopia (pituitary tumors). Lesion pressing on the lateral aspect of the chiasm produce nasal hemianopia in the ipsilateral eye, and lesions proximal to the chiasm produce homonymous hemianopia (loss of contralateral fields). Pupils should be checked in all neurosurgical patients.

   (c) III—Oculomotor nerve. This nerve controls pupillary size and response to light and all intrinsic eye muscles except the external rectus and superior oblique. Complete IIIrd nerve palsy causes ptosis, a divergent squint (affected eye looks down and out), pupillary dilatation, loss of accommodation and light reflexes, and double vision. It is commonly affected in uncal and temporal lobe herniation.

   (d) IV, V, VI—Trochlear, trigeminal, and abducens nerves. Cavernous sinus lesions may produce IIIrd, IVth, Vth, and VIth cranial nerve lesions as they all travel inside (IIIrd) or in the lateral wall of the cavernous sinus. Lesions of the ophthalmic branch of the Vth nerve produce loss of the corneal reflex, which renders the patient more likely to sustain corneal damage. The VIth nerve has a long intracranial course and is often affected by raised ICP and injuries to the base of the skull. The patient will complain of diplopia and will be unable to look laterally with the involved eye (convergent squint).

(e) **VII—Facial nerve.** The VIIth nerve supplies the muscles to the face and taste to the anterior two thirds of the tongue. It is sometimes affected by large cerebellopontine tumors, and facial paralysis is one of the common complications of surgery for these tumors. A proper preoperative assessment is vital in determining if a change related to surgery has occurred.

(f) **VIII—Auditory nerve.** Unilateral hearing loss is the usual presentation for cerebellopontine angle tumors, e.g., acoustic neuromas. Certain operations, e.g., microvascular decompressions of cranial nerves, have a significant incidence of postoperative deafness and preoperative evaluation of hearing is important in determining if surgery is the cause.

(g) **IX, X—Glossopharyngeal and vagus nerves.** The IXth nerve supplies sensation to the posterior third of the tongue and pharynx. The gag reflex uses the IXth nerve as its afferent limb and the Xth nerve as its efferent limb. Its absence increases the risk of aspiration. Ninth nerve dysfunction is rare in isolation. Tenth nerve dysfunction often gives symptoms of speech changes that are nasal in nature due to paralysis of the palate.

(2) **Peripheral nervous system.** Testing for touch sensation can elicit the level of damage in patients with spinal cord injuries or compression. The phrenic nerve is supplied by C_3, C_4, and C_5. Patients who have low cervical myelopathy or low cervical lesions can breath quite adequately without the intercostal and abdominal assistance to breathing due to continued diaphragmatic function although respiratory reserve will be impaired. Once the level of the cord lesion gets to C_5 or above, breathing is rapidly compromised.

The testing of reflexes is also useful in determining the level of the lesion, e.g., biceps ($C_{5/6}$), triceps ($C_{6/7}$), upper abdominal ($T_{7/8/9}$), lower abdominal ($T_{11/12}$), knee ($L_{2/3/4}$), and ankle ($S_{1/2}$).

The plantar reflex—the response of the toes to stroking of the lateral aspect of the sole of the foot—is normally downgoing. The Babinski sign is an abnormal response and consists of an upgoing toe and fanning of the toes. It is present in upper motor neuron disease or pyramidal tract damage.

A simple screen for gross motor function is to check bilateral grasp and bilateral dorsiflexion noting differences between sides and upper and lower limbs. This simple check should be performed on all neurosurgical patients.

3. **Cardiac.** General examination should include measurement of the BP and heart rate, examination for peripheral edema and raised jugular venous pressure, auscultation of the heart (heart sounds and presence of valve lesions) and chest (basal crepitations), and assessment of the peripheral pulses (at least the upper limbs). In patients with vascular disease it is important to compare the pulses in both radial arteries; if any difference is detected, the BP in both arms is measured. These patients may have subclavian stenosis with quite different BPs in each arm. The arm with the higher BP is the one used for BP measurement. The patient should be told about this difference. Hypertension is very common in patients with vascular disease, Cushing's disease, and acromegaly.

4. **Respiratory.** General examination should include respiratory rate and effort, the presence of cyanosis, and auscultation of the chest. Specifically asking the patient to breath in and out maximally gives an indication of vital capacity that is often decreased in patients with scoliosis, cervical myelopathy, and a history of smoking.

5. **Endocrine.** The manifestations of Cushing's disease (moon facies, central obesity, hirsutism, striae, easy bruising, proximal muscle weakness, plethora) and acromegaly (coarse facial features, prognathism, large tongue, large feet/hands) may be seen. Both are also associated with DM.

6. **Airway.** The airway must always be carefully assessed. Among neurosurgical patients, acromegalics have large jaws, faces, and tongues, which may make airway management and intubation difficult. Patients having temporal decompressions might have limited mouth opening due to temporomandibular joint fibrosis. Trauma patients may have facial, neck, and larynx injuries that require careful assessment.

7. **Volume status.** The intravascular volume needs to be carefully assessed in patients with trauma, DM, DI, and aneurysm, obtunded patients, and patients who had a recent angiogram or were fasting.

8. **Nasal passages when nasal intubation planned.** If a nasal intubation is planned it is important to exclude fractures to the base of skull and CSF leaks; both are contraindications. Assessing which nostril is more patent is useful in the elective patient.

I. **Laboratory studies**

1. **Neurodiagnostic studies.** Ideally one should have direct access to the neurodiagnostic studies. As these are often not available to us, at least the reports should be reviewed. Valuable information will be missed if this is not done.

   a. **Computed tomography/magnetic resonance imaging**

      (1) **Hemorrhage.** Hemorrhage shows as an area of high density (white) on computed tomography (CT) scan. Extraaxial bleeding (epidural, subdural, and subarachnoidal) is commonly associated with trauma. Subarachnoid and intraventricular bleeding is associated with aneurysm rupture. Computed tomography will detect 90% of all subarachnoid bleeds in the first 24 hours. Isolated parenchymal bleeding is likely to be nontraumatic in nature (hypertension, tumors, or vascular lesions). Cerebral contusions that consist of parenchymal microhemorrhages will coalesce to become visible on CT as ill-defined areas of high attenuation involving the gyral crests.

      (2) **Fractures.** Computed tomography is superior to the magnetic resonance imaging (MRI) in diagnosis of skull fractures and is the imaging modality of choice in head trauma. The digital lateral scout view of the CT scan should always be assessed for skull or upper cervical spine fractures that may not be seen on the axial views.

      (3) **Cerebral edema** (brain swelling due to excess water and sodium accumulation). There are three types: vasogenic, cytotoxic, and interstitial. However, except for location, the CT and MRI changes are similar. Edema shows on CT scans as a decrease in density and appears dark. The MRI shows increased water as deceased signal (black) on T1-weighted studies and increased signal

(white) on T2-weighted studies. Contrast enhancement occurs early in vasogenic edema and later in cytotoxic edema.

(4) **Herniation syndromes.** Herniation of the brain may occur when there are nonuniform increases in ICP.

   (a) **Subfalcine (under the falx).** This is associated with effacement of ipsilateral lateral ventricle. Occasionally there may be an increase in the size of the contralateral lateral ventricle because of obstruction of the foramen of Monro. The falx will be shifted over ("midline shift"). There will be asymmetry of the six-pointed star representing the suprasellar cistern which progresses to complete obliteration of this space.

   (b) **Transtentorial (through the tentorial notch).** This is more ominous and may be descending (supratentorial lesions) or ascending (infratentorial, e.g., cerebellar lesions). The ascending type may be associated with enlarged ventricles due to aqueduct obstruction. The descending type can be unilateral or bilateral. Initially the uncus is displaced medially initially progressing to downward herniation.

   (c) **Tonsillar (through the foramen magnum).** When there is increased pressure in the posterior fossa or transmitted pressure from the supratentorial space, the cerebellar tonsils may herniate inferiorly through the foramen magnum. This is associated with medullary compression and death. Decerebrate posturing, respiratory disturbance, and cardiac irregularities are common. Performing a lumbar puncture in this setting can be fatal as it increases the herniation by decompressing the CSF from below.

   (d) **Transcalvarial (through a defect in the skull).** If the skull is no longer contiguous, brain may herniate through the defect. This is usually associated with a severe head injury.

(5) **Tumors.** The CT scan and MRI will demonstrate the specific location and size of

the lesion as well as giving some indication of its nature, e.g., glioma, meningioma, metastasis. From this can be determined the likely operative position and the need for brain shrinkage (for deep lesions). The degree of tumor vascularity, hydrocephalus, surrounding edema, midline shift, and some indication of raised ICP can also be determined.

(6) **Hydrocephalus.** In communicating hydrocephalus the obstruction occurs at the point of CSF absorption and all of the ventricles (lateral, third, and fourth) are dilated in proportion on CT. There may also be indistinct areas of symmetrical low density around the periventricular regions indicative of interstitial edema. Herniation syndromes are not seen. In noncommunicating hydrocephalus the obstruction occurs within the ventricular system and a portion of it will be dilated out of proportion to the rest. Herniation syndromes may then be seen.

(7) **Pneumocephalus.** This may be seen on CT after skull fractures, operations (either from air left *in situ* or via CSF leaks), pneumoencephalograms, or lumbar punctures. The presence of intracranial air is a contraindication to the use of nitrous oxide.

(8) **Raised ICP.** The signs of raised ICP on the CT are effacement of the cortical sulci, basal cisterns, and interhemispheric fissures, compressed ventricles (if hydrocephalus is not the cause), and herniation syndromes. There may also be a decrease in the size of the pituitary gland and even potential enlargement of the sella turcica associated with a partially empty sella.

b. **Plain skull films.** Plain skull films, although good for diagnosing fractures, are much less sensitive in diagnosing intracranial pathology. The indications are limited to the investigation of penetrating injuries (especially for the course, location, and number of gunshot fragments), the location of other foreign bodies, and the presence and relationships of depressed skull fractures.

c. **Positron emission tomography (PET).** The PET scan allows *in vivo* assessment of brain physiology and biochemistry, and is useful in diagnosing grades of glioma and in differentiating recurrent tumor from radiation-induced necrosis. The spatial resolution of PET is not a good as that of CT or MRI.

d. **Angiogram, embolization, balloon occlusions,** and **the Wada test.** It is always worth reviewing the angiogram report (if done) prior to anesthesia. Valuable information can be obtained about the vascularity of the lesion, whether any vessels are involved or at risk during the procedure (which helps decide whether evoked potential monitoring is indicated and, if so, which type), the general state of the intracranial vasculature, and the presence of cross-filling. Intracranial stenosis and the absence of cross-filling increase the risk of cross-clamp-related cerebral ischemia in carotid endarterectomies. The venogram gives information about the risk of bleeding (in arteriovenous malformation, or AVM) and the general nature of the cerebral venous system.

Very vascular tumors and AVMs often have major feeding vessels embolized at the time of the angiogram. This substantially reduces the bleeding associated with surgery but carries the risk of hemorrhage, inadvertent occlusion of functional vessels, and cerebral edema. It is important to know the extent to which the embolization has or has not been effective. This aids in the planning for vascular access and the types of blood warmers and rapid infusion devices needed.

Sometimes when the surgeon wants to know if it is safe to occlude a major vessel, e.g., in a cavernous sinus aneurysm, the radiologist will occlude the vessel with a balloon when the patient is awake and see if any neurologic changes occur. With the Wada test, the radiologist injects a fast-acting barbiturate into the cerebral circulation (intracarotid or posterior cerebral) and assesses the effect on each temporal lobe. Typically, the test is used to determine the suitability of a patient for temporal lobectomy for epilepsy. The aim is to identify which lobe is dominant with regard to language and memory.

e. **Carotid ultrasounds.** It is important to know the degree of carotid artery stenosis when a patient presents for carotid endarterectomy. The presence of contralateral stenosis or occlusion makes it more likely that ischemia (however detected) will occur with cross-clamping of the carotid. Patients scheduled for other types of neurosurgical procedures should also have preoperative carotid ultrasounds should a bruit be detected preoperatively over the carotids. The presence of an asymptomatic stenosis if severe may warrant this being addressed prior to other procedures. If left untreated a carotid stenosis makes it more likely that hypotension during surgery will cause cerebral ischemia.

    f.   Transcranial Doppler. This is done commonly on patients who have had a subarachnoid hemorrhage in order to detect the presence of vasospasm. The diagnosis is made on the basis of increased flow velocity. The presence of vasospasm, even if subclinical, is a relative contraindication to induced hypotension and a risk factor should inadvertent hypotension occur perioperatively.

    g.   Visual fields (pituitary surgery). Pituitary tumors will often affect the visual fields and this may be worsened by surgery (often temporarily). Visual fields are evaluated routinely prior to this type of surgery.

J.   What tests do we need? Much is written about the need to be selective in the tests we order preoperatively. In general, however, the neurosurgical patient is different. The disease processes mandate the following routine tests:

    1.   Electrolytes—Na^+/K^+/Cl^-/TCO2/Glucose/Ca^{2+} (albumin if low). Electrolyte disturbances are common both pre- and postoperatively. Changes in serum sodium (Na^+) are associated with marked changes in brain volume. Potassium (K^+) loss is common with diuretics and steroids. Chloride (Cl^-) and total CO_2 (TCO_2) help delineate common electrolyte disturbances. Glucose measurement is needed as hyperglycemia is common with steroids and endocrine abnormalities and may exacerbate neurological damage should cerebral ischemia occur.

        Hypo- and hypercalcemia are common in malignancy and hypocalcemia is a risk factor for seizures. If the calcium is low, then one needs to check the albumin concentration as hypoalbuminemia will produce artifactual hypocalcemia (50% is bound to albumin).

    2.   Liver function tests. These are needed in patients taking anticonvulsants, especially phenytoin as hepatic toxicity is not uncommon.

    3.   Full blood count should be determined for all neurosurgical patients. Platelet count helps determine the risk of bleeding. Hemoglobin indicates the risk of cerebral and cardiac ischemia and provides a baseline should bleeding occur. The white cell count is useful as a guide to infection but is often elevated with steroid usage and postoperatively.

    4.   Coagulation tests. If the patient gives a history suggestive of a bleeding disorder, a prothrombin time (PT) and partial thromboplastin time (PTT) should be measured to assess coagulation. If these are abnormal, further tests are needed to elucidate the exact nature of the coagulation disorder and the most appropriate perioperative management.

A hematologist's advice should be sought. Because of the major consequences of postoperative hemorrhage, these tests are often done as screening tests for intracranial and spinal surgery. No evidence to support or refute this practice exists for neurosurgical patients.

5. **Platelet function tests.** Patients who have had drugs that interfere with platelet function should be tested if the consequences of bleeding are great (intracranial surgery) or if the procedure cannot be delayed until the drugs and their effects have passed. Even if one proceeds, the tests are useful because if bleeding occurs intraoperatively and the platelet function tests are normal, then no indication exists to give platelets unless major bleeding has occurred. Platelet function tests take hours to perform and cannot be done emergently.

6. **Cardiac studies**
   a. **ECG.** Patients requiring preoperative ECG include men over 40, women over 50, and any patient with a history of cardiac disease or at increased risk of cardiac disease, e.g., hypertension, hypercholesterolemia, diabetes, cerebral aneurysm, vascular disease in other sites, or electrolyte abnormalities. Patients in whom induced hypotension may be used, e.g., AVMs, who might not have other indications should also have an ECG.

   b. **Echocardiography (two-dimensional), dobutamine echo.** Echocardiography is indicated for patients who have or may have impaired cardiac function or valvular disease. An echocardiogram may also be part of the workup for patients having operations in the sitting position to detect the presence of a patent foramen ovale.

   c. **Stress ECG tests, exercise thallium scans, dipyramidole thallium scans.** These are all used to delineate the nature of chest pains or the significance of ECG changes. Elective patients who can exercise would usually have a stress ECG first (possibly combined with a thallium scan). Those who cannot exercise are given dipyramidole to induce intracoronary steal and simulate exercise. Consultation with a cardiologist is suggested if significant cardiac disease is suspected.

   d. **Coronary angiography.** This is the gold

standard to diagnose coronary artery disease. Left ventriculography also gives an indication about left ventricular function and aortic and mitral valve function. Angioplasty might be possible at the same time if a suitable lesion is present.

7. **Respiratory function tests**
   a. **Spirometry.** Spirometry is indicated for any patient with pulmonary disease or in whom respiratory reserve may be compromised (cervical myelopathy, scoliosis).
   b. **Blood gases.** These should be done where the patient has marked pulmonary disease. Diagnosis of patients with carbon dioxide retention warns of a group with minimal respiratory reserve. Patients with preexisting hypoxemia will need pulse oximetry monitoring for a least 48 hours after operation.
   c. **Chest x-ray.** This is indicated only in patients with cardiovascular disease, significant pulmonary disease, abnormal anatomy of the tracheobronchial tree, and where there is a suspicion of tuberculosis or intrathoracic malignancy.
   d. **Sleep apnea.** Patients with a history of this condition need to have their continuous positive airway pressure (CPAP) systems available for them in the postanesthesia care unit (PACU) and need postoperative pulse oximetry monitoring. Those with a history suggestive of this condition should be evaluated prior to elective surgery due to the risks of postoperative hypoxemia.

8. **Implications of disorders of:**
   a. **Hemoglobin (Hb).** Hb <10 g/dL can lead to a greater incidence of myocardial or cerebral ischemia (unless chronic). Routine administration of blood to raise Hb preoperatively is no longer justifiable. An Hb > 16 (polycythemia) is associated with a greater risk of complications; reducing Hb below 16 appears to reduce the risk of complications.
   b. **Platelets.** Platelet counts <75,000 necessitate preoperative platelet transfusions. When platelet function tests demonstrate mildly impaired function and the surgery has a low risk of bleeding, then it may be reasonable not to order platelets preoperatively and only give them if inappropriate bleeding occurs intraoperatively.

   If the platelet function is markedly impaired, the surgery involves a significant risk of bleeding, and there is not enough time to allow a drug-induced effect to resolve, then platelets should be given immediately preoperatively. The platelet transfusion must be repeated in the postoperative period.

c. **Coagulation (PT, PTT).** Abnormalities of these tests preoperatively need to be elucidated with more detailed testing. Vitamin K deficiency and liver disease will elevate the PT; hemophilia and lupus inhibitors will elevate the PTT. Once the specific cause is found, the deficiency should be treated perioperatively.

d. **Bleeding times.** Increased bleeding times are associated with drugs that interfere with platelet function. However, the test's ability to predict which patients will or will not have bleeding problems is poor and there is little place for its use.

e. **Serum/urine osmolality.** These usually form a baseline for further changes. Rapid correction of chronic hyperosmolality secondary to hypernatremia will lead to cerebral edema. Hyperosmolality due to uremia is without importance in the genesis of cerebral fluid shifts as urea is relatively freely permeable to the blood–brain barrier and hence has no osmotic effects. Hypoosmolality should be correctly preoperatively to reduce the likelihood of cerebral edema formation.

f. **Fluid balance.** Hypovolemia will make vasospasm more likely to become clinically apparent and will lead to a greater risk of intraoperative hypotension. Ideally, the patient should have a normal volume state preoperatively.

g. **Electrolytes.** Hyper- and hyponatremia are associated with hyper- and hypoosmolality. Hypokalemia should have some correction preoperatively as the use of diuretics will lead to further potassium loss. It is important to recognize that hypokalemia usually represents a substantial (200 to 300 mmol) potassium deficit and cannot be rapidly corrected safely. There is little or no increase in anesthetic risk with a potassium ≥ 3.0 mmol/L. Chloride deficits are associated with nonrespiratory alkalosis. Hypocalcemia and hypomagnesemia increase the likelihood of seizures. Hypercalcemia may occur in patients with bony metastases or tumors that secrete parathyroid hormone.

9. **Blood products.** Each hospital needs to determine its policy regarding the use of blood products. In general, except where blood may be needed immediately (cerebral aneurysms or very vascular tumors/AVMs), type and screening is appropriate when a blood transfusion might be needed but not emergently.

All intracranial surgery and major spinal surgery should have a type and screen. In the absence of antibodies, the risk of a transfusion reaction to type-specific blood is less than 1 in 10,000 units. Some hospitals now do computerized cross-matches where no physical cross-match is done; others only cross-match the first unit as a check that the ABO grouping has been done correctly.

II. **Communication with surgeon.** Unless one is completely familiar with a particular surgeon's practice, then it is wise to clarify the following with a member of the surgical team:

A. **Patient's position.** Ideally the surgeon will indicate on the operating room schedule the position of the patient. Knowledge of the patient's position will facilitate plans for location of monitoring and infusion catheters and for extra items that may be needed for this position. Sitting position cases involve additional preoperative investigations and special operating table equipment.

B. **Position of equipment and instruments.** Knowledge of the position of equipment and instruments will help in the planning of access to the patient and the position of the anesthetic machine. Ideally, the position of the anesthetic equipment and the surgeon's equipment will be a compromise that meets both parties' needs and not just those of the surgeon.

C. **Temporary occlusion versus induced hypotension for aneurysms.** This is a topic of much debate. One needs to know which particular technique will be used as this will partially determine the blood pressure during aneurysm dissection. In addition, cerebral vasospasm, coronary artery disease, and renal disease are relative contraindications to induced hypotension.

D. **Intraoperative studies.** If an intraoperative study, such as angiogram or ultrasound, is planned, then access to the groin and other sites must be provided.

E. **Plans for postoperative care.** After intracranial surgery, patients spend the first postoperative night in an area that allows close monitoring including invasive blood and ICP monitoring. Patients who have other illnesses that mandate careful postoperative care might also need a similar area.

Pain management should be discussed with the patient, especially if a specialized form of pain management is to be used, e.g., patient-controlled analgesia. The acute pain service may need to be contacted in such cases.

If postoperative intubation is planned, e.g., after high cervical surgery in a patient with poor respiratory function preoperatively, then this must be carefully explained to patients so that they will not become unduly distressed upon awakening.

F. **Awake techniques.** In surgery near eloquent areas

of the brain it is sometimes the practice to perform the procedure under local anesthesia to allow cerebral mapping, e.g., during epilepsy and AVM surgery. The entire process should be clearly explained to the patient so that he or she fully understands what is going to happen and what his or her own responsibilities are. The patient is likely to be extremely anxious and require considerable explanation and reassurance. Often the single best way to alleviate this (as with all fears of anesthesia) is the simple reassurance that you will be present during the entire procedure and will be immediately available to help should problems arise.

Patients having scoliosis surgery might also need to be awakened during their procedure if evoked potential monitoring is equivocal. Again, a full explanation of what will happen is needed.

G. **Anesthetic techniques and neuromonitoring.** If neuromonitoring is employed, then it is necessary for the anesthesiologists to know what types are being used and how this is affected by the anesthetic technique. In general, if one is trying to infer that changes relating to surgery or blood pressure are causing the monitoring to change, then it is necessary to ensure that the concentrations of drugs that affect this monitoring remain constant. Most neuromonitoring is very sensitive to drugs that affect the central nervous system.

If a motor response is needed, e.g., facial nerve monitoring, then paralysis is avoided or limited to allow a response to be measured.

Centers that use neuromonitoring will usually have developed anesthetic protocols that have the minimum effect on these techniques. Anesthesiologists should be aware of these since failure to follow the protocols may cause the surgery to be unsuccessful.

H. **Availability of ICP monitoring during induction of anesthesia.** Unless the patient has an ICP monitor in place prior to induction, I do not believe there is any indication to insert a monitor for induction of anesthesia. If it is *in situ*, then the anesthesiologist should ensure that ICP is monitored during induction.

III. **Monitoring.** It is necessary to plan what monitoring modalities will be used in the case so that the patient can be informed and the more complex monitoring can be arranged ahead of time.

It is important to understand why we are monitoring a patient. All monitoring is dangerous and this ranges from the real (rupturing pulmonary arteries with Swan-Ganz catheters) to the theoretical (microelectrocution) to the practical (it may distract the anesthesiologist from more important concerns). Monitoring does not of itself confer a benefit; it may warn us of important changes but does not usually of itself make the appropriate response. Benefit is

Table 5-3.   Monitoring for surgical cases[a]

Arterial catheter
   Intracranial surgery
   Operations in the sitting position
   Craniofacial reconstructions
   Surgery on the cervical spine in the prone position
   Carotid endarterectomy
   Transsphenoidal hypophysectomy
   Operations lasting longer than 4 hr
   Operations in which major blood loss is expected

Central venous catheter
   Intracranial surgery
   Craniofacial reconstructions
   Carotid endarterectomy
   Operations in which major blood loss is expected
   Operations in which vasopressors are needed
   Operations with a risk of air embolus[b]

Swan-Ganz catheter
   Cerebral aneurysm surgery and poor left ventricular function

Somatosensory evoked responses
   Cerebral aneurysm surgery
   Tumors involving major intracranial arteries
   Tumors involving the brain stem
   Spinal distraction surgery
   Surgery for spinal fractures, especially cervical

Brain stem auditory evoked potentials
   Microvascular decompression of cranial nerves
   Tumors around 8th nerve, e.g., acoustic neuromas
   Vestibular nerve sections
   Pontine brain stem tumors

Electroencephalogram
   Surgery on the extracranial carotid, e.g., carotid endarterectomy
   Cerebral aneurysms of the ICA/MCA
   When cerebral protection with barbiturates is planned

Cortical mapping
   Epilepsy surgery
   AVMs, tumors in eloquent areas

Precordial Doppler
   When air embolus is a risk, e.g., sitting position

Transesophageal echocardiography
   Cerebral aneurysm surgery with femoral-femoral bypass
   When air embolus is a risk and the patient has a patent fora-
      men ovale

Transcranial Doppler
   Carotid endarterectomy
   Cerebral aneurysms (when spasm is present)

ICA, internal carotid artery; MCA, middle carotid artery; AVM, arteriovenous malformation; NIPB, noninvasive blood pressure; SpO_2, pulse oximetry or oxygen saturation.
[a]Assumes that all patients will have pulse oximetry, end-tidal CO_2, ECG, temperature, esophageal stethoscope, and noninvasive blood pressure as well.
[b]In this case, the catheter is a single-lumen multiorifice catheter with its tip at the junction of the superior vena cava and right atrium (done with ECG or x-ray guidance).

therefore gained by making the correct management changes as a result of the information obtained. This also means that if we make the wrong decision we may harm the patient. Monitoring is fundamentally about gaining sufficient information to make the appropriate management decisions about the patient. Only when the benefit of gaining this information outweighs the risks should a particular type of monitoring be used. Table 5-3 outlines monitoring for typical cases.

Suggested Readings

Fischer SP. Preoperative evaluation of the adult neurosurgical patient. *Int Anesthesiol Clin* 1996;34(4):21–32.

Laine JL, Smoker WR. Neuroradiology. In: Cottrell JE, Smith DS, eds. *Anesthesia and neurosurgery*, 3rd ed. St. Louis: Mosby, 1994:175–209.

Roizen MF. Anesthetic implications of concurrent diseases. In: Miller RD, ed. *Anesthesia*, 4th ed. New York: Churchill Livingstone, 1994:903–1014.

Roizen MF. Preoperative evaluation. In: Miller RD, ed. *Anesthesia*, 4th ed. New York: Churchill Livingstone, 1994:827–882.

Smith RR, Caldemeyer KS. Increased intracranial pressure and cerebrospinal fluid spaces. *Semin Ultrasound Comput Tomogr Magn Res Imag* 1996;17(3):206–220.

Complications in the Postanesthesia Care Unit

Jean G. Charchaflieh

I. **Complications after operation for supratentorial tumor**
  A. **Increased intracranial pressure (ICP).** The cranial cavity has a limited capacity to accommodate increased intracranial volume without a significant increase in pressure. Increased volume of any of the three components of the intracranial cavity—brain cells, blood, and cerebrospinal fluid (CSF)—may increase ICP. Increased ICP causes injury to the brain by compression, herniation, and ischemia. Brain ischemia in turn enhances brain edema, propagating a cycle of vascular insufficiency and swelling.

    Intracranial hemorrhage, hydrocephalus, and cerebral edema are the most common postoperative causes of increased ICP. Intracranial hypertension leads to headache, nausea, vomiting, decreased level of consciousness, and neurologic dysfunction. These signs are not specific for increased ICP and are not uncommon postoperatively. Detection relies on clinical signs and symptoms, direct measurement of ICP, and computed tomography (CT) scanning. Prevention and treatment aim at avoiding and alleviating factors that can aggravate intracranial hypertension such as arterial hypertension, impaired cerebral venous drainage, blocked or malfunctioning surgical drains, postoperative pain, respiratory depression, nausea and vomiting, shivering, and seizures. The treatment of edema might require hyperventilation and the use of diuretics. The head is elevated 30°, blood pressure permitting, to facilitate venous drainage.
  B. **The adequacy of ventilation and oxygenation** is demonstrated by respiratory monitoring, including pulse oximetry, with supplemental oxygen as needed. Pain after craniotomy is usually mild and can be treated with small doses of codeine (0.25 mg/kg i.m. every 2 to 3 hours) or morphine (0.025 to 0.05 mg/kg i.v. every 1 to 2 hours) as needed.
  C. Ondansetron (4 to 8 mg i.v.) may be used intraoperatively to prevent nausea and vomiting or postoperatively to prevent recurrence of nausea and vomiting. An advantage of this medication is its lack of sedative side effects.
  D. Postoperative shivering is treated with gradual rewarming of the patient and small doses of meperidine (12.5 mg i.v.). Phenytoin controls **seizures**

(loading dose of 15 mg/kg followed by 5 to 7 mg/kg/day in 3 divided doses).

II. **Complications after operation for infratentorial tumor**

A. **Increased ICP.** The elastance of the infratentorial compartment is greater than that of the supratentorial compartment: a smaller increase in volume causes a more significant increase in pressure. Furthermore, increased pressure in the posterior fossa is more life threatening because it can compress or herniate the brain stem. Brainstem herniation can occur downward through the foramen magnum or upward through the tentorium, which is most common after resection of tumors of the cervical medullary junction. Brainstem compression is manifested by a decreased level of consciousness and respiratory and cardiovascular abnormalities including collapse.

Measures to control ICP should be continued in the postoperative period: head elevation, prevention and treatment of hypertension, treatment of pain, nausea and vomiting, prevention and treatment of shivering, and maintenance of adequate ventilation and oxygenation. Decreased level of consciousness or the development of respiratory or cardiovascular abnormalities should prompt surgical consultation.

B. **Brain stem injury** can occur intraoperatively. In the postoperative period there may be failure to regain consciousness or resume spontaneous respiration, along with the presence of cardiovascular abnormalities such as bradycardia and hypertension/hypotension. Pharmacologic causes should be ruled out by ensuring adequate reversal of anesthetic agents and muscle relaxants. Supportive care in the form of mechanical ventilation and hemodynamic therapy is indicated.

C. **Injury to cranial nerves** IX, X, and XII may compromise the patient's ability to maintain a patent protected airway due to difficulty in swallowing and clearing secretions. The trachea is extubated only after the integrity of protective upper airway reflexes is evident. Respiratory monitoring is continued postoperatively, and intubation and mechanical ventilation are reinstituted if the patient fails to maintain adequate ventilation and a patent protected airway. Injury to the ophthalmic division of the trigeminal nerve (cranial nerve V) may impair protective reflexes of the cornea and require external protection with an eye patch.

D. **Edema of the mucosa** of the upper airway may occur after prolonged surgery, especially in the sitting position. It is more significant in children due to the small diameter of their airways. Tracheal extubation should be performed only after absence of airway edema is ascertained by deflating the cuff of the endotracheal tube and confirming the ability of the patient to breath around the tube. If airway edema is suspected, the trachea should remain intubated and the patient sedated, if needed, until the edema resolves. Inhaled racemic epinephrine (0.5 mL of 2% solution in 3 mL saline) decreases localized mucosal edema and might relieve upper airway obstruction. Macroglossia may accompany upper airway edema causing complete airway obstruction. If this occurs, cricothyroidotomy or tracheotomy or laryngeal mask may be the fastest means of reestablishing the airway.

E. **Pneumocephalus** occurs after craniectomy, especially in the sitting position, and is usually of little clinical consequence. Tension pneumocephalus, which may decrease the level of consciousness due to brain compression, is more common in patients after ventricular shunting and aggressive drainage of CSF; this allows air to be trapped in the space surrounding the brain that had been drained of CSF. Pneumocephalus is diagnosed by a CT scan or x-ray of the head and is effectively treated with a burr hole to release the trapped air. Done under local anesthesia, this procedure produces rapid recovery of consciousness.

F. Patients who had intraoperative air embolism may develop pulmonary edema requiring mechanical positive pressure ventilation and diuresis. Extubation is accomplished after resolution of pulmonary edema as documented by clinical examination, chest x-ray, and arterial blood gases. New neurologic deficits, decreased level of consciousness, and cardiac abnormalities can also be sequelae of venous air embolism.

III. **Complications after operation for pituitary tumor**

A. **Endocrine complications** include adrenocortical insufficiency, diabetes insipidus (DI), and hypothyroidism. Thyroid hormone replacement is reserved for patients who were hypothyroidic preoperatively. All patients receive corticosteroid coverage until testing indicates an intact pituitary-adrenal axis.

Diabetes insipidus occurs in 10% to 20% of patients, usually develops within 12 to 24 hours after surgery, and lasts for a few days. Decreased release of antidiuretic hormone (ADH) results in the excretion of excessive amounts (4 to 14 L/day) of dilute urine and leads to dehydration, hypernatremia, increased serum osmolality (>300 mOsm/kg), decreased urine osmolality (<200 mOsm/kg), and decreased urine-specific gravity (<1.005). Symptoms of hypernatremia are nonspecific and include decreased level of consciousness, tremulousness, muscle weakness, irritability, ataxia, spasticity, confusion, seizures, coma, and possibly intracranial bleeding due to increased serum osmolality.

Treatment of DI consists of hydration and hormonal supplementation. The amount and content of intravenous fluids are guided by urine volume and serum electrolytes and osmolality. Free water (H_2O) deficit can be estimated using the formula:

Free H_2O deficit =
$$\frac{(\text{Serum Na}_a^+ - 140)\,\text{body weight (kg)} \times 0.6}{140}$$

If fluid is replaced early, it is not necessary to administer free water (D_5W). Rather, a hypotonic solution such as 0.45% NaCl or lactated Ringer's may be given. Insulin and potassium supplementation might be required when dextrose-containing fluids are used, especially if corticosteroids are used concomitantly.

1-Deamino-8-D-arginine vasopressin (DDAVP), a synthetic analog of the natural hormone arginine vasopressin, can be given intravenously, subcutaneously, or intranasally when hormonal replacement is required. Intranasal administration might not be feasible, however, after transnasal transsphenoidal pituitary surgery. The usual intravenous or subcutaneous dose is 0.3 μg/kg once daily or in two divided doses. The dose is adjusted according to the patient's sleep pattern and water turnover. Thiazide diuretics (e.g., hydrochlorothiazide 50 to 100 mg daily) can be given to treat hypernatremia, but only after intravascular volume has been restored.

B. **Rhinorrhea** of CSF may develop after transnasal transsphenoidal operation. Spontaneous resolution occurs commonly and clinical observation is sufficient in most cases. If signs of infection develop, antibiotic therapy and surgical repair are indicated.

C. **Airway obstruction** from bleeding and accumulation of blood and secretions in the pharynx sometimes occurs after transnasal transsphenoidal surgery. Frequent assessment of the patency of the airway and adequacy of ventilation is important. Excessive bleeding might require reintubation and surgical consultation.

D. **Nausea and vomiting** might develop due to swallowing of blood during transsphenoidal resection of pituitary tumors. The pharynx and the stomach are suctioned at the conclusion of surgery to decrease the risk of nausea and vomiting. Ondansetron (4 mg i.v. over 2 to 5 min) may be given postoperatively to prevent recurrence of nausea and vomiting.

IV. **Complications after operation for head trauma.** Systemic sequelae of head trauma frequently become apparent in the postoperative period. These include adult respiratory distress syndrome (ARDS), neurogenic pulmonary edema (NPE), cardiac arrhythmias, electrocardiographic (ECG) changes, disseminated intravascular coagulation (DIC), diabetes insipidus (DI), syndrome of inappropriate antidiuretic hormone secretion (SIADH), hyperglycemia, nonketotic hyperosmolar hyperglycemic coma, and gastrointestinal ulcers and hemorrhage.

A. **Neurogenic pulmonary edema** is a fulminant form of pulmonary edema that progresses rapidly (within hours to days) toward either resolution or death. The pathologic characteristics of NPE are marked pulmonary vascular congestion, pulmonary arteriolar wall rupture, protein-rich edema fluid, and intraalveolar hemorrhage. Neurogenic pulmonary edema results from a massive transient central sympathetic discharge due to an increase in ICP and is particularly associated with hypothalamic lesions. The pathophysiology includes systemic vasoconstriction and left ventricular failure, redistribution of blood from the systemic to the pulmonary vessels, pulmonary venous constriction, and increased pulmonary-capillary permeability. Treatment is aimed at reducing ICP, reducing sympathetic hyperactivity, mainly by using α-adrenergic blockers such as diazoxide (1 to 3 mg/kg i.v. q 5 minutes up to 150 mg) or phentolomine (5-mg i.v. increments) and providing respiratory supportive care and inotropic therapy as needed.

B. **The syndrome of inappropriate antidiuretic hormone** causes water retention with continued urinary excretion of sodium. This leads to dilutional hyponatremia, decreased serum osmolality, increased urine osmolality, and decreased urinary output. Water retention and serum hypoosmolality might progress to water intoxication, which leads to nonspecific symptoms such as nausea, vomiting, headache, irritability, disorientation, seizures, and coma. Treatment consists of water restriction, loop diuretics, and hypertonic saline. In mild cases, fluid restriction (1 to 1.5 L/day) is sufficient to correct hyponatremia. Furosemide may be added because it impairs renal ability to concentrate urine. Hypertonic saline is usually reserved for serum sodium of less than 120 to 125 mEq/L. It is given in small amounts for a short time (1 to 2 mL/kg/hour for 2 to 3 hours), after which serum sodium and osmolality are measured.

During the acute phase of SIADH, urine output is measured hourly and urine osmolality and specific gravity and serum sodium and osmolality are measured every 6 to 8 hours. Serum sodium should be increased at a rate of no more than 0.5 mEq/L/hour or 12 mEq/L/day. Faster rates of correction may cause osmotic demyelination which develops over several days. It is associated with nonspecific signs such as behavioral changes, movement disorders, seizures, pseudobulbar palsy, quadriparesis, and coma.

C. **Trauma to other organs** occurring in conjunction with head injury might become apparent only in the postoperative period. Up to 15% of patients with head injury sustain cervical spine injury as well. Precautions to avoid exacerbation of spinal cord injury are continued in the postoperative period until cervical spine injury is ruled out. Patients who do have spinal cord injury receive methylprednisolone within 8 hours of injury (intravenous loading dose of 30 mg/kg followed by an infusion of 5.4 mg/kg/hour for 23 hours). Acute phase spinal shock is treated with fluids, inotropes, and pressors. During the chronic phase of spinal injury adequate analgesia is provided before somatic or splanchnic stimulation in patients with injury above T_6 to avoid the risk of autonomic hyperreflexia.

D. **Cardiovascular and respiratory monitoring,** with the appropriate laboratory tests, is aimed at detecting extracranial injuries and complications such as pneumothorax, hemothorax, intraabdominal or retroperitoneal hemorrhage, and fat embolism.

E. **Prevention of secondary brain injury** is continued in the postoperative period. Hypotension, hypoxia, hyperthermia, hyperglycemia, hypoglycemia, increased ICP, and any aggravating factors such as pain, nausea, vomiting, seizures, hypertension, hypercarbia, and impaired cerebral venous drainage should all be prevented and treated.

Conscious, mechanically ventilated patients are sedated with short-acting agents, such as propofol (10 to 30 μg/kg/minute i.v.) or midazolam (0.5 to 2 mg/hour i.v.), to allow intermittent neurologic assessment. Pain due to the operative procedure or the primary or associated injury is relieved with opioids such as morphine (0.05 mg/kg) or fentanyl (0.5 to 1 μg/kg). Nausea and vomiting are treated with stomach suctioning (after ruling out skull base fracture) and pharmacologic means such as ondansetron (4 to 8 mg i.v.), metoclopramide (10 mg i.v.), or droperidol (0.625 mg i.v.).

Seizure prophylaxis after head trauma is somewhat controversial. Many institutions give phenytoin (loading dose 15 mg/kg i.v. followed by 5 to 7 mg/kg/day in 3 divided doses) for 2 weeks after injury if there have been no seizures or longer if there have.

F. **Clotting** may be impaired because of the release of tissue thromboplastin and a trauma-induced decrease in platelets, prothrombin (factor II), proaccelerin (factor V), and plasminogen, and a decrease in fibrin degradation products.

V. **Complications after operation for aneurysm**

A. **Vasospasm.** Angiographic narrowing of blood vessels occurs in about 30% of patients between days 4 and 14 after subarachnoid hemorrhage (SAH). Neurologic dysfunction (disorientation, decreased level of consciousness, focal deficit) occurs in about 50% of patients who have angiographic narrowing. The risk for developing vasospasm correlates with the amount of blood around the circle of Willis, the preoperative use of antifibrinolytic therapy, and the postoperative development of the cerebral salt wasting (CSW) syndrome.

The calcium channel blocker nimodipine (60 mg p.o. q4h) is given prophylactically to patients within 96 hours of SAH and is continued for at least 21 days. "Triple-H" therapy (hypervolemia, hypertension, and hemodilution) for treatment of vasospasm includes the administration of crystalloid and colloid (pulmonary capillary wedge pressure of 15 mm Hg and hemoglobin level of 11 g/dL) and the use of inotropes and vasopressors [mean arterial pressure (MAP) of 120 mm Hg or more]. Antidiuretic therapy is sometimes necessary to prevent the diuresis induced by volume loading. Hypotension, heart failure, myocardial ischemia, and pulmonary edema are occasional sequelae of therapy.

B.   Obstructive hydrocephalus due to subarachnoid blood-induced disturbances in CSF circulation occurs after SAH. The patient's level of consciousness might be decreased from the increase in ICP. Computed tomography scan is diagnostic and ventriculostomy with CSF drainage is the effective therapy.

C.   Hyponatremia after SAH can be due to the syndrome of CSW or, less commonly, to SIADH. Cerebral salt wasting is caused by increased secretion of atrial natriuretic peptide (ANP), brain natriuretic peptide (BNP), and C-type natriuretic peptide (CNP). These suppress aldosterone synthesis and lead to natriuresis, diuresis, and vasodilatation. Hyponatremia in the CSW syndrome results from increased renal excretion of sodium (150 to 200 mEq/L), which is followed by water with resultant hypovolemia. Hyponatremia of SIADH is mainly due to water retention in conjunction with renal excretion of sodium in a range of 20 to 30 mEq/L.

Treatment of the two forms of hyponatremia is completely different. Patients with CSW require sodium replacement and fluid administration, whereas patients with SIADH require fluid restriction and diuresis. Fluid restriction and diuresis in a patient with CSW can be fatal due to the possibility of severe hypovolemia and cerebral infarction; fluid and salt administered to a patient with SIADH may lead to osmotic demyelination. Hypertonic saline may be used with close monitoring of serum sodium in either case.

D.   Diabetes insipidus occurs less frequently than CSW and SIADH after SAH (see III.A). Treatment includes hypotonic fluids in the form of enteral free water or parenteral D_5W, D_5, $2NaCl$, or 0.45% NaCl. 1-Deamino-8-D-arginine vasopressin is given intravenously or subcutaneously in a dose of 0.3 $\mu g/kg$ once daily or in two divided doses.

E. **Intracranial hematomas** might develop at the operative site or at the bridging dural veins due to overzealous CSF drainage. Manifestations are those of increased ICP, which may be associated with focal deficit. Computed tomography scan and treatment with surgical evacuation may be required.

F. **Seizure prophylaxis** is continued in the postoperative period due to the high risk of seizures after SAH, especially in hypertensive patients. Phenytoin is usually given for 3 to 6 months after SAH.

G. **Neurogenic pulmonary edema** occurs in some patients after SAH due to the sudden increase in ICP, which produces intense sympathetic activation, catecholamine release from the hypothalamus and the medulla, and increased pulmonary vascular pressure and permeability (see IV.A). Diagnosis depends on the exclusion of other causes of pulmonary edema such as Triple-H therapy and aspiration pneumonia. Treatment includes oxygen, positive end-expiratory pressure, and reduction of ICP.

H. After SAH, patients are at moderate risk for the development of **deep venous thrombosis (DVT)** and **pulmonary embolus (PE)**. Mechanical DVT prophylaxis is instituted in all patients after SAH and continued postoperatively in the form of graduated stockings or intermittent pneumatic compression of the lower extremities. Anticoagulation is contraindicated in the acute postoperative phase. During this period, recurrent PE is treated by the insertion of a filter into the inferior vena cava (IVC) to prevent further embolization.

I. **Cardiac complications** are common after SAH. Electrocardiographic changes of arrhythmia, ischemia, or infarction, detected in more than 50% of patients, occur within 48 hours of SAH but may be first noted in the early postoperative period. Evidence of myocardial injury is detected by echocardiography, thallium scintigraphy, and autopsy. These ECG changes may be due to hypothalamic injury and high catecholamine levels. Treatment depends on the severity of the complications, the hemodynamic stability of the patient, and concomitant vasospasm. Infarcted, stunned, or hibernating myocardium might exclude these patients from Triple-H therapy.

VI. Complications after ablation of arteriovenous malformation

After surgery for arteriovenous malformation (AVM), patients are at risk of developing complications similar to those found after aneurysm surgery (vasospasm, hy-

drocephalus, and seizures). In addition, these patients
are at high risk of developing hyperemic complications.

A. **The syndrome of normal perfusion-pressure
   breakthrough or cerebral hyperperfusion** is a
   hyperemic state characterized by cerebral edema,
   swelling, and/or hemorrhage that develops after resection of AVM. This condition results from the restoration of cerebral blood flow (CBF) to chronically
   hypoperfused areas or from venous outflow obstruction after AVM ablation. The ensuing cerebral
   swelling and hemorrhage cause neurologic dysfunction and are a major cause of postoperative morbidity and mortality. Patients who have ischemic
   rather than hemorrhagic symptoms pre-operatively
   or certain angiographic features such as high or inverse flow in a large, deep, border zone AVM are
   particularly at risk.

   Staged repair and strict control of blood flow
   through the AVM may decrease the risk of hyperemic complications. Treatment of the manifestations of cerebral hyperemia includes mechanical hyperventilation, osmotic diuresis, and barbiturate
   coma.

VII. **Complications after carotid endarterectomy**

A. **Cardiac ischemia and infarction** are the leading
   cause of mortality after carotid endarterectomy
   (CEA). Coronary artery disease (CAD) is common
   among patients undergoing CEA. Perioperative
   tachycardia, hypertension, and hypotension increase the risk of perioperative myocardial ischemia
   and infarction. The α agonists, such as phenylephrine, are preferable in the treatment of hypotension
   in this setting because they raise blood pressure
   without significantly increasing heart rate. However, the ensuing hypertension may be detrimental.
   Combined α and β agonists, such as ephedrine, increase heart rate and have been associated with
   myocardial ischemia and infarction in this setting.

B. **Occlusion of the operated carotid artery** should
   be suspected whenever new neurologic symptoms
   develop postoperatively. This is one cause of postoperative cerebral ischemia that is amenable to surgical intervention. Early diagnosis and treatment significantly alter outcome. A Doppler flow study can
   detect cessation of flow in the involved vessel, and
   angiography will confirm vascular occlusion. Surgical reexploration need not await angiographic con-
   firmation but may be undertaken on the basis of the
   clinical picture and the ultrasound examination.

C. **The cerebral hyperperfusion syndrome** may develop after CEA due to the sudden increase in CBF
   in a maximally dilated vascular bed that has lost
   its ability to autoregulate because of longstanding
   hypoperfusion. This hyperperfusion can lead to cerebral edema or hemorrhage with headache, sei-

zures, decreased level of consciousness, and focal neurologic deficit. Severe carotid stenosis and hypertension contribute to the development of this syndrome. Careful control of blood pressure is essential in preventing hyperperfusion.

Mild elevation of blood pressure need not be treated in the postoperative period, whereas moderate to severe hypertension should be reduced to avoid the cerebral hyperperfusion syndrome. Titratable, short-acting agents such as sodium nitroprusside (SNP) (0.25 to 8 μg/kg/minute) and esmolol (loading dose 500 μg/kg over 1 minute followed by 50 to 300 μg/kg/minute) are preferable in this setting. The β-blocking effects of esmolol offset the sympathetic hyperactivity from SNP.

D. Hypotension is poorly tolerated by hypertensive patients who have a rightward shift in their autoregulatory curve. Hypotension can lead to cerebral and cardiac hypoperfusion and can increase the risk of thrombus formation in the operated vessel. Blood pressure is usually kept at 20% above baseline. Hypotension is treated with volume expansion and infusion of a short-acting α agonist such as phenylephrine (40 to 180 μg/minute, 20 mg in 250 mL D_5W at 30 to 160 mL/hour).

E. Treatment of stroke after CEA consists of blood pressure management, supportive care, and treatment of complications. Intravenous thrombolytic therapy is contraindicated in the postoperative period. Intraarterial thrombolytic therapy may be considered in institutions that have the expertise. Neuroprotective therapy, still the subject of clinical trials, has not been approved for clinical use.

F. Airway obstruction can result from hematoma formation and can be aggravated by laryngeal edema and cranial nerve injury. Reestablishing airway patency might require suture removal and drainage of the hematoma. This is best accomplished by a surgeon, in conjunction with tracheal intubation and racemic epinephrine. If the patient is in extremis, the first person to reach the bedside opens the wound to secure the airway.

VIII. Complications after vertebral column procedures

A. Complications after anterior cervical discectomy. The patient's trachea is extubated in the operating room after an uncomplicated discectomy. However, tracheal intubation may be maintained postoperatively if upper airway edema is anticipated after a prolonged operation or one associated with infusion of large volumes of fluid. It is important to prevent the patient from coughing and straining while the trachea is intubated. This may cause the newly placed bone graft to dislodge, which can compress the trachea or the esophagus and require reoperation. After extubation, the patient's voice is evaluated to detect recurrent laryngeal nerve injury, a benign complication that usually resolves over days to weeks.

B. Complications after cervical corpectomy and stabilization. These procedures are usually more invasive, more prolonged, associated with more fluid administration, and therefore more likely to cause airway edema at the conclusion of surgery. The patient's trachea usually remains intubated until the airway edema resolves, as evidenced by the ability of the patient to breath around the endotracheal tube after the cuff has been deflated. Sedation is provided as needed while the trachea is intubated.

C. Complications after transoral resection of the odontoid and occipitocervical fusion. Operation is usually performed in two steps: anterior transoral resection of the odontoid and posterior occipitocervical fusion. Airway management involves either tracheotomy or an oral endotracheal tube draped out of the surgical field as for tonsillectomy. The procedure is associated with significant posterior pharyngeal swelling, which requires postoperative intubation for several days. The patient is usually awakened at the conclusion of surgery to undergo a neurologic examination and then sedated again. The degree of resolution of the airway edema is evaluated by deflating the cuff of the endotracheal tube and establishing the patient's ability to breathe around the endotracheal tube.

D. Complications after posterior cervical spine procedures. Complications are related to the patient's intraoperative position and the degree of airway edema and pulmonary dysfunction at the conclusion of surgery. The operative positions include prone, sitting, and three quarters prone. Complications of the prone position include injury at pressure points: eyes, cheeks, lips, breasts, and genitalia. Injury to these structures requires appropriate surgical consultation. Airway edema is dependent on the duration of surgery, the amount of blood loss, and fluid administration.

Respiratory dysfunction may exist preoperatively due to involvement of C_3 to C_5 nerve roots or may result from resection of intramedullary spinal cord tumors. These patients are evaluated before extubation to demonstrate the patency of the airway (lack of airway edema) and adequacy of respiratory function (tidal volume, vital capacity, negative inspiratory force). Postoperative intubation and mechanical ventilation might be required until airway edema resolves and respiratory function recovers.

E. Complications after scoliosis surgery. These procedures are performed with the patient in the prone or lateral position or a combination of a lateral position operation followed immediately or 1 to 2 weeks later by a prone-position instrumentation. Complications related to the prone position are those of pressure point injury, particularly the eyes. Ischemic optic neuropathy is correlated with intraoperative hypotension and ischemia, regardless of position. Central retinal artery occlusion can occur during prone-position procedures due to improper protection of the eyes.

Scoliosis surgery patients are thus particularly vulnerable to ischemic optic neuropathy, which is manifested postoperatively by varying degrees of unilateral or bilateral decreases in visual acuity or defects in the visual field. The decrease in visual acuity may resolve over time, but the defects in the visual field usually persist. Postoperative visual examination is performed routinely in these patients; ophthalmologic consultation is requested if any abnormality is detected.

Scoliosis patients may have respiratory dysfunction preoperatively due to skeletal deformities, muscular weakness, CNS dysfunction, or a combination of factors. This respiratory dysfunction might be aggravated postoperatively by the residual effect of anesthetics, inadequate reversal of muscle relaxants due to hypothermia, restrictive effect of pain, and pneumothorax. Airway edema from positioning, prolonged surgery, and administration of a large volume of fluids contributes to the respiratory compromise. Extubation of the trachea is undertaken only after adequacy of respiratory function and airway patency have been established. Pain control is essential for patient comfort and the maintenance of adequate respiratory function.

Postoperative hemorrhage can continue externally via surgical drains or internally into the operative site. Monitoring of systemic blood pressure, urinary output, central venous pressure, if present, and hemoglobin and hematocrit is necessary. Excessive blood loss is treated with volume expansion, blood transfusion, hemodynamic support, and surgical consultation.

Central and peripheral neurologic function is monitored postoperatively. Patients might develop spinal cord injury due to instrumentation or hematoma formation and CNS dysfunction due to pharmacologic or hemodynamic factors. Neurologic dysfunction should prompt a thorough examination of the patient, review of medication, hemodynamic and laboratory workup, surgical consultation, and supportive therapy as needed.

F. Complications after lateral extracavitary and percutaneous endoscopic procedures. A factor common to these two operations is the intraoperative use of double-lumen endotracheal tubes or other forms of one-lung ventilation. Pulmonary edema may develop with reexpansion of the lung after one-lung ventilation for more than 3 hours, most likely within 1 hour of reexpansion. If mechanical ventilation is to be maintained in the postoperative period, the double-lumen tube is exchanged for a single-lumen one. Alternatively, a univent tube, which is a single-lumen tube with a movable endobronchial blocker, may be used intraoperatively and postoperatively during weaning and until extubation.

IX. **Complications after spinal cord procedures**

A. **Complications after syringomyelia repair.** Respiratory complications are the main concern. Preoperative respiratory dysfunction is due to skeletal deformities, autonomic dysfunction, and chronic aspiration and pneumonia from depressed gag reflex and vocal cord paralysis. This may be exacerbated in the postoperative period by airway edema, residual anesthetic effects, and incomplete reversal of muscle relaxants, which could be aggravated by the hypothermia of autonomic dysfunction. Extubation is performed only after the adequacy of respiratory function and airway patency have been established. Respiratory monitoring and support are maintained in the postoperative period as needed.

B. **Complications after resection of spinal cord tumors.** Significant cord edema may develop up to 24 hours after resection. The edema-induced respiratory dysfunction associated with resection of upper cervical cord tumors might not become apparent in the immediate postoperative period. Respiratory monitoring of these patients in an intensive care setting for at least 24 hours postoperatively is therefore necessary.

C. **Complications after spinal cord injury.** Patients with spinal cord injury develop complications related to sympathectomy, skeletal muscle denervation, immobilization, chronic instrumentation, decreased respiratory force, and coexisting injuries involving other organs. About 50% of patients with cervical spine injury have concurrent head trauma and about 25% have injuries to the chest, abdomen, or extremities.

The severity and mechanism of the initial spinal shock, which lasts for 2 to 3 weeks after injury, are related to the level of the injury. With midthoracic lesions (T_{6-7}), hypotension may not be severe and is mainly due to vasodilatation. With higher lesions (T_4 or above), hypotension may be profound when vasodilatation is added to a decrease in heart rate, contractility, and compliance from loss of cardiac accelerator fibers (T_{1-4}).

Succinylcholine may cause hyperkalemia in denervated patients due to the increased number and sensitivity of their neuromuscular cholinergic receptors. These receptor changes start 3 days after the injury and remain for 6 to 8 months. Succinylcholine is therefore avoided in spinal cord injury patients from 48 hours to 8 months after the injury.

Autonomic hyperreflexia is caused by noxious stimulation below the level of the lesion in a patient with a sympathectomy at or above T_6. The risk of autonomic hyperreflexia is highest during the 4th week after injury but continues thereafter. At this time, while the patient is recovering from the spinal shock phase which lasts for 2 to 3 weeks after the initial injury, the flaccid paralysis changes to spastic paralysis because of the absence of the effect of central inhibitory pathways. The efferent sympathetic fibers recover from the initial injury but remain unaffected by central inhibitory input from the brain stem and hypothalamus.

The severity and manifestations of autonomic hyperreflexia are affected by the level of the sympathectomy. With midthoracic lesions below the level of cardiac accelerator fibers, hypertension is accompanied by reflex bradycardia transmitted via cardiac accelerator fibers and the vagus. In patients whose sympathectomy is above the level of the thoracic cardiac accelerator fibers, tachycardia may occur because cardiac accelerator fibers become part of the efferent sympathetic activity rather than part of the central inhibitory input from the brain stem and hypothalamus. Arrhythmias and occasionally heart block may accompany changes in heart rate.

Clinical manifestations of autonomic hyperreflexia include vasodilatation, decreased sympathetic activity, and increased vagal activity above the level of the lesion such as nasal congestion, flushing, headache, dyspnea, nausea, and visceral muscle contraction. Vasoconstriction and increased sympathetic activity below the level of the lesion cause vasoconstrictive pallor, sweating, piloerection, and somatic muscle fasciculation. Patients also develop hypertension with headache, blurred vision, myocardial infarction, and retinal, subarachnoid, and cerebral hemorrhages that can lead to syncope, convulsions, and death.

Autonomic hyperreflexia may be prevented or attenuated by regional or deep general anesthesia, but this is usually impractical in the postanesthesia care unit. Instead, local anesthetic (60 to 90 mL of pontocaine 0.25%) installation into the bladder 20 minutes before cystoscopy may be used to prevent autonomic hyperreflexia. Pharmacologic means of preventing and treating autonomic hyperreflexia include alpha blockers such as diazoxide (1 to 3 mg/kg i.v. q 5 min up to 150 mg) or phentolamine (5-mg i.v. increments), vasodilators such as SNP (0.25

to 8 μg/kg/minute i.v.), and selective beta blockers such as esmolol (loading dose 500 μg/kg followed by 50 to 300 μg/kg/minute i.v.) for supraventricular tachycardia.

SUGGESTED READINGS

Charchaflieh J. *Management of acute ischemic stroke: general care and thombolysis*. Progress in Anesthesiology, Vol. 12, 1998, Chapter 11.

Giffin JP, Grush K, Karlin A, Cottrell JE, Newfield P. Spinal cord injury. In: Newfield P, Cottrell JE, eds. *Neuroanesthesia: handbook of clinical and physiologic essentials*. Boston: Little, Brown and Company, 1991, Chapter 14.

Layon AJ, Stachniak JB, Day AL. Neurointensive care. In: Cucchiara RF, Black S, Michenfelder JD, eds. *Clinical neuroanesthesia*. New York: Churchill Livingstone, 1998, Chapter 18.

Newfield P, Weir BDA, Hamid RKA, Lam AM. Intracranial aneurysms and A-V malformations. In: Albin MS, ed. *Textbook of neuroanesthesia with neurosurgical and neuroscience perspectives*. New York: McGraw-Hill, 1997.

Petrozza PH, Prough DS. Postoperative and intensive care. In: Cottrell JE, Smith DS, eds. *Anesthesia and neurosurgery*. Chicago: Mosby-Year Book, 1994.

Perioperative Pain Management in the Neurosurgical Patient

Timothy R. Deer

The unpleasant experience of pain has long been deemed a necessity of surgical procedures. Recent advances in pain treatment and emphasis on pain as a social issue have led to a renewed focus on the successful attenuation of perioperative suffering. Successful management of acute surgical pain requires a careful team approach from both the anesthesiologist and the surgeon to maximize the ability to decrease the stress response and reduce pain. The importance of the anesthesiologist in decreasing anxiety, creating a treatment plan, and executing the plan is crucial to a successful surgical experience.

The pain pathway consists of the initial impulse (transduction), the transfer of information (transmission), and the interpretation of the signal (modulation). The cortex then processes this pathway into an emotional interpretation. The goal of acute pain management is to change the pathway at one or more of these important steps. The method of analgesia selected will depend on the disease process and the proposed treatment of the problem.

The challenge to maintain a stable hemodynamic condition in the neurosurgical patient presents a difficult problem. The undertreatment of pain can lead to an unstable postoperative course and adversely affect an otherwise successful procedure. The uncontrolled pain stimulus causes changes in vital signs, hormonal responses, clotting studies, immunologic status, and intracranial pressure (ICP). This may also adversely affect morbidity and mortality, patient satisfaction, and surgeon satisfaction. The purpose of this chapter is to focus on the appropriate pain treatment care plan of the patient undergoing a variety of neurosurgical procedures.

I. **Preoperative assessment**
    A. **Preadmission or presurgical considerations**
        1. **Reducing anxiety.** The neuroanesthesiologist should devote a portion of the preanesthetic evaluation to the discussion of the treatment of pain after the procedure. Important considerations at this time include the patient's past experience with pain and the response to previous treatments. A focus is placed on the patient's expectations and fears. The plan of treatment should be reviewed with the patient and all questions addressed prior to ending the assessment. The time spent at this phase of treatment might prove significant in the reduction of peri-

operative stress and might enhance the success of pain treatment modalities.

2. **Pain treatment history.** Many patients undergoing neurologic surgery have had a history of acute pain treatment. The outcome of the previous method of treatment might be helpful in the plan of treatment for the proposed surgery. A focused discussion should occur regarding any history of complications with previous pain techniques, bleeding disorders, and adverse reactions to pain medications. The preoperative neurologic dysfunction might greatly influence the method of perioperative pain treatment. A thorough assessment of the perioperative function and expected postoperative function should be detailed. An explanation of what pain treatment option will be utilized should be discussed. Patient reassurance will receive high priority during this period of treatment.

3. **Understanding the procedure.** It is critical to understand the surgical implications of the scheduled surgical procedure. The patient's postoperative mental status will influence the pain management technique to be utilized. Techniques such as patient-controlled analgesia (PCA) may be contraindicated in a patient with mental status changes. Regional anesthesia may not be possible if the surgical procedure involves the surgical instrumentation of the spine and is usually avoided. A discussion with the neurosurgical team is essential to establish a pain treatment plan.

4. **Role of coexisting disease.** The patient's nonsurgical disease processes must be considered when tailoring a pain treatment plan. The review of systems is critical in determining what recommendations should be made. The following factors should be considered when doing a presurgical assessment.

   a. **Neurologic system.** The site of surgery and the perioperative morbidity should be considered. The patient's baseline cognitive function also determines whether a PCA system can be put into use. Patient controlled analgesia can be used in children as young as 5 years, but should be instituted with caution and requires the education of both patients and their parents.

   b. **Renal system.** A patient with renal disease will be prone to complications from drugs with metabolites removed by the kidneys. Meperidine, for example, breaks down to normeperidine, which can cause seizures in the patient with renal impairment.

Table 7-1. Preoperative pain treatment checklist

Understand the pain pathway
Understand the proposed procedure
Understand possible pain treatment options
Review previous records of pain treatment
Identify contraindications to treatments
Review the impact of coexisting disease processes
Discuss options with the patient
Discuss options with the surgeon
Explain the risks/benefits for each option
Create a written treatment plan

    c. **Infectious disease.** Neuroaxial procedures may be contraindicated in the patient with systemic infection or local infection at the site of the proposed procedure.

    d. **Hematological system.** The clotting cascade must be considered in a patient undergoing regional anesthesia. This may be evaluated both historically and by laboratory values. A history of bleeding during dental procedures or easy bruising may influence the pain management protocol. Another concern is the use of low molecular weight heparin and regional anesthesia, which may lead to epidural hematoma.

    e. **Cardiovascular system.** Patients with tenuous blood pressure may not tolerate an infusion of local anesthetics. These patients will also be at risk for myocardial ischemia if pain is untreated. This increases cardiac work load, since both pulse and blood pressure might increase with catecholamine surges.

    f. **Gastrointestinal system.** A history of ileus may lead to concerns by the surgeon in regard to a local anesthetic infusion and use of narcotics.

B. **Summary of the preoperative period**

    1. The preoperative period is crucial in the overall success of the neurosurgical pain treatment program. The clinician should develop a mental checklist of assessment points prior to bringing the patient to the operating theatre (Table 7-1).

II. **The importance of pain treatment**

    A. The patient undergoing neurosurgical intervention may develop many perioperative changes that can affect the overall outcome if allowed to occur without attempts at intervention. The stress response, which is somewhat dependent on the complexity and site of surgery, can affect the immunologic response, coagulation, cardiac function, hormonal response, and other systems crucial to the perioperative recovery of the neurosurgical patient. Several options are available to the anesthesiologist to blunt the stress response, but unfortunately few of these methods are successful.

B. Studies of patients undergoing epidural infusion therapy for procedures involving the upper abdomen and thorax have demonstrated both improved clinical outcomes and cost effectiveness. Neurologic surgery patients were not included in these groups and no current peer-reviewed studies exist in this population.

III. The stress response: an overview

A. The patient undergoing neurosurgical surgery is often very sensitive to subtle changes in other organ systems. The pathophysiologic changes associated with the stress response from surgical trauma can greatly affect the outcome from procedures with high risk of morbidity and mortality.

B. **Physiological effects of the stress response.** The stress response is made up of an initial depressed phase and a subsequent hyperdynamic phase.

    1. **The depressed phase.** In the initial portion of the response, the body responds by depressing most physiologic functions. This phase is brief in the surgical patient and might be unidentifiable in some patients.

    2. **The hyperdynamic phase.** The portion of the stress response of most concern to the anesthesiologist and most involved in morbidity and mortality in the neurosurgical patient is the period of recovery after surgery. This lasts for a period of time that is directly proportional to the amount of tissue trauma. A characterization of this response is outlined below.

        a. **Endocrinologic changes.** Both catabolic and anabolic responses are seen during this phase of response.

            (1) **Catabolic changes** include increases in several hormones: catecholamines, renin, angiotensin II, aldosterone, glucagon, cortisol, tumor necrosis factor, adrenocorticotropic hormone (ACTH), growth hormone, and interleukin (primarily IL-1 and IL-6).

            (2) **Anabolic changes** include decreases in insulin and testosterone.

        b. **Metabolic changes.** Several metabolic changes are important to understand when considering the importance of the stress response on outcomes.

            (1) Important changes are created by the endocrinologic factors noted above: insulin resistance, muscle breakdown, glucose intolerance, fat breakdown, increased tissue oxidation with the creation of free radicals, sodium and water retention, hyperglycemia, increased acute phase proteins, and fluid shifts and third spacing.

(2) These changes will adversely affect fluid balance, protein metabolism, fat metabolism, and carbohydrate metabolism.

C. **Body system responses to the stress response**
1. The uninhibited stress response has been shown to increase cardiac workload; increase vascular tension; adversely affect platelet function; decrease fibrinolysis; decrease renal perfusion; decrease the urinary excretion of water, wastes, and electrolytes; decrease hepatic function; increase oxygen consumption; decrease immunocompetence; and decrease the centrally mediated temperature regulation mechanisms.
2. Considering the enormous changes noted above in the unbridled stress response, the importance of blunting this response in enhancing outcomes becomes critical. Pain treatment mechanisms utilized in limiting this systemic response are detailed.

IV. **Mechanisms of blunting the stress response to surgery**
A. **General anesthesia.** The use of inhalational anesthetics and total intravenous anesthetic techniques have been responsible for tremendous advances in improving the surgical experience and reducing pain at the time of surgery. Unfortunately, the success has not been encouraging in the ability to block the metabolic and endocrine response to tissue trauma. Despite this overall failure, a few agents have had some ability to change the clinical response.
1. **Etomidate.** This intravenous drug does affect the ability of the adrenocortical system to respond to stress. The effect of this inhibitory response is a decreased ability to increase cortisol levels. This is achieved by an inhibition of enzymes in the cortisol synthesis pathway. The net effect of this inhibition is debatable and this drug is often avoided as a sedative in the patient who has a prolonged recovery period after surgery.
2. **Inhalational agents.** Ether and cyclopropane are no longer used clinically in the United States on a regular basis. Both drugs have the characteristic of increasing the response of the sympathetic nervous system to tissue trauma.

This stimulatory response also affects the adrenocortical system.

3. **High-dose opioids.** The use of high doses of intravenous opioids is helpful in blunting many aspects of the initial stress response. Unfortunately, this ability to decrease or eliminate the stress response is very short-lived; once the serum level of opiate decreases, the effect diminishes rapidly.

B. **Regional anesthesia**
1. **Neuroaxial.** Regional anesthetic techniques appear to have the greatest ability to block the stress response. In multiple studies the use of epidural or intrathecal analgesia has improved postoperative nitrogen balance, renal function, glucose metabolism, oxygen consumption, coagulation and fibrinolysis, and hepatic and immunologic function, and decreased cardiac workload. Other beneficial effects may include a decrease in blood loss and thromboembolic events and improved pulmonary function. Unfortunately, these data are largely based on studies in the thoracic, abdominal, and pelvic surgery population. The data suggests less success in blocking the stress response to surgery in the upper abdomen and thorax than in the lower abdomen and extremities. The use of local anesthetics and opioids in combination appears to be better than either agent alone. Continuous spinal might also be superior to epidural techniques. The use of continuous spinal and epidural analgesia in the postoperative management of pain appears limited in the neurosurgical patient, although the data pertaining directly to neurosurgical patients is sparse.

C. **Peripheral nerve blockade.** A single blockade of a peripheral nerve may improve the initial response to surgery but has no proven benefit. The goal of therapy would be to block the sensation of the area without creating a motor blockade in the postoperative period. Common selections of infusion include bupivacaine 0.25% or less, ropivacaine 0.2% or less. Common locations for peripheral nerve blockade include the brachial plexus, the cervical plexus, the femoral nerve, and peripheral nerves of the lower extremities.

D. **Adrenergic blockade.** The use of spinal or epidural α-adrenergic blockade is showing some promise in reducing the stress response. The most commonly used drug in this regard is clonidine. It is uncertain if the reduction in adrenergic response with epidural or intrathecal clonidine is a direct effect of the α-adrenergic blockade or a response to the clonidine-induced analgesia. The use of systemic β-adrenergic and α-adrenergic agents has also been examined. They may have some mild beneficial effect on the stress response, but this may be transient. More study is needed.

E. Nonsteroidals. The perioperative use of nonsteroidal anti-inflammatory drugs (NSAIDs) may enhance the ability of other techniques such as regional analgesia and anesthesia in blocking the stress response. This is thought to be directly related to their action at peripheral receptors involved in the tissue trauma cascade.

F. Intravenous opioids. The use of PCA has led to markedly improved patient satisfaction and improved pain scores. Unfortunately, this does not correlate with any change in the overall stress response.

G. Transcutaneous electrical nerve stimulation (TENS). There are no current studies that show any significant reduction in the stress response with the use of this intervention.

H. Psychological counseling. The use of biofeedback, relaxation, and other neuromodulation techniques has found a role in the treatment of acute and chronic pain. Unfortunately, there are no data to suggest any change in the stress response as a result of these techniques.

V. Intraoperative and postoperative pain treatment interventions

A. Preemptive analgesia

1. **Preoperative local anesthetic infiltration of the surgical field.** The blunting of the response to incision may be crucial to the overall ability to provide a stable postoperative pain treatment course, the amount of anesthetic involved, and the initial stage of the surgical stress response.

2. **Neuroaxial anesthetic techniques.** By utilizing a spinal or epidural technique the initial response to surgery may be blunted, as well as the detrimental response in the perioperative period. A combined opioid and local anesthetic technique may be most effective, as noted above.

3. **Anesthetics and systemic opioids.** There is no evidence that the administration of high-dose systemic opioids to a patient under general anesthesia blunts the stress response to pain in the postoperative period. There may be short-term benefit to these agents, but most likely this does not influence the outcome.

B. Neuroaxial infusion therapy: epidural. The use of epidural infusion therapy has grown in recent years as a primary method of acute pain control in patients undergoing surgical procedures involving peripheral nerves. The proper use of an epidural infusion requires a working knowledge of dermatomal anatomy, drug pharmacokinetics, drug synergies, and postoperative follow-up requirements.

1. **Epidural location** is important in the dosage requirement and infusion rate required for proper analgesia. Epidural placement ideally should be within two levels of the nerve root of primary focus of the surgical procedure.

2. **Lipophilia** is crucial in drug selection for postoperative pain. A lipophilic drug such as fentanyl would require placement of the catheter at a level near the nerve innervation of the surgical site. With morphine, which is much less lipid-soluble, the catheter placement is less critical since the drug may cover several interspaces prior to being absorbed. Hydromorphone has intermediate properties.

3. **Drug synergies.** The combination of local anesthetics and opioids offers a synergistic effect that leads to better analgesia than either drug infused alone. Local anesthetic infusion therapy has been shown to be the most effective method of blunting the stress response to tissue trauma. The addition of opioids helps eliminate the problem of tachyphylaxis that may develop with local anesthetics alone.

C. **Neuroaxial infusion therapies: subarachnoid.** The use of spinal blockade in neurosurgical procedures is somewhat limited. Continuous spinal infusion therapy is generally discouraged because of the risk of CSF leaks and infection, and the confusion of the neurologic exam.

D. **Peripheral nerve blockade.** In the patient undergoing surgery on peripheral nerves (e.g., schwannoma), a peripheral nerve continuous infusion of bupivacaine or ropivacaine might be helpful in controlling the pain and might affect the stress response. Common sites for continuous infusion include the brachial plexus and the femoral nerve. Catheters are often placed via the paresthesia technique and a nerve stimulator may be used to reduce the risk of nerve injury as compared with the paresthesias for placement. In general, a blunt-tipped needle is preferable to a sharp beveled needle, and again might reduce the risk of nerve injury. A wire-reinforced catheter might reduce the failure rate of this method as opposed to a standard infusion catheter.

E. **Patient-controlled analgesia.** The use of patient-controlled narcotic delivery may be applied to either intravenous opioid delivery or epidural infusion medications such as local anesthetics, opioids, or clonidine. The neurosurgical patient presents a dilemma in the decision making process. Careful attention must be given to the baseline preoperative function in regard to the ability to understand the use of a PCA system and equally to the expected postoperative cognitive function and the ability to utilize the system. A team approach involving surgeon, anesthesiologist, and patient is needed when this mode of treatment is considered.

F. **Nurse-administered intermittent analgesia.** The classic method of postoperative pain relief in the neurosurgical patient is to have a nurse administer intravenous medications. This involves either administration on the demand of the patient or at scheduled times at the request of the surgeon or anesthesiologist. This mode of treatment is most appropriate in the patient with altered preoperative or postoperative cognitive function. The disadvantages of this method include delay in treatment, creating unnecessary suffering, and excessive sedation. It is also labor-intensive.

G. **Transcutaneous electrical nerve stimulation.** There are no current data to support any change in postoperative outcome with the use of TENS for incisional pain. This is a difficult method to use in the neurologic surgery population because of the technical difficulties of application.

H. **Psychological counseling.** The addition of a psychologist to the postoperative acute pain team is helpful in improving the patient's ability to cope with the emotional stress of pain and disease. Unfortunately, since no good studies exist on the cost effectiveness of adding this service, reimbursement may be difficult to obtain.

I. **Adjuvant drugs.** The use of NSAIDs may greatly improve the ability to control breakthrough pain in the patient with incidental pain or pain with movement. Intramuscular or intravenous ketorolac is generally the drug of choice; however, this drug should be avoided if the patient is at high risk of hemorrhage. The addition of antiemetics might also be helpful in controlling nausea that can accompany postoperative analgesics. Ondansetron is an attractive choice because it does not tend to potentiate the neurologic cognitive changes of the opioids and other pain medications.

VI. **Creating a case-specific pain management plan**

A. **Intracranial procedures.** The patient who has had an intracranial procedure presents one of the most difficult problems in pain management. The use of regional anesthesia is not an option. Oversedating the patient can lead to hypercarbia and hypoxemia. The cognitive function might be impaired because of the surgical area involved. Despite these limitations, it is crucial to control pain in this group because of the increased morbidity and mortality associated with uncontrolled hemodynamic function and its intracranial sequelae (e.g., hemorrhage, edema). Multiple factors must be considered when treating pain in this patient population.

B. **Procedures of the extremities.** The patient requiring surgery of the extremities gives the anesthesiologist many options. A discussion should occur regarding the patient's postoperative neurologic function and the need for serial functional checks. If the issue of sensory loss is minimal, the use of regional anesthesia is optimal because of the blunting of both pain and the stress response. Other techniques are also acceptable in this population.

C. **Procedures involving the spine.** When neurologic surgery is performed on the structures of the neuroaxis, regional anesthesia should be avoided. The exception to this would be the patient in whom the surgeon specifically requests neural blockade. Since cognitive function is normally at baseline, these patients are often ideal candidates for PCA.

VII. **Complications of neuroanesthesia pain management**

A. **Mental status changes.** Serial neurologic checks are often an essential part of the postoperative course. If pain treatment interferes with this assessment the overall benefit of the pain treatment may be lost. It is crucial to establish a team approach with the surgical team and the nursing team to balance the risks and benefits of pain therapies.

B. **Elevation of arterial carbon dioxide (CO_2).** The importance of ICP is variable in the neurosurgical population. In patients in whom this is an important factor, it is crucial to have some method of monitoring postsurgical CO_2. Despite the benefits of improved hemodynamics in assuring the stability of the patient with elevated ICP, the risk of excessive sedation and hypercarbia is real, and the patient must be watched closely.

C. **Reduction of arterial O_2.** Hypoxemia may create multiple problems in the patient with neuronal tissue trauma. Anaerobic metabolism occurs when neurons do not have enough oxygen substrate. This can result in a reduction of ATP and subsequent cell death. The use of supplemental oxygen and oxygen saturation, as well as serial arterial blood gas monitoring, is essential in patients receiving systemic opioids.

D. **Hypotension.** In the patient with possible spinal cord trauma the use of regional anesthesia can be helpful in controlling the stress response and subsequent systemic changes. The resultant decrease in mean arterial pressure can decrease perfusion to the neurologic tissue and create ischemia. Careful attention to blood pressure is crucial when using local anesthetics postoperatively.

E. **Cerebrospinal fluid leak.** The possibility of subarachnoid puncture when placing an epidural catheter must be weighed against the benefit of the catheter. The risks of brain herniation must also be discussed with the surgeon if there is any intracranial disease process.

F. Nerve injury. When using regional techniques in those with coexisting neurologic disease, a risk of nerve injury exists if the patient has abnormal nociception in the area of the proposed procedure. This also holds true for the patient under general anesthesia or heavy sedation who may be unable to respond to inadvertent intraneural injection.

G. Infection

1. In the sedated patient aspiration precautions should be ordered. This should be accompanied by frequent neurologic checks.

2. Regional anesthesia should be avoided in the patient with local infection at the site of the proposed regional procedure, or in the patient with untreated or uncontrolled systemic infection.

3. With indwelling regional catheters the site of the catheter should be checked regularly for infection.

VIII. Anesthesia in procedures for pain treatment

A social emphasis on the importance of treating patients with chronic pain has led to a growth in the number of practitioners performing procedures requiring anesthesia. Neurosurgeons, anesthesiologists, physiatrists, orthopedic surgeons, and neurologists now perform these surgeries. Regardless of the practitioner involved, the anesthetic issues are important for a stable course.

A. Spinal cord stimulation. This procedure is most commonly performed for pain involving the extremities. The procedure is often separated into stages.

1. **The percutaneous trial.** A temporary stimulation system may be placed under fluoroscopic guidance in either the operating room or radiology suite. Anesthesia in this group is difficult because many of these patients have been taking oral opioids for long periods and are very tolerant to this class of drugs. The patient may require heavy sedation to place the lead in either the lumbar or cervical region, but then must be cognitively functional for the computer screening. Computer screening involves connecting the epidural lead to the hand-held computer and creating electrical stimulation of the nerve tissue in order to obtain a paresthesia. This requirement for varying levels of sedation makes propofol and remifentanil attractive choices in this group of patients.

2. **The surgical lead.** In some patients with more anatomically difficult spines or in whom a percutaneous lead has failed, a surgical lead must be placed. This procedure also usually requires a wake-up period to discuss the perception of

stimulation. This may lead to a more difficult task since the procedure itself requires a hemilaminectomy. Some surgeons may request a general anesthetic with evoked potential testing for this procedure. This is controversial because of the risk of undetected nerve injury, but it is the decision of the surgeon.

3. **The permanent lead.** The lead placed for the trial procedure is often used as a permanent lead if successful. If that is the case, the patient is brought back to the operating room 1 to 4 weeks later for connection to a permanent generator. This procedure is most often performed under monitored anesthesia care or general anesthesia. There is no period of discussion at this stage of the case. Thus, the anesthetic is much less complex. In some cases, both the lead and generator are placed on the same day. This is the case in the patient in whom a temporary lead is placed and secured only to the skin without tunneling. Repositioning from the prone to lateral decubitus position will be required, as well as changes in the level of sedation. A discussion with the surgeon prior to initiating the procedure will help with the anesthetic plan.

B. **Intrathecal and epidural drug infusion systems.** The use of neuroaxial infusions to treat pain that is unresponsive to oral or transdermal medications is becoming more common. Catheters may be tunneled and connected to an external infusion source or may be connected to an implantable system which is placed in the subcutaneous tissue.

1. **Totally implantable infusion systems.** When an intrathecal or epidural pump is placed in the subcutaneous tissue, the procedure involves two steps. First, a catheter must be placed in the epidural or intrathecal space. Once this is successfully completed, the catheter is connected to an infusion source. Anesthesia for these procedures might consist of sedation with local infiltration, subarachnoid or epidural block at the time of catheter placement, or general anesthesia. Each method has its risks and benefits. By using general anesthesia the patient is less likely to move, and the risk of nerve injury is diminished. With the spinal or epidural technique, the general anesthetic is avoided, which may be advantageous for someone at high risk for pulmonary or cardiac complications. By using sedation with local anesthetic infiltration, the risk of undiagnosed nerve injury at the time of catheter insertion is reduced. In some patients, the stimulation involved in the tunneling

and pocketing component of the procedure might not be successfully blunted with sedation and local infiltration alone, and a conversion to general anesthesia might be required during the course of the procedure.

2. **Externalized infusion systems.** In patients in whom the need for infusion is short term or in those with a life expectancy of less than three months, an externalized system is often selected. The need for general anesthesia in this population is rare because of the lack of pocket creation. Although this procedure could be completed under neuroaxial blockade or general anesthesia, the more common scenario is to use monitored anesthesia care with local infiltration.

C. **Radiofrequency nerve ablation.** The cost effectiveness of radiofrequency ablation of the spinal joints has led to a vast increase in the number of procedures performed annually in the United States and Europe. This technique is also being utilized more commonly in ablating the sympathetic nervous system and selected peripheral nerves. The anesthetic in these cases is inherently difficult. The patient must be sufficiently sedated to permit placement of a large radiofrequency cannula, and then rapidly allowed to awaken and become conversant to answer important stimulation questions involving sensory, motor, and nociceptive input. The risks of nerve injury are greatly increased in the patient who is not fully able to discern the computer stimulation pattern. Because of these issues, the infusion of quick-acting and rapidly-waning drugs is often utilized. Propofol and remifentanil are the drugs of choice.

D. **Spinal endoscopy.** In 1997, the U.S. Food and Drug Administration approved the use of spinal endoscopy. In this method, the physician uses a fiberoptic scope to visualize and treat disease processes of the spine by an epidural route. This procedure is very stimulating and requires sedation to be tolerated in most cases. The use of general anesthesia should be avoided because of the risks of nerve damage in the patient who is unable to report paresthesias.

IX. **Summary**

The patient with neurologic disease requiring surgery presents a tremendous challenge. Weighing the functional impairment with the treatment options leads to the optimal treatment plan. More studies are needed to further evaluate the role of pain control techniques in this group. The pain treatment plan should be developed in every case as a routine portion of the preoperative evaluation.

Suggested Readings

Kehlet H, Cousins M, Bridenbaugh P. Modification of responses to surgery by neutral blockade. In: Cousins M, Bridenbaugh P, eds. *Neural blockade in clinical anesthesia and management of pain*, 5th ed. New York: Lippincott-Raven Publishers, 1998:129–165.

Long SP. The management of post-operative pain and the rationale for pre-emptive analgesia. *J Back Musculo Rehab* 1997;9:279–297.

Morgan M. Epidural and intrathecal opioids. *Anaesth Inavere* 1978; 15:60–67.

Spencer L, Carpenter R, Neal J. Epidural anesthesia and analgesia: their role in postoperative outcome. *Anesthesiology* 1995;82(6): 1474–1586.

Wall P. The prevention of postoperative pain. *Pain* 1988;33:289–290.

II

Anesthetic Management

8

Anesthetic Management of Head Trauma

Takefumi Sakabe

Head trauma (traumatic brain injury) is one of the most serious, life-threatening conditions in trauma victims. Prompt and appropriate therapy is mandatory to obtain a favorable outcome. Anesthesiologists are involved in managing these critically ill patients in the emergency room, in neuroradiology suites, and in the operating room, as well as in the neurointensive care unit (NICU).

Management of these patients requires an understanding of the pathophysiology of head injury including injury-associated conditions such as cardiopulmonary disturbances and intracranial hypertension, which produce secondary brain injury and thus contribute to adverse outcome.

It is impossible to save the brain tissue destroyed by the primary impact. Thus, the major goal of the management of head trauma patients is to improve the functional outcome either by surgical procedures (elevation of depressed skull fracture; evacuation of epidural, subdural, or intracerebral hematoma; decompression craniotomy; etc.) or medical therapy, mainly focusing on prevention of secondary brain injury.

It must also be considered that head trauma is often associated with spinal cord injury and trauma to other organs, which may produce various problems during the perioperative period. Anesthesiologists should be aware of these problems for the better management of these severely injured patients.

I. **Classification of head injury.** Head injury is classified in several ways, but a classification into primary injury and secondary injury is useful when considering therapeutic strategies.

   A. **Primary injury** is the damage produced by a direct mechanical impact and/or acceleration–deceleration stress onto the skull and brain tissue including skull fractures (cranial vault, skull base) and the resultant intracranial lesions. The intracranial lesions are further classified into two types: diffuse injury and focal injury.

   1. **Diffuse brain injury** includes:
      a. **Brain concussion.** Loss of consciousness lasting less than 6 hours.
      b. **Diffuse axonal injury.** Traumatic coma lasting longer than 6 hours.

   2. **Focal brain injury** includes:
      a. **Brain contusion.** Usually located either below or opposite the region of impact.
      b. **Epidural hematoma.** Often caused by skull fracture and laceration of the middle meningeal artery.

        c. **Subdural hematoma.** Usually caused by torn bridging veins between the cerebral cortex and draining sinuses. Acute subdural hematoma is often associated with high mortality.

        d. **Intracerebral hematoma.** Usually located in frontal and temporal lobes and visualized as hyperdense mass on a computed tomography (CT) scan.

   3. **Indication for surgery.** Presently there is no definite therapeutic measure to treat diffuse axonal injury. Most depressed fractures and open or compound skull fractures with dural laceration require early surgical repair. Uncomplicated basal fractures usually do not require surgery. Brain contusions with compression of basal cisterns and with a greater risk of developing herniation (usually in the temporal lobe) are surgical indications. Intracranial hematomas are the most common pathology requiring surgical treatment.

B. **Secondary injury.** The primary injury initiates a variety of disorders that provoke secondary injury including ischemic brain damage. The most common disorders that provoke secondary injury include:

   1. Respiratory dysfunction (hypoxemia, hypercapnia)

   2. Cardiovascular instability (hypotension, low cardiac output)

   3. Elevation of intracranial pressure (ICP)

   4. Biochemical derangements

II. **Pathophysiology of head trauma**

A. **Systemic effects of head trauma**

   1. **Cardiovascular responses to head trauma,** commonly observed at the early stage, include hypertension, tachycardia, and increased cardiac output. However, in severely head-injured patients or patients suffering from multiple trauma with substantial blood loss, hypotension and decreased cardiac output can occur. Systemic hypotension (systolic blood pressure < 90 mm Hg) at the time of admission to the hospital is well recognized as a major determinant of adverse outcome.

   2. **Respiratory responses** to head trauma include apnea or abnormal respiratory pattern associated with severe ventilatory insufficiency or spontaneous hyperventilation. Patients may suffer from aspiration of vomitus and central neurogenic pulmonary edema.

   3. **Temperature regulation** might be disturbed, and hyperthermia, if it occurs, can provoke further brain damage.

B. **Changes in cerebral circulation and metabolism** In focal brain injury, cerebral blood flow (CBF) and cerebral metabolic rate for oxygen ($CMRO_2$) decrease in the core area as well as in the perifocal area of the injured tissue. When ICP increases, diffuse and more marked hypoperfusion and hypometabolism ensue.

In diffuse brain injury hyperemia may occur, but in most cases CBF usually decreases within a few hours after trauma. Autoregulation of CBF is often impaired, and if blood pressure decreases, brain ischemia is easily induced. Chemical-metabolic regulation of CBF may also be impaired, which makes management of these patients more complicated.

C. Acute brain swelling and brain edema

1. **Acute brain swelling** is provoked by a decrease in vasomotor tone and a marked increase in the volume of the cerebral vascular bed. In this situation, blood pressure increases can easily produce further brain swelling and increases in ICP. Brain swelling after head trauma occurs more commonly in children than in adults.

2. **Brain edema** after trauma often exhibits a mixture of vasogenic and cytotoxic types caused by blood–brain barrier disruption and ischemia, respectively.

   After head trauma, both acute brain swelling and edema occur concurrently. These pathologic conditions in association with intracranial hematoma cause intracranial hypertension and result in further reduction of CBF and eventually in brain herniation.

D. Excitotoxicity. In head trauma, it is known that the glutamate concentrations in cerebrospinal fluid (CSF) are increased due to excessive release from neurons and glia. Thus, the biochemical changes associated with excessive glutamate release might occur. Activation of glutamate receptors can induce various events such as activation of phospholipase, protein kinase, protease, nitric oxide synthase, etc., all of which are closely related to an increase in intracellular calcium ion. These enzyme activations can produce lipid peroxidation, proteolysis, free radical formation, DNA damage, and so forth, and finally result in neuronal death (Fig. 8-1).

E. Inflammatory cytokines and mediators. The cytokines are known to be major mediators initiating inflammatory and metabolic responses to injury. In cerebral ischemia, cytokines have been shown to increase. Interleukin-6 (IL-6) and tumor necrosis factor α (TNF-α) are known to be released after traumatic brain injury. Patients with Glasgow Coma Scale (GCS) scores of less than 8 show a higher and sustained elevation of IL-6. The cytokines released after traumatic brain injury stimulate the production of free radicals and arachidonic acids, and upregulate the activity of the adhesion molecules, all of which contribute to the secondary brain injury. In head injury an increase in adhesion molecules, e.g., intercel-

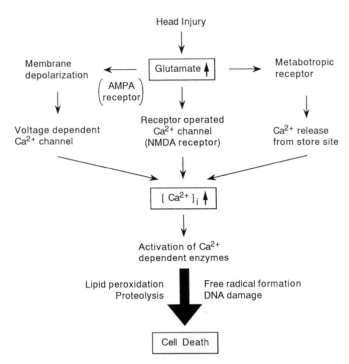

Fig. 8-1. Excitotoxicity in head injury. AMPA, α-amino-3-hydroxy-5-methyl-4-isoxazoleproprionate; NMDA, N-methyl-D-aspartate; $[Ca^{2+}]_i$, intracellular Ca^{2+}.

lular adhesion molecule (ICAM-1), has been observed which can produce disturbances of microcirculation.

III.   **Emergency management**
    A.   **Assessment of the patient's conditions**
        1.   **Neurologic assessment.** Usually there is not much time to evaluate the patient's condition thoroughly. However, while stabilizing the patient's condition (adequate oxygenation and CO_2 elimination, stabilizing blood pressure), a quick neurologic assessment should be performed.
            a.   **Glasgow Coma Scale** (Table 8-1) is a simple and universally accepted method for the assessment of the consciousness and neurologic status in head-injured patients. The GCS has low interobserver variability and is a good predictor of outcome.
                1.   A GCS score of less than 8 characterizes severe head injury.
                2.   A GCS score of 9–12 represents moderate injury.

Table 8-1. Glasgow Coma Scale

Adult scale		Pediatric scale		
Parameter	Score	Parameter	Score	
Eye opening		Eye opening		
Spontaneously	4	Spontaneously	4	
To speech	3	To speech	3	
To pain	2	To pain	2	
None	1	None	1	
Best verbal response		Best verbal response[a]		
Oriented	5	Oriented to place	5	>5 yr
Confused	4	Words	4	>12 mo
Inappropriate	3	Vocal sounds	3	>6 mo
Incomprehensible	2	Cries	2	>6 mo
None	1	None	1	
Best motor response		Best motor response in upper limbs[a]		
Obeys commands	6	Obeys commands	6	>2 yr
Localizes to pain	5	Localizes to pain	5	6 mo–12 yr
Withdraws from pain	4	Normal flexion to pain	4	>6 mo
Flexes to pain	3	Spastic flexion to pain	3	<6 mo
Extends to pain	2	Extension to pain	2	
None	1	None	1	

[a] Score highest appropriate for age.

3. A GCS score of 13–15 represents mild injury.

   b. Assessment of pupillary responses (size, light reflex) and symmetry of motor function in the extremities also should be performed quickly.

2. **Assessment of other organ injury.** Trauma patients often suffer from multiple organ injuries. Particular attention should be paid to intrathoracic and intraperitoneal (intrapelvic) hemorrhage. If these are suspected, exploration of the thorax or abdomen should be performed without delay.

   Treatment of hemorrhagic shock takes precedence over neurosurgical procedures. Hemoglobin levels should be checked and a sufficient number of units of typed and cross-matched blood ordered.

B. **Establishment of airway and ventilation**

1. **Tracheal intubation.** To maintain a secure airway quickly, orotracheal intubation with a cuffed endotracheal tube is the best choice. Since all trauma patients are considered to have a full stomach and not infrequently (about 10%) a cervical spine injury, cricoid pressure and in-line stabilization of the cervical spine should be used during laryngoscopy and intubation.

2. **Blind nasal intubation.** If laryngoscopic visualization is presumed to be difficult or impossible for any reason, blind nasal intubation may be a choice unless the patient is apneic. However, blind nasal intubation may cause coughing and straining, and hence a marked elevation of systemic blood pressure and ICP.

   Nasal intubation carries some risk in patients with basilar skull fractures because this procedure can introduce contaminated materials into the brain. Basilar skull fractures are strongly suspected when hemorrhage of tympanic cavity, otorrhea, petechiae on the mastoid process (Battle's sign), and petechiae around the eyes (panda sign) are observed.

3. **Drugs to facilitate laryngoscopy and intubation** (see IV.B.1.a.).

4. **Mechanical ventilation.** As soon as the trachea is intubated, a nondepolarizing muscle relaxant, preferably vecuronium (0.1 mg/kg), is given and hyperventilation ($PaCO_2$ around 30 mm Hg) is instituted. Hypoxemia, if present, should be corrected immediately. If massive aspiration is suspected, bronchial suctioning using a fiberscope is advisable before transferring the patient to the neuroradiology suite or operating room.

C. **Cardiovascular stabilization.** Systemic hypotension is one of the major contributors to poor outcome after head trauma. Thus, it should be quickly corrected by fluid resuscitation and, if necessary, with inotropic and vasopressor agents.

1. **Fluid resuscitation.** Hypovolemia is often masked by a relatively stable blood pressure secondary to sympathetic hyperactivity or the reflex response to increased ICP. Thus fluid resuscitation should be guided not only by blood pressure but by urinary output and central venous pressure (CVP).

   a. **Crystalloid and colloid solution.** Isotonic or hypertonic crystalloid and/or colloid solutions are given to maintain adequate intravascular volume.

      (1) **Lactated Ringer's solution** can be used but it is slightly hypotonic to plasma. If a substantial amount of lactated Ringer's solution is used, serum osmolarity should be periodically monitored or another crystalloid (normal saline) administered.

      (2) **Hypertonic saline** (3%, 7.5%) is beneficial in smaller volumes for traumatic brain injury. Large volumes may produce a lethal increase in serum sodium concentration.

      (3) **Hydroxyethyl starch** (HES) and human plasma products are useful to maintain intravascular volume for longer periods. No more than 1.5 L of HES is to be used with careful monitoring of blood coagulation, since the incidence of coagulopathy in head-injured patients is high (approximately 20%) and HES itself can disturb blood coagulation. The incidence of coagulation disturbance appears less with pentastarch than with hetastarch.

   b. **Blood transfusion.** In patients with a low hematocrit, blood transfusion is necessary to optimize oxygen delivery; the hematocrit should be maintained above 30%. Children require special attention because they can frequently lose large volumes of blood into an intracranial or subgaleal hematoma or through a scalp laceration without loss in other organ systems.

   c. **Adverse effect of glucose-containing solutions.** Routine use of glucose-containing solutions is not advised because hyperglycemia might aggravate neurologic damage, possibly because of enhancement of lactic acidosis which may be neurotoxic. Glucose should only be used to treat hypoglycemia. The plasma level of 80 to 150 mg/dL is desirable;

values above 200 mg/dL should be avoided
and treated with insulin.

2. **Inotropics and vasopressors.** If blood pressure
and cardiac output cannot be restored with fluid
resuscitation, administration of intravenous inotropics and vasopressors is necessary; phenylephrine or dopamine infusion might be the choice. A
cerebral perfusion pressure (CPP) above 70 to 80
mm Hg should be maintained.

D. **Management of elevated ICP** (see also IV.B.2.c).
Management of elevated ICP and blood pressure support are crucial because both directly determine CPP:
mean arterial pressure (MAP) − ICP.

1. **Hyperventilation.** In severely head-injured patients, hyperventilation to a partial pressure of
carbon dioxide ($PaCO_2$) of 30 mm Hg should be
instituted since hyperventilation is a quick and
effective measure for reducing ICP.

Hyperventilation is more effective in children
than in adults because acute brain swelling from
hyperemia occurs more frequently in children
than in adults. However, hyperventilation might
cause ischemia through excessive vasoconstriction with resultant reduction in CBF. To avoid
this risk, additional measures, including diuretic
therapy, should be initiated immediately. Prolonged hyperventilation is best avoided. Cerebrovascular sensitivity to CO_2 may in some patients
be blunted or absent, and the expected beneficial
effect of hyperventilation in reducing CBF, cerebral blood volume (CBV), and ICP might not occur. In such cases other interventions to reduce
ICP must be exercised.

2. **Diuretic therapy.** Mannitol 1 g/kg (i.v. bolus)
is given in patients with suspected transtentorial
herniation. An infusion can be given in most
other cases, 0.25 to 1 g/kg over 10 to 20 minutes,
and repeated every 3 to 6 hours.

3. **Posture.** Head-up tilt by 10 to 30° aids cerebral
venous drainage and reduces ICP.

4. **Corticosteroid.** Corticosteroids have long been
believed to be of value in reducing brain edema
and hence ICP in head trauma, but some reports
demonstrated even worse outcomes with the use
of corticosteroids. They also increase blood glucose levels, which can adversely effect the injured
brain. Corticosteroids therefore have no place in
the treatment of head injury despite the proven
efficacy in spinal cord injury.

IV. **Anesthetic management**

A. **Preoperative evaluation and preparation.** See
Chapter 5.

B. **Anesthesia.** The major goals of anesthetic management are to (a) optimize cerebral perfusion and oxygenation, (b) avoid secondary damage, and (c) provide

adequate surgical conditions for the neurosurgeons. Basically, general anesthesia is the choice because of better control of respiratory and circulatory function.

1. **Induction of anesthesia.** The majority of patients with severe head injury already have endotracheal tubes in place from the emergency room or the neuroradiology suite for CT examination. If patients come to the operating room without tracheal intubation, immediate oxygenation and securing of the airway is in order. As discussed earlier (see III.B.1), anesthesiologists must be aware of the existence of full stomach, decreased intravascular volume, and potential cervical spine injury.

   Direct arterial pressure monitoring via an indwelling arterial catheter is recommended, if possible before induction of anesthesia. A cannula is inserted into the radial artery or, alternatively, into the dorsalis pedis artery, depending on other sites of injury. Several induction techniques are available.

   a. **Rapid sequence induction** might be desirable in hemodynamically stable patients, although this procedure can produce an elevation of blood pressure and ICP. During administration of 100% oxygen, a small dose of nondepolarizing muscle relaxant (vecuronium 1 mg) is given. Then, an induction dose of thiopental (3 to 4 mg/kg) or propofol (1 to 2 mg/kg) and succinylcholine (1.5 mg/kg) is administered and the trachea is intubated. Etomidate (0.2 to 0.3 mg/kg) may also be used. The induction dose is substantially decreased or even omitted in hemodynamically unstable patients.

      Succinylcholine has been shown to increase ICP. Prior administration of small doses of nondepolarizing muscle relaxant cannot predictably prevent this increase. However, succinylcholine is a good choice to facilitate laryngoscopy and rapid securing of the airway. Rocuronium is an alternative because of its rapid onset of action and lack of effect on intracranial dynamics.

   b. **"Modified" rapid sequence induction.** In the situation where the patient is stable and does not have a full stomach, anesthesia can be induced by titrating the dose of the induction agent to minimize circulatory instability.

      A large dose of vecuronium (0.3 mg/kg), administered with or without a priming dose, can provide fairly satisfactory intubating conditions within 2 minutes.

      Because of its rapid onset, rocuronium (0.6 to 1 mg/kg) might be the drug of choice. Intubating conditions can be obtained within 60 to 90 seconds.

Intravenous lidocaine (1.5 mg/kg), given 90 seconds before laryngoscopy, can prevent the elevation of ICP produced by the intubation procedure. Small doses of fentanyl (1 to 4 μg/kg) might also be helpful.

c. A large-bore orogastric tube is inserted after intubation and gastric contents aspirated and drained during surgery. Nasal gastric tubes should be avoided in the patient with a basilar skull fracture.

2. **Maintenance of anesthesia.** The ideal maintenance drug does not elevate ICP, maintains adequate oxygen supply to the brain tissue, and protects the brain against the ischemic-metabolic insult.

There is no gold standard anesthetic for head injury that fulfills these requirements. The selection of anesthetic drugs is based on a consideration of the intracranial pathology as well as systemic conditions such as cardiopulmonary disturbances and multi-system trauma.

a. **Anesthetics**

(1) **Intravenous anesthetics**

(a) **Barbiturates** (thiopental and pentobarbital). Thiopental and pentobarbital decrease CBF, CBV, and ICP. Since ICP reduction with these drugs is related to the reduction of CBF and CBV coupled with metabolic depression, these drugs are expected to have an effect even in patients who have impaired CO_2 response.

Thiopental and pentobarbital have been demonstrated to have a protective effect against focal ischemia. In head injury, ischemia is a common sequela and thus these drugs might be effective. However, no randomized clinical trial has demonstrated that barbiturates definitely improve outcome after head trauma. In small doses, thiopental is a short-acting drug, but when used for prolonged periods its duration of action is increased.

(b) **Etomidate.** Etomidate's effects on CBF, $CMRO_2$, and ICP are similar to those of barbiturates. Systemic hypotension occurs less frequently than with barbiturates.

(c) **Propofol.** Propofol also has cerebral hemodynamic and metabolic effects similar to those of barbiturates. This drug might be useful in patients with intracranial pathology provided that hypotension is avoided. Since the context-sensitive half-life is short, emergence from anesthesia is rapid, even after prolonged administration. This may offer an advantage over other intravenous anesthetics in providing the opportunity for early postsurgical neurologic evaluation. However, because of propofol's potent circulatory depressive effect, meticulous care should be exercised to maintain adequate CPP. Hypovolemia must be corrected prior to the use of propofol.

(d) **Benzodiazepines.** Benzodiazepines (diazepam, midazolam) may be useful for sedating patients or as induction anesthetics since these drugs may not perturb systemic circulation and are less likely to impair cerebral circulation. Diazepam, 0.1 to 0.2 mg/kg as an induction dose, is given and repeated if necessary up to a total dose of 0.3 to 0.6 mg/kg. Midazolam, 0.2 mg/kg, is used for induction and repeated as needed.

(e) **Narcotics.** In general, narcotics, in clinical doses, produce a minimal to moderate decrease of CBF and $CMRO_2$ and probably have a minimal effect on ICP when ventilation is adequately maintained. Fentanyl may or may not increase ICP. However, this drug provides satisfactory analgesia and avoids unnecessary use of high concentrations of inhalational anesthetics. Some reports have shown that sufentanil increases ICP in severely head-injured patients. Thus, should these drugs be used, measures to reduce ICP such as hyperventilation and barbiturates should be implemented.

(2) **Inhalational anesthetics**

(a) **Halothane.** Among inhalational agents, halothane may be the most potent in increasing CBF and ICP. Its effect is dose-related. The elevation of ICP can be attenuated by prior institution of hyperventilation (hypocapnia) and by concomitant use of intravenous anesthetics such as barbiturates. However, the beneficial effects of hypocapnia might not be realized when the initial ICP is very high or reactivity to CO_2 is lost globally.

(b) **Isoflurane.** Isoflurane is a potent metabolic depressant and has less effect on CBF and ICP than halothane. Because it depresses cerebral metabolism isoflurane might have a cerebral protective effect when the ischemic insult is not severe. The data favor the use of isoflurane over either halothane or enflurane.

(c) **Sevoflurane.** Limited data are available for sevoflurane. In the rabbit cryogenic brain injury model, ICP elevation in association with blood pressure elevation was greater in the animals anesthetized with sevoflurane than with halothane. However, clinical studies demonstrated that sevoflurane's effect on cerebral hemodynamics is similar to that of isoflurane. The disadvantage of sevoflurane is that this drug is biodegraded and the metabolite may be toxic in high concentrations. However, there is no evidence of adverse effect at clinically-used concentrations unless sevoflurane is administered in a low-flow circuit for prolonged periods.

Rapid emergence after sevoflurane anesthesia may be an advantage because it facilitates early postoperative neurologic evaluation. Sevoflurane thus may have a place in the management of head trauma patients.

(d) **Desflurane.** Desflurane at high concentrations appears to increase ICP.

(e) **Nitrous Oxide (N_2O).** Nitrous oxide should not be given to patients with intracranial hypertension or decreased intracranial compliance because of its ability to dilate cerebral vessels and increase ICP. It should also be avoided in the presence of pneumocephalus or pneumothorax because N_2O diffuses into an airspace more rapidly than nitrogen diffuses out and, as a consequence, increases the volume.

(3) **Local anesthetic.** Infiltration of lidocaine 1% or bupivacaine 0.25% in the skin around the scalp incision is helpful to avoid the use of unnecessarily deep anesthesia.

(4) **Muscle relaxants.** Adequate muscle relaxation will facilitate hyperventilation and reduce ICP. Coughing and straining should be avoided because both can produce cerebral venous engorgement.

   (a) **Vecuronium** appears to have no or minimal effect on ICP, blood pressure, or heart rate, and would be effective in head-injured patients. This drug is given as a initial dose of 0.08 to 0.1 mg/kg, followed by infusion at a rate of 1 to 1.7 μg/kg/minute.

   (b) **Pancuronium** does not produce an increase in ICP. However, this drug is not recommended when hypertension and tachycardia will be a risk to the patient.

   (c) **Atracurium** has no effect on ICP. Because of its rapid onset and short duration of action, bolus dose (0.5 to 0.6 mg/kg) followed by continuous infusion (4 to 10 μg/kg/minute) is used with monitoring of neuromuscular blockade.

b. **Intraoperative respiratory and circulatory management**

(1) **Mechanical ventilation.** Mechanical ventilation should be adjusted to maintain $PaCO_2$ around 30 to 35 mm Hg. The FiO_2 should be adjusted to avoid hypoxemia, maintaining a PaO_2 above 100 mm Hg.

   Patients, especially those with pulmonary contusion, aspiration, or central neurogenic edema, may require positive end-expiratory pressure (PEEP) to maintain adequate oxygenation. Excessive PEEP is avoided, however, because the elevation in intrathoracic pressure can compromise cerebral venous drainage and increase ICP.

(2) **Circulatory management.** Cerebral perfusion pressure should be maintained above 70 to 80 mm Hg. The

transducer for direct blood pressure monitoring is zeroed at the level of mastoids to reflect the cerebral circulation.

When hypotension persists despite adequate oxygenation, ventilation, and fluid replacement, careful elevation of the blood pressure with a continuous infusion of inotrope or vasopressor may be necessary. Phenylephrine (0.1 to 0.5 μg/kg/minute) and dopamine (1 to 10 μg/kg/minute) by infusion are appropriate drugs in this setting. A bolus dose of vasopressor must be used cautiously because abrupt increases in blood pressure can elevate ICP to dangerous levels, especially in patients with disturbed autoregulation.

Treatment of hypertension must be carried out with extreme caution because hypertension could be due to compensatory hyperactivity of the sympathetic nervous system in response to elevated ICP. Adequacy of oxygenation, ventilation, volume replacement, and analgesia should first be assessed and corrected if necessary. Then administration of antihypertensive drugs (preferably the drugs with fewer cerebral vasodilating properties such as labetalol, 5 to 10 mg i.v.) is instituted. When treating hypertension, maintenance of CPP should be a major concern.

c. **Intraoperative management of elevated ICP** (see III.D)

   (1) **Patient's posture.** Slight head-up tilt (15 to 30°) is desirable. When surgeons request head and neck rotation, meticulous care not to interfere with venous return is necessary.

   (2) **Ventilation.** Maintain mild to moderate hypocapnia ($PaCO_2$ 30 to 35 mm Hg).

   (3) **Circulation.** Correct hypotension (< 100 mm Hg) and hypertension (>160 mm Hg).

   (4) **Diuretics**

      (a) **Mannitol** will decrease cerebral volume and reduce ICP (see III.D.2).

      (b) **Furosemide** may be coadministered in severe cases as well as in the patient with compromised cardiac function and the potential for heart failure. Furosemide, 0.1 to 0.2 mg/kg, is given 15 minutes before mannitol administration.

When furosemide and mannitol are coadministered, careful monitoring of intravascular blood volume by CVP or pulmonary arterial pressure (PAP) is necessary.

If brain protrusion is observed after craniectomy despite adequate ventilation, oxygenation, anesthetic selection, and diuretics, additional thiopental (or pentobarbital) or propofol might be required and more vigorous hyperventilation might be considered.

    (5) CSF drainage. CSF drainage can be helpful to reduce ICP if an intraventricular catheter is in place.

C. Monitoring

  1. Standard monitoring includes ECG, noninvasive and direct arterial pressure measurement, heart rate and rhythm, pulse oximetry, end-tidal CO_2 monitoring, body temperature, urinary output, CVP, and neuromuscular blockade. Arterial blood gases, hematocrit, electrolytes, glucose, and serum osmolarity should be measured periodically.

  2. Monitoring of air embolism. Detection of venous air embolism by Doppler ultrasound should be considered for surgical procedures in which veins in the operative site are above the level of the heart.

  3. Brain monitoring such as electroencephalogram (EEG), evoked potentials, jugular venous bulb oxygen saturation (SjO_2), flow velocity measured by transcranial Doppler (TCD), and ICP may be used.

    a. SjO_2. The SjO_2 provides continuous information about the balance between global cerebral oxygen supply and demand. An SjO_2 below 50% for more than 15 minutes is a poor prognostic sign and is often associated with a poor neurologic outcome. The decrease in SjO_2 could be caused by excessive hyperventilation, decreased perfusion pressure, cerebral vasospasm, or a combination. Major causes of a decreased SjO_2 and treatment are listed in Table 8-2.

    b. Flow velocity of basal cerebral arteries (measured by TCD technique). Flow velocity measurement of basal cerebral arteries is of great help in assessing the cerebral circulatory state at the bedside, although it does not provide an absolute value for the CBF. High-normal values might indicate hyperemia or vasospasm. These two conditions can be differentiated by the TCD waveform. A disad-

Table 8-2.   Major causes of decreased SjO_2^a and treatment

Cause	Clinical condition	Treatment
$CaO_2 \downarrow$	Hypoxemia	Correction of hypoxemia
	Anemia	Blood transfusion
$CBF \downarrow$	Hypotension	Fluid replacement; inotropics and vasopressors
	Hyperventilation	Correction of $PaCO_2$
	Intracranial hypertension	Mannitol, furosemide, barbiturate, propofol
$CMRO_2 \uparrow$	Hyperthermia	Cooling
	Seizures	Barbiturate, propofol

CaO_2, oxygen content in arterial blood; CBF, cerebral blood flow; $CMRO_2$, cerebral metabolic rate for oxygen.
a $SjO_2 \propto [CaO_2 - CMRO_2/CBF]$.

vantage of this monitor is that the application of Doppler probe is not always possible during the surgical procedure.

   c. **Near-infrared refrectance spectroscopy (NIRS)** is currently available in clinical practice. It provides relative information about changes of oxy- and deoxyhemoglobin and cytochrome oxidase redox status in the brain tissue of interest noninvasively and continuously.

   d. **Intracranial pressure.** The association between severity of ICP elevation and poor outcome has been reported. Monitoring of ICP is therefore useful not only as a guide to therapy but also for assessment of the response to the therapy and determination of prognosis.

V. Cerebral protection

   A. **Hypothermia.** Temperature reduction to 33°C to 35°C is not harmful and might even have beneficial effects. The protective mechanisms include reducion of metabolic demand, excitotoxicity, free radical formation, and edema formation. In an animal ischemia model, mild hypothermia (temperature decreased by 2°C to 3°C) markedly attenuated ischemic injury. Hypothermia has also been reported to be effective in head-injured patients.

   Locations for monitoring include tympanic membrane, nasopharyngeal area, esophagus, or blood. Monitoring at two or more sites is recommended.

VI. Postoperative management

   A. **Emergence and extubation.** Anesthesiologists often receive requests to awaken patients in order for them to be available for early neurologic assessment postoperatively. Patients whose preoperative level of consciousness was normal and who underwent evacuation of an epidural or subdural hematoma can be awakened in the operating room if their awake airways are patent, and adequate spontaneous ventilation and oxygenation are maintained at the end of surgery. After reversal of the remaining effects of neuromuscular blockade, the trachea is extubated. Smooth emergence and extubation are important.

B. Contraindications to extubation. For patients whose consciousness level was decreased preoperatively and in whom brain swelling is marked during surgery or expected to occur postoperatively, extubation in the operating room is discouraged. Patients with multiple trauma are also candidates for postoperative ventilatory care. Regarding patients who are hypothermic, it is better to maintain mechanical ventilation postoperatively. Patients are slowly rewarmed and their tracheas are extubated when their condition improves.

VII. Summary

The major goal of perioperative management of head-injured patients is to prevent secondary damage. Control of intracranial hypertension, prevention of brain edema, and amelioration of biochemically induced secondary damage are the main goals of therapy. Appropriate selection of anesthetics and meticulous general management of respiration, circulation, metabolism, fluid replacement, and temperature are all essential to improve outcome.

References

1. Martin NA, Patwardhan RV, Alexander MJ, et al. Characterization of cerebral hemodynamic phases following severe head trauma: hypoperfusion, hyperemia, and vasospasm. *J Neurosurg* 1997;87:9–19.
2. Hudspith MJ. Glutamate: a role in normal brain function, anesthesia, analgesia and CNS injury. *Br J Anaesth* 1997;78:731–747.
3. Vassar MJ, Fischer RP, O'Brien RE, et al. A multicenter trial for resuscitation of injured patients with 7.5% sodium chloride. *Arch Surg* 1993;128:1003–1013.
4. Warters RD, Allen SJ. Hyperventilation: new concepts for an old tool. *Curr Opin Anesthesiol* 1994;7:391–393.
5. Doppenberg EMR, Bullock R. Clinical neuro-protection trials in severe traumatic brain injury: lessons from previous studies. *J Neurotrauma* 1997;14:71–80.

9

Anesthesia for Supratentorial Tumors

Patrick A. Ravussin and O. H. G. Wilder-Smith

I. **Anesthesia for supratentorial tumors**
   A. **Background.** About 35,000 new brain tumors are diagnosed per year in the United States. In adults, 85% are primary (9% of all primary tumors); 60% are primary and supratentorial (gliomas about 35%; meningiomas about 15%; pituitary adenomas about 8%). Approximately 12% of intracranial tumors are metastases. Their incidence increases with age and about one sixth of cancer patients develop a brain metastasis. Thus, more than 100,000 cancer patients have a brain metastasis, symptomatic in the majority of cases and often the controlling variable for survival.
   B. **General considerations**
      1. **Concerns and problems**
         a. **Patient symptoms** result from local and generalized intracranial pressure (ICP) effects.
         b. **Main surgical concern.** Brain exposure without retraction/mobilization damage.
         c. **Main anesthesia concern.** Avoidance of secondary brain damage (Table 9-1). Thus, understanding of the following is vital: pathophysiology of ICP and intracerebral perfusion; effects of anesthesia on ICP, perfusion, and metabolism; therapeutic options for decreasing ICP, brain bulk, and tension perioperatively.
         d. **Specific problems.** Massive intraoperative hemorrhage, seizures, air embolism (head-elevated/sitting position or if venous sinuses are traversed), monitoring brain function and environment, rapid versus prolonged anesthetic emergence. A concurrence of intra- and extracranial pathologies could also occur (e.g., cardiovascular or pulmonary disease; paraneoplastic phenomena with metastases; chemo-/radiotherapy effects).
      2. **Pathophysiology of rising ICP.** The usual intracranial space-occupying components—brain tissue, intravascular blood, cerebrospinal fluid (CSF)—are contained in an unyielding skull. Any volume increase must be compensated by parallel volume reduction of one or more of these components, mainly CSF or blood (the brain is largely incompressible). The ability to compensate for the presence of a mass and maintain homeostasis de-

Table 9-1.   Secondary insults to the already injured brain

Intracranial	Systemic
• Increased intracranial pressure	• Hypercapnia/hypoxemia
• Epilepsy	• Hypo-/hypertension
• Vasospasm	• Hypo-/hyperglycemia
• Herniation: falx, tentorium, foramen magnum, craniotomy	• Low cardiac output
	• Hypoosmolality
• Midline shift: tearing of cerebral vessels	• Shivering/pyrexia

pends on the volume of the mass and its rate of growth (the ICP–volume curve shifts to the left for rapidly expanding masses). Homeostatic mechanisms: *early* (limited capacity)—intracranial to extracranial blood shift; *late* (larger capacity)—CSF displacement (ineffective if CSF flow obstructed); *exhaustion*—rapid ICP rise → impaired cerebral circulation → brain herniation (end stage of compensation).

3. **Intracerebral perfusion and cerebral blood flow (CBF)**
    a. **Regulation of CBF.** Via gradients in wall pressure of cerebral arterioles [result of cerebral perfusion pressure (CPP)] and $PaCO_2$ concentration (result of ventilation) (Fig. 9-1).

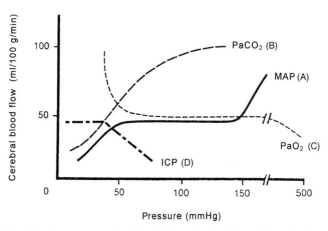

Fig. 9-1.   Pressure–cerebral blood flow relationships. A: Cerebral blood flow (CBF) autoregulation. CBF is maintained at 50 mL/100 g/minute for mean arterial pressure (MAP)/cerebral perfusion pressure (CPP) = 50 to 150 mm Hg. B: Linear relationship between $PaCO_2$ and CBF for $PaCO_2$ = 20 to 80 mm Hg. C: PaO_2 and CBF. D: ICP and CBF.

b. **Autoregulation of CBF** keeps the CBF constant despite changing CPP via alterations in cerebral vasomotor tone, i.e., cerebrovascular resistance (CVR). Characteristics: dominant to ICP homeostasis; normally functional for CPP of 50 to 150 mm Hg; impaired/affected by intracranial (e.g., blood in CSF, trauma, tumors, etc.) and extracranial (e.g., chronic systemic hypertension) pathologies and anesthesia drugs.

c. **Formulas.** CBF = CPP/CVR, CPP = MAP − ICP [N.B.: normally, ICP ≈ CVP (central venous pressure)].

d. **Inadequate perfusion.** Ischemia occurs around CBF of less than 20 mL/100 g/minute; CPP of less than 50 mm Hg (autoregulation intact). Action: restore CPP, CBF [↑ MAP (mean arterial pressure), ↓ ICP, ↑ cardiac output]; reduce cerebral metabolic demand (deepen anesthesia, hypothermia).

e. **Vasodilatory and vasoconstrictive cascades.** ↑ ICP → ↓ CPP → cerebral arteriolar relaxation, → ↑ MAP via systemic autonomic response. However, particularly for impaired intracranial homeostasis, cerebral vessel relaxation → ↑ CBV (intracerebral blood volume) → ↑ ICP (vicious circle!). Note also that acute ↓ CPP (or ↓ MAP) → ↑ ICP (therefore hypovolemia is dangerous); conversely, ↑ CPP → ↓ ICP via cerebral vasoconstriction.

f. **PaCO$_2$.** Hypocarbia results in vasoconstriction, reducing CBF, CBV, and thus ICP, making hyperventilation a favorite tool for the acute control of intracerebral hyperemia and elevated ICP.

4. **Anesthesia and intracerebral pressure, perfusion, and metabolism.** Anesthesia affects the intracranial environment via drug and nondrug effects, all sensitive to the intra- and extracranial state (e.g., cerebral compliance, intracranial pathology, volemic state, etc).

a. **Intravenous anesthetics** (barbiturates, propofol, etomidate) reduce cerebral metabolic rate (CMR) dose-dependently by depressing electrical (not basal metabolic) activity of the neurons with a ceiling effect at electroencephalogram (EEG) burst suppression. They are cerebral vasoconstrictors → ↓ CBF, CBV, and ICP. Cerebral flow–metabolism coupling, autoregulation, and PaCO$_2$ vessel reactivity remain intact. In contrast to volatile anesthetics, propofol suppresses the cerebrostimulatory effects of nitrous oxide.

b. **Volatile anesthetics** (e.g., isoflurane, sevoflurane, desflurane) decrease CMR (only isoflurane similarly to intravenous anesthetics), vasodilate cerebrally (worst: halothane) → ↑ ICP (particularly if ↓ cerebral compliance), and impair autoregulation. For less than 1 minimum alveolar concentration (MAC) and normal brain, $PaCO_2$ reactivity is intact permitting hypocapnic control of vasodilatation. A situation to avoid would be brain pathology + high volatile MAC → impaired/abolished CO_2 reactivity.

c. **Nitrous oxide** is cerebrostimulatory → ↑ CMR, CBF, and sometimes ICP, particularly with volatile anesthesia. For the normal brain, cerebral vasodilatation can be controlled by hypocapnia or intravenous anesthetics (volatiles—*no* attenuating effect). CMR and CBF are higher for 1 MAC anesthesia with nitrous oxide—volatile versus volatile only.

d. **Opioids** have been associated with short-term ↑ ICP (especially sufentanil, alfentanil). However, no direct opioid cerebral vasodilator effect is proven; thus, reflex cerebral vasodilatation after ↓ MAP/CPP probably causes the transient ↑ ICP. Opioids modestly ↓ CMR without affecting flow–metabolism coupling, autoregulation, or vessel CO_2 sensitivity.

e. **Other drugs.** Avoid vasodilating antihypertensive agents (nitroglycerin, nitroprusside, hydralazine) → cerebral vasodilatation. Theophylline constricts cerebral vessels, but it increases CSF production and is a potent central nervous system (CNS) stimulant.

5. **Reducing ICP, brain bulk, and tension** (cf. Table 9-2). The effectiveness of these instruments depends on intact intracerebral homeostatic mechanisms and/or structures.

a. **Intravenous anesthetics** → ↓ CMR, CBF → ↓ CBV, ICP → ↓ brain bulk. Cerebral vasoconstriction depends upon intact CMR–CBF coupling (Fig. 9-2) and is dose-related up to neuronal electrical silence (EEG burst suppression). Like autoregulation, CMR–CBF coupling is impaired by brain contusion and other intracerebral pathologies.

b. **Hyperventilation** → hypocarbia → cerebral vasoconstriction (acute effect lasting for a maximum of 24 hours). For intact autoregulation, CBF is linearly related to $PaCO_2$ from 20 to 70 mm Hg. Factors impairing CO_2 reactivity are as follows: head injury, other intracerebral pathology, high inspired volatile anesthetic concentrations, nitrous oxide (es-

**Table 9-2. Intracranial hypertension
and brain bulging: prevention and treatment**

Prevention	Treatment
• Preop: adequate anxiolysis and analgesia	• CSF drainage (lumbar catheter or ventricle)
• Preinduction: hyperventilate on demand, head-up position, head straight, no jugular vein compression	• Osmotic diuretics
	• Hyperventilation
• Avoid overhydration	• Augment depth of anesthesia using intravenous anesthetics (propofol, thiopental, etomidate)
• Osmotic diuretics (mannitol, hypertonic saline); steroids for tumor	• Muscle relaxation
• Optimize hemodynamics: MAP, CVP, PCWP, HR; use beta-blockers, clonidine, or lidocaine if necessary	• Improve cerebral venous drainage: head-up, no PEEP, reduce inspiratory time
• Ventilation: $PaO_2 > 100$; $PaCO_2 \sim 35$ mm Hg, low intrathoracic pressure	• Mild controlled hypertension if cerebral autoregulation intact (MAP $\sim$ 100 mm Hg)
• Use of intravenous anesthetics for induction and maintenance	

MAP, mean arterial pressure; CVP, central venous pressure; PCWP, pulmonary capillary wedge pressure; HR, heart rate; CSF, cerebrospinal fluid; PEEP, positive end-expiratory pressure.

pecially already dilated vessels). Typical target: $PaCO_2$ of 30 to 35 mm Hg; based on arterial blood gas analysis rather than end-tidal CO_2 ($ETCO_2$; possibility of large arterio-alveolar CO_2 gradients in neurosurgical patients). Side effects of hyperventilation include linear reduction in coronary artery flow and cardiac venous return, as well as hypokalemia.

   c. **Diuretics.** Osmotic diuretics (e.g., mannitol, hypertonic saline) → acutely ↑ blood osmolality → ↓ brain water content (mainly healthy brain tissue with intact blood–brain barrier) → ↓ brain bulk, ICP, ↑ compliance. Also: better blood rheology (↓ endothelial edema; ↓ erythrocyte edema → ↑ erythrocyte deformability). Typical regimen: 0.5 to 1 g/kg mannitol i.v. (split between rapid precraniotomy dose and slower infusion until brain dissection complete). ICP effect: prompt, lasts for 2 to 3 hours, removes about 90 mL brain water at peak effect. Problems: hypernatremia, acute hypervolemia. Loop diuretics

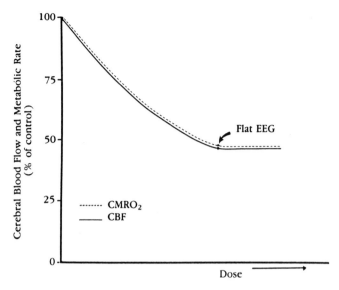

Fig. 9-2. Cerebral blood flow (CBF)–cerebral metabolic rate for oxygen (CMRO$_2$) coupling during increasing doses of an intravenous anesthetic. A normal CMRO$_2$ of 4 mL/100 g/minute is coupled to a CBF of approximately 50 mL/100 g/minute.

(e.g., furosemide) achieve a small ICP reduction via isosmotic contraction of the extracerebral extracellular space.

d. **CSF drainage.** Either by direct puncture of the lateral ventricle (surgeon) or lumbar spinal catheter (by anesthesiologist preoperatively; effective only without caudal block to CSF outflow). Acute brain herniation might occur; therefore, lumbar CSF drainage should be used cautiously and only when dura is open and patient is at least mildly hyperventilated. Draining 10 to 20 mL CSF effectively reduces brain tension; up to 50 mL can be drained if necessary.

e. **Use the vasoconstrictive cascade.** Mild ↑ MAP → ↑ CPP → ↓ CBV.

f. **Avoid other factors** causing cerebral vasodilatation: hypovolemia, hypoxia, patient positioning (head-down, extreme turning of the neck → ↓ cerebral venous drainage).

C. **General anesthetic management**

1. **Preoperative assessment.** Anesthetic strategy is based on the patient's neurologic and general state and the planned surgery; both should be discussed with the neurosurgeon.

Table 9-3. Preoperative neurologic evaluation

History
- Seizures, level of consciousness
- ↑ ICP: headache, nausea, vomiting, blurred vision
- Focal neurology: hemiparesis, sensory deficits, etc.
- Hydration: duration of bed rest, fluid intake, diuretics, syndrome of inappropriate secretion of antidiuretic hormone
- Medication: steroids, antiepileptic drugs
- Associated illnesses, trauma

Physical examination
- Mental status, level of consciousness
- Papilledema (↑ ICP), Cushing's response (hypertension, bradycardia)
- Pupil size, speech deficit, Glasgow Coma Scale score, focal signs

Investigations (CT/MRI scan)
- Size and location of the tumor, e.g., silent or eloquent area? near major vessel?
- Intracranial mass effects: midline shift, ↓ ventricle size, temporal lobe herniation, CSF space surrounding the brain stem, edema, hydrocephalus

ICP, intracranial pressure; CT, computed tomography; MRI, magnetic resonance imaging.

a. **Neurologic state of patient.** Assess (Table 9-3): ICP increase; size of ICP/CBF homeostatic reserve (margin before brain ischemia/neurologic impairment); intracranial compliance; autoregulation impairment; presence of neurologic damage (permanent/reversible); present drug therapy; neurodiagnostic studies.

b. **General state of patient.** Cardiovascular system: brain perfusion/oxygenation depends on it; intracranial pathologies affect its function (↑ ICP versus cardiac conduction); supratentorial surgery (meningiomas, metastasis) may result in significant bleeding (hypovolemia, hypotension → ↓ CPP/CBF and ↑ ICP). Respiratory system: hyperventilation to ↓ ICP, CBF, CBV and brain tension depend on it; 40% of brain metastases are from lung (primary tumor, its chemo-/radiotherapy). The head-up/sitting position affects the cardiac and respiratory systems. Other systems: paraneoplastic or chemo-/radiotherapy-associated syndromes (hematology, coagulation); renal system, diuretics and decreased fluid intake; altered endocrine system (intracranial processes; pituitary adenoma or its therapy; steroids); gastrointestinal tract (steroids and mucosa; motility effects of ↑ ICP).

c. **Planned operative intervention.** Clarify surgical approach (tumor size/position, proximal structures and likelihood of vascular involvement, radical excision); resultant patient positioning (typical for supratentorial masses: pterional, temporal, frontal craniotomy—bifrontal approach and sagittal venous sinuses → bleeding, venous air embolism), and tumor type.

   (1) **Meningiomas.** The combination of large size, difficult location, and radical excision (total resection is virtually curative) makes for long, technically demanding operations, often with significant bleeding (surrounding structures, meningioma vascularity). Anesthetic priority: maximal brain tension reduction to facilitate surgical access.

   (2) **Gliomas.** Often simple debulking with easy surgical access and little risk of bleeding.

   (3) **Others.** Third ventricle colloid cysts, which may result in obstructive hydrocephalus and thus ↑ ICP at induction. Colloid cysts, basal cistern epidermoids, and transcranially resected pituitary tumors need maximal brain relaxation for exposure at skull base.

   (4) **Pituitary adenoma by transsphenoidal resection.** Essentially an extracranial operation.

d. **Determination of anesthetic strategy.** Points to be addressed:

   (1) **Vascular access.** Consider risk of bleeding or venous air embolism, hemodynamic and metabolic monitoring, and infusion needs for vasoactive and other substances.

   (2) **Fluid therapy**. Target normovolemia/normotension; avoid hyposmolar (Ringer's lactate) and glucose-containing solutions (hyperglycemia → ↑ ischemic brain injury).

   (3) **Anesthetic regimen.** "Simple" procedures (low risk of ICP problems or ischemia, little need for brain relaxation): volatile-based technique okay. "High-risk" procedures (anticipated ICP problems, significant risk of intraoperative cerebral ischemia, need for excellent brain relaxation): use total intravenous anesthesia (TIVA).

(4) **Extracranial monitoring**, such as cardiovascular or renal, venous air embolism.

(5) **Intracranial monitoring.** General environment versus specific functions: metabolic (jugular venous bulb), neurophysiologic (EEG/evoked potential), functional (transcranial Doppler).

2. **Preoperative preparation**

a. **Premedication.** Risk assessment: *sedation* → hypercapnia, hypoxemia, upper airway obstruction → ↑ICP; *stress* → ↑CPP/CBF/CMR, ↑ICP and the development of vasogenic edema with impaired autoregulation. Best: titrated intravenous analgesia/sedation (e.g., midazolam 0.5 to 2 mg ± fentanyl 25 to 100 μg or sufentanil 5 to 20 μg) under direct anesthesiologic supervision for vascular access placement, etc. Patients without signs of ↑ICP can benefit from oral ward premedication with a small benzodiazepine dose (e.g., 5 mg midazolam). Continue steroids (supplement with pituitary axis suppression) and other regular medication (anticonvulsants, antihypertensives, other cardiac drugs). Consider starting anticonvulsant therapy if not already initiated (e.g., loading dose of phenytoin 10 to 15 mg/kg over 30 minutes) and H_2 blockers (for ↓gastric emptying, ↑acid secretion with steroids, ↑ICP).

b. **Vascular access.** Two large-bore peripheral intravenous catheters are typical for full craniotomy.

(1) **Central venous access.** Recommended for significant risk of venous air embolism (radiographically control catheter tip position at transition of vena cava/right atrium) or bleeding, major cardiovascular compromise (if severe, consider pulmonary artery catheter or transesophageal echocardiography), and continuous infusion of vasoactive drugs. Jugular cannulation technique (conventional or retrograde) must be meticulous and avoid impairment of cerebral venous drainage (hematoma, head-down position → ↑ICP!).

(2) **Arterial cannulation.** Obligatory for full craniotomy due to need for close monitoring and control of CPP (obtain by transducing arterial pressure at midear/circle of Willis level, CPP = MAP − ICP); frequent determination of arterial $PaCO_2$ (hyperventilation) and plasma glucose, potassium, etc., values.

N.B.: ETCO$_2$ monitoring is no substitute for PaCO$_2$ measurement (correlate poorly, especially with ventilation-perfusion mismatch).

(3) **Jugular venous bulb monitoring (JVBM).** Permits monitoring (continuous with fiberoptic oximetry) of cerebral oxygen extraction (SaO$_2$-SjvO$_2$), allowing conclusions about the adequacy of global cerebral perfusion (assuming CMR constant or observing its alterations by EEG monitoring). Technique: retrograde cannulation of jugular vein; catheter tip must be radiographically verified to be in the jugular venous bulb.

c. **Monitoring**

(1) **Cardiovascular.** Electrocardiographic (myocardial ischemia, arrhythmias); arterial and central venous pressures (cf. above); pulse oximetry. Others: ETCO$_2$ (*trend* monitor for PaCO$_2$, detection of venous air embolism); temperature via esophageal thermistor [modest, passive hypothermia (about 35°C) might confer significant neuronal protection during focal ischemia at small systemic cardio-respiratory risk]; urinary catheter.

(2) **Air embolism.** Sensitively detected by precordial Doppler, end-tidal nitrogen (alternative: transesophageal echocardiography).

(3) **Neuromuscular block.** Do not monitor on hemiplegic extremities (↑ acetylcholine receptor density of lower motor neuron units innervated by dysfunctional or nonfunctional upper motor neurons → resistance to nondepolarizing myorelaxants → effective overdose for normal neuromuscular units). Contralateral hemiparesis to a supratentorial tumor is *not* associated with hyperkalemia as in paraplegic or burn patients; succinylcholine is therefore not contraindicated.

(4) **Blood chemistry.** Monitor glucose regularly; hyperglycemia → ↑ neuronal damage during ischemia. During general anesthesia, steroids → ↑ blood glucose levels; brain retraction → focal cerebral ischemia. Others: K$^+$, hematocrit, coagulation.

(5) **Intracranial environment, cerebral function.** Jugular venous bulb monitoring (cf. above); EEG monitoring (information on CMR, cerebral ischemia, "depth of anesthesia"). Others: evoked

potentials (intactness of specific CNS pathways); transcranial oximetry (by near-infrared spectroscopy; holds promise of noninvasive information on regional cerebral oxygenation, but needs full validation).

   (6)   ICP monitoring. Rare today for elective neurosurgery due to improvements in perioperative ICP control but still has an important role in neurotraumatology.

3.   Induction of anesthesia

   a.   Goals. Ventilatory control (early mild hyperventilation; avoid hypercapnia, hypoxemia); sympathetic/blood pressure control (avoid CNS arousal: adequate antinociception, anesthesia); optimal position on ICP–volume curve (avoid venous outflow obstruction).

   b.   Typical induction scheme. Detailed in Table 9-4.

   c.   Myorelaxants. Modern nondepolarizing drugs have minimal effects on intracerebral hemodynamics. *Caution:* atracurium (↑ laudanosine with prolonged use); succinylcholine (may → transient ↑ CMR, CBF, ICP secondary to muscle spindle activation; reserve for

Table 9-4.   Suggested anesthesia induction and maintenance scheme

Induction	Maintenance
• Adequate preoperative anxiolysis	• Propofol 50–150 μg/kg/min or isoflurane 0.5–1.0% (or sevoflurane, desflurane)
• ECG, capnometer, pulse oximeter, NIBP	• Maintain analgesia: fentanyl 1–2 μg/kg/h (or alfentanil, sufentanil, remifentanil)
• Venous, arterial lines: insert under LA	• LA, fentanyl 2 μg/kg (skullpin head holder placement, skin incision)
• Preoxygenation, then fentanyl 1–2 μg/kg (or alfentanil, sufentanil, remifentanil)	• Position: head up, jugular veins free
• Propofol 1.25–2.5 mg/kg or thiopental 3–6 mg/kg, then nondepolarizing myorelaxant	• Mannitol 0.5–0.75 g/kg, insert lumbar drain
• Control ventilation (PaCO$_2$ ≈ 35 mm Hg)	• If propofol, possibly N$_2$O when dura open
• Lidocaine 1.5 mg/kg	• Ensure adequate volemia (NaCl 0.9% or HES 6%—not Ringer's lactate!)
• Intubation	

ECG, electocardiogram; NIBP, noninvasive blood pressure; LA, local anesthesia; HES, hydroxyethyl starch.

difficult intubation or rapid sequence induction); myorelaxant antagonization (undesirable CNS arousal). Interaction ($\uparrow$ doses by 50% to 60%) between pancuronium/vecuronium (not atracurium) and chronic (more than 7 days) phenytoin/carbamazepine treatment can occur; no neuromuscular transmission monitoring on hemiplegic extremities (cf. above). [N.B.: Since neurosurgical patients are susceptible to myorelaxant hangover (difficult to detect by manual relaxometry), avoid long-acting myorelaxants (e.g. pancuronium); use middle to short-acting drugs (e.g., vecuronium, cisatracurium, mivacurium, rocuronium)].

d. **Patient positioning.** Pin holder application is a maximal nociceptive stimulus. Block by deeper anesthesia (e.g., propofol bolus 0.5 mg/kg) or analgesia (fentanyl bolus 1 to 3 μg/kg, alfentanil 10 to 20 μg/kg, remifentanil 0.25 to 1 μg/kg), and local anesthetic infiltration of the pin site. Alternative: antihypertensives (esmolol 0.5 mg/kg, labetalol 0.075 to 0.15 mg/kg). Remember that pin insertion can introduce venous air embolism! Avoid extreme positions; pad and/or fix regions susceptible to pressure, abrasion, or movement injury. Fix the endotracheal tube securely to avoid accidental extubation and abrasions with movement and tape eyes occlusively to avoid corneal damage. Mild head-up position helps venous drainage; mild knee flexion decreases back strain. Avoid severe lateral extension/flexion of head on neck (maintain more than two fingers' space between chin and nearest bone). If the head is turned laterally, elevate contralateral shoulder (wedge/roll) to prevent brachial plexus stretch injury. Lateral/sitting position: specific precautions.

4. **Maintenance of anesthesia (Table 9-4)**
   a. **Goals**
      (1) **Controlling brain tension via control of CMR and CBF.** Preventing CNS arousal (depth of anesthesia, antinociception); treating consequences of CNS arousal (sympatholysis, antihypertensives); the "chemical brain retractor concept" (Table 9-5).
      (2) **Neuroprotection.** Maintenance of an optimal intracranial environment (matching cerebral substrate demand and supply); attempts at specific neuroprotection.
   b. **Choice of technique.** Controversy: Intravenous or volatile anesthesia for neurosurgery?

Table 9-5.   The chemical brain retractor concept

• Mild hyperosmolality[a]	• Intravenous anesthetic agent
• Mild hyperventilation	(propofol)
	• Mild controlled hypertension[b]
Combined with:	
• Adequate head-up positioning	• Avoidance of brain retractors
• Lumbar CSF drainage	• Venous drainage: jugular
	veins free

[a] Before bone flap removal, give mannitol (1,319 mosmol/kg) 0.5–0.75 g/kg or 7.5% NaCl (2,533 mosmol/kg) 3–5 ml/kg. N.B.: NaCl 0.9% = 304 mosmol/kg.
[b] Mean arterial pressure ~100 mm Hg.

No study to date has shown significant outcome differences for intravenous versus volatile-based neuroanesthesia.

(1) **Volatiles.** *Con:* CBF-CMR uncoupling; ↑ CBF/ICP/brain bulk. *Pro:* easy, extensive, successful use; control, predictability (early awakening). *Recommendation:* use for "simple" cases (no ischemia, ICP, or brain bulk problems); early moderate hyperventilation; Fi less than 1 MAC; avoid combination with N_2O (↑ cerebrostimulation).

(2) **Intravenous techniques.** *Con:* onerous use; prolonged/unpredictable awakening [mitigated by: computer-controlled infusion (CCI), short-acting, infusion duration–insensitive drugs, e.g., propofol, remifentanil]. *Pro:* intact CBF–CMR coupling; ↓ CBF/ICP/brain bulk; propofol blunts N_2O cerebrostimulation; probably better specific neuroprotection. *Recommendation:* use for cases with risk of ICP/brain bulk problems or intraoperative cerebral ischemia; use CCI and short-acting drugs.

c. **Management of increases in ICP and brain bulk** (see Table 9-2)

d. **Other measures.** When CNS and hemodynamic arousal are evident despite adequate anesthesia/analgesia, consider sympatholysis (esmolol 0.5 mg/kg; labetalol 0.075 to 0.15 mg/kg). Moderate hypothermia (~34°C to 35°C) may provide some neuroprotection during ischemia.

e. **Fluid therapy.** Goals: normovolemia, normotension, normoglycemia, hematocrit ~ 30%, mild hyperosmolality (≤320 mOsm/L at end of procedure). *Recommendations:* avoid glucose-containing solutions, Ringer's lactate (hypoosmolar); use 0.9% NaCl or 6% hydroxy-ethyl starch (HES).

5. **Emergence from anesthesia** causes respiratory, cardiovascular, metabolic/endocrine, and neurologic changes. Emergence is associated with hemodynamic arousal lasting 10 to 25 minutes, weakly correlating with rises in oxygen consumption and mediated by elevated catecholamine levels and nociceptive stimuli. Treatment: sympatholysis, antinociception. Oxygen consumption is increased (up to 5 times) by rewarming (shivering/nonshivering thermogenesis) and pain. As a result of all of these factors, 20% of elective craniotomy patients develop raised ICP in the early postoperative period.

   a. **Aims of emergence** Maintain intra-/extracranial homeostasis (MAP-CPP-CBF-ICP, CMR, $PaCO_2$, PaO_2, temperature). Avoid factors leading to intracranial bleeding and/or an increase in CBF/ICP (e.g., coughing, intratracheal suctioning, ventilator fight, ↑ airway pressure). The patient should be calm, cooperative, and responsive to verbal commands soon after emergence.

   b. **Early versus late emergence.** Ideal: rapid emergence to permit early assessment of surgical results and postoperative neurologic follow-up. However, there are still some categories of patients where early emergence is not appropriate (below and Tables 9-6 and 9-7).

Table 9-6. Early vs. delayed awakening: pro and con

Early awakening	Delayed awakening
Pro	*Pro*
• Earlier neurologic exam and reintervention	• Less risk of hypoxemia and/or hypercarbia
• Baseline neurology for subsequent exams	• Better respiratory, hemodynamic control
• Less hypertension, catecholamine burst	• Easier to transfer to the ICU
• Performed by anesthesiologist who knows patient	• Stabilization in same state as during surgery
• Surgery/recovery period separated, ↓ costs	• → Better late hemostasis
Con	*Con*
• Increased risk of hypoxemia, hypercarbia	• Less neurologic monitoring
• Respiratory monitoring during transfer to ICU	• More hypertension, catecholamine release

ICU, intensive care unit.

Table 9-7.   Checklist before trying an early landing

- Adequate preop state of consciousness
- Cardiovascular stability, normal body temperature and oxygenation
- Limited brain surgery, no major brain laceration
- No extensive posterior fossa surgery involving cranial nerves IX–XII
- No major arteriovenous malformation removal (avoiding malignant postoperative edema)

   c.   **Indications for late emergence.** Obtunded consciousness or inadequate airway control preoperatively; intraoperative catastrophe; significant risk of brain edema, ↑ ICP, or deranged intracerebral hemo- or homeostasis postoperatively. Risk factors for latter: long (greater than 6 hour) and extensive surgery (particularly with bleeding), repeat surgery, glioblastoma surgery, surgery involving or close to vital brain areas, and surgery associated with significant brain ischemia (e.g., long vascular clipping times, extensive retractor pressure). If delayed emergence is chosen, adequate sedation and analgesia should be assured, preferably with short-acting drugs.
   d.   **Preconditions for early emergence.** Anesthesiologic: should be planned (see Table 9-7); use pharmacologically adequate anesthetic technique for early awakening; pay meticulous attention to intraoperative homeostasis (oxygenation, temperature, intravascular volume, cardiovascular function, CNS metabolism); avoid trauma of mechanical brain retraction (pharmacologic ICP/brain bulk control; see Table 9-5). Neurosurgical: minimization of blood loss (obsessive hemostasis), minimal surgical invasiveness (microsurgery, small operative fields). Under these conditions, early emergence can be associated with less hemodynamic, metabolic, and endocrine activation than for delayed emergence.
   e.   **Differential diagnosis of unplanned delayed emergence.** In 20 to 30 minutes after cessation of pharmacologically adequate anesthesia, the patient should be awake enough to obey simple verbal commands. If not, consider and treat or rule out nonanesthetic causes (include seizure, cerebral edema, intracranial hematoma, pneumocephalus, ves-

sel occlusion/ischemia, metabolic or electrolyte disturbances). Suspected opioid over-
hang: try carefully titrated antagonization
with small doses of naloxone or naltrexone.

D. Specific anesthetic management

1. **Difficult airway.** Avoiding hypoxia is more important than preventing ICP increases. Method of
choice: awake fiberoptic intubation. Technique:
well-prepared, informed, cooperative patient;
good local anesthesia (nasopharynx, airways);
supplemental judicious light sedation (bolus midazolam 0.5 to 1 mg ± fentanyl 25 to 50 μg; alternatively: low-dose propofol infusion at 1 to 2 mg/
kg/hour); treat hypertension promptly (esmolol,
labetalol).

2. **Infectious tumors (abscesses)** are part of the
differential diagnosis of supratentorial mass lesions. They are often accompanied by low-grade
fever. Risk factors: contiguous infections (sinus,
ear); right-to-left cardiac shunt; immunosuppres-
sion (extrinsic/intrinsic); intravenous drug abuse.
Initial treatment: antibiotics (infection); corticosteroids (brain swelling). Definitive diagnosis/
treatment: craniotomy, abscess aspiration. Surgical and anesthetic management: as for supratentorial neoplasms; aseptic precautions and sterile
technique are vital for immunocompromised [ac-
quired immunodeficiency syndrome (AIDS)] patients. [N.B.: Association between human immunodeficiency virus (HIV) infection and cerebral
non-Hodgkin's lymphomas.]

3. **Craniofacial/skull base surgery:** Increasingly
used for orbital, posterior nasal sinus wall tumors. *Particularities:* complex, multidisciplinary
surgery; tracheostomy/oral intubation frequent.
Extensive bony involvement → ↑ bleeding, hemorrhagic diathesis, venous air embolism (head-up
position). Sensory ± motor neurophysiologic cranial nerve monitoring is common (motor monitoring: avoid neuromuscular blockade). Repeat
procedures may be necessary and a difficult intubation (skull base exposure requires extensive
temporalis muscle mobilization which can lead to
mandibular pseudoankylosis and limited mouth
opening) may result.

II. Anesthesia for intracranial hematomas

A. **General considerations.** The effects of intracranial
hematomas on neurostatus and ICP depend particularly on the speed with which they arise. *Slow:*
chronic subdural hematomas- subtle neurologic signs,
small ↑ ICP; anesthetic technique: similar to supratentorial tumors. *Fast:* acute epidural or subdural he-
matoma- massive neurologic impairment, potentially
acutely life-threatening ↑ ICP; anesthetic technique:
aggressive ↓ ICP and measures to preserve brain ox-

ygenation and perfusion, followed by urgent surgical decompression.

B. **Anesthetic management of acute intracranial hematoma**

1. **Induction.** For a detailed discussion, see Chapter 8.

   a. **Basics.** Assure oxygenation, then secure airway and mildly hyperventilate with 100% oxygen. Swift, atraumatic intubation (always dangerous if a fractured cervical spine is suspected or confirmed by x-ray); aim for a minimal ICP rise by avoiding coughing and arterial hypertension due to light anesthesia. In polytraumatized, hypotensive, hypovolemic patients one should decrease hypnotic, analgesic doses and restore circulating volume. If a full stomach, aspiration prophylaxis and cricoid pressure (cautiously if fractured cervical spine).

   b. **Pharmacologic range of options.** Intubation without further use of drugs in the deeply unconscious patient; judicious sedative use (e.g., etomidate 0.2 to 0.5 mg/kg, propofol 0.2 to 0.5 mg/kg) together with myorelaxation for a semiconscious, struggling patient; "classical" rapid sequence induction for the (still) conscious and stable patient. *Controversy:* What myorelaxant scheme to use? Succinylcholine, perhaps preceded by a small dose of nondepolarizing myorelaxant, remains the classical and time-tested scheme. Alternatives include the "priming option:" a priming dose of a non-depolarizing myorelaxant is followed 3 minutes later by full dose of the myorelaxant; or "megadose myorelaxation:" a 1.5 to 2 times the ED_{95} dose of a short- to medium-acting nondepolarizing myorelaxant (e.g., vecuronium, mivacurium) usually permits intubation 1 minute later (not recommended for difficult airways!).

   c. **Control of ICP and brain swelling.** Next priority after securing ventilation and airway; should be started as early as possible and continued through to intensive care treatment.

2. **Anesthesia maintenance.** Aims: control of ICP and brain swelling; maintenance of cerebral perfusion and oxygenation by matching CMR and CBF.

   a. **Monitoring**

      (1) **Cardiovascular monitoring** for these frequently hemodynamically unstable patients should include invasive arterial pressure monitoring, preferably commenced before induction (close hemo-

dynamic control, repeated laboratory determinations). Electrocardiographic monitoring: changes due to cerebral (blood in CSF → ↓ T waves) or cardiac (heart contusion → conduction problems, precordial ST segment change) causes.

(2) **ICP monitoring.** Generally installed once hematoma is evacuated, mainly for use in intensive care unit.

(3) **Laboratory analyses.** Blood gas analysis (acid–base balance, ventilation, etc.); glucose (hyperglycemia and brain ischemia), coagulation profile (N.B.: brain tissue damage → ↑ circulating thromboplastin); blood osmolality (guidance for use of osmotic diuretics: e.g., with mannitol, maximum should be 320 mOsm/kg).

b. **Anesthetic technique.** Intravenous anesthetics (→ ↓ CMR, ↓ CBF, ↑ CVR) are the mainstay of anesthesia for acute intracranial hematoma. Volatile anesthetics are *not* recommended because of risk of ↑ ↑ ICP/brain tension (to the point of acute transtentorial/craniotomy herniation, even with preexisting hypocapnia) and much smaller CMR reduction and neuroprotection against focal ischemia than with intravenous anesthetics (propofol, barbiturates, etomidate).

c. **Cardiovascular control.** Avoid arterial hypotension (by using too large doses of intravenous anesthetics, opioids) to prevent ↓ CPP (→ cerebral ischemia and/or reflex cerebral vasodilatation → ↑ ICP not controlled by hypocapnia; cf. I.B.3.e). *Controversy:* Control of arterial hypertension and acute intracranial hematoma (see Table 9-2): carefully balance maintenance of CPP to areas of brain rendered ischemic due to compression by hematoma against risk of more vasogenic brain edema or bleeding. Jugular venous bulb oxygen saturation monitoring may help assess adequacy of global CPP. Globally adequate CPP does not rule out regional CPP inadequacies → regional ischemia. If arterial pressure requires reduction, first improve analgesia (i.e., opioids) and/or depth of anesthesia (propofol, barbiturates, etomidate) before instituting specific antihypertensive treatment (usually antisympathetic drugs, e.g., esmolol, labetalol, clonidine). Vasodilating antihypertensives (nitroprusside, nitroglycerin, hydralazine) → ↑ ICP via cerebral vasodilatation, which parallels ↓ MAP/CPP!

  d. **Emergence.** Patients with acute cerebral hematoma have significant brain injury with significant actual and potential brain swelling. They should thus undergo slow weaning and delayed extubation in the neurointensive care unit. Chronic subdural hematoma patients frequently have minimal neurologic impairment preoperatively and can therefore often be awakened and their tracheas extubated immediately after surgery.

III. **Conclusions.** The main objectives of anesthesia for excision of a cerebral tumor include:

 •Preserving uninjured cerebral territories by global maintenance of cerebral homeostasis and cardiovascular stability as well as neuroprotection.

 •Balancing CBF autoregulation and MAP and preserving cerebral vasoreactivity to $PaCO_2$.

 •Achieving and maintaining brain relaxation by means of:

  - ↓ CMR, CBF, and CBV
  -moderate hyperventilation ($PaCO_2 < 35$ mm Hg)
  -strict maintenance of CPP
  -osmotherapy
  -CSF drainage

 •Timely awakening to facilitate early and continuing neurologic assessment and permit prompt diagnosis and treatment of complications

REFERENCES

1. Rosner MJ, Daughton S. Cerebral perfusion pressure management in head injury. *J Trauma* 1990;30:933–940.
2. Grubb RL, Raichle ME, Eichling JO, Terpogossian MN. The effects of changes in $PaCO_2$ on cerebral blood volume, blood flow, and vascular mean transit time. *Stroke* 1974;5:630–639.
3. Miller JD, Leech HP. Effects of mannitol and steroid therapy on intracranial volume–pressure relationships in patients. *J Neurosurg* 1975;42:274–281.
4. Leonov Y, Sterz F, Safar P, et al. Mild cerebral hypothermia during and after cardiac arrest improves neurologic outcome in dogs. *J Cereb Blood Flow Metab* 1990;10:57–70.
5. Todd MM, Warner DS, Sokoll MD, et al. A prospective, comparative trial of three anesthetics for elective supratentorial craniotomy. *Anesthesiology* 1993;78:1005–1020.

10

Anesthesia for Posterior Fossa Surgery

Deborah J. Culley and Gregory Crosby

Surgery in the posterior fossa is often demanding, delicate, and long. Anesthesia for these cases is also challenging; in addition to the anesthetic management issues that apply to supratentorial surgery, posterior fossa surgery presents special problems related primarily to positioning, cranial nerve dysfunction, and prevention of and monitoring for venous air embolism.

I. Preoperative considerations

    A. The reticular activating system, cranial nerves, and structures vital for control of the airway and cardiovascular and respiratory systems are contained within a very small space in the posterior fossa. Accordingly, patients may present with dysphagia, laryngeal dysfunction, respiratory irregularities, or altered consciousness. In some cases, chronic aspiration due to loss of airway reflexes can further compromise respiratory function.

    B. Intracranial hypertension is less of a concern than for supratentorial surgery, but hydrocephalus caused by obstruction of ventricular outflow is a common cause of increased intracranial pressure (ICP). This will be evident on the preoperative computed tomography (CT) or magnetic resonance imaging (MRI) scan, and can be treated by ventricular drainage or hypertonic osmotherapy such as mannitol and lasix both pre- or intraoperatively.

II. Positioning

    A. General issues

        1. Posterior fossa surgery often requires unusual patient positioning. The prone, lateral, park bench, and sitting positions are commonly used. Regardless of the position chosen, care in positioning is of utmost importance since most problems are presumably avoidable with careful positioning and padding of vulnerable areas.

        2. In the prone position, facial skin ulcerations can occur from uneven pressure distribution when the horseshoe headrest is used, and blindness can result from pressure on the globe of the eye.

        3. In the lateral and park bench positions, there is a risk of brachial plexus injury if the up arm is pulled caudally to gain access to the retromastoid area.

        4. Excessive neck rotation can also stretch and damage the brachial plexus and extreme neck flexion is associated with a risk of quadriplegia.

     5. Also possible is injury to the ulnar nerve at the elbow or peroneal nerve at the knee.

B. The sitting position

    1. Advantages of the sitting position include good surgical exposure, improved ventilation, better access to the airway, greater comfort for the surgeon, and possibly reduced blood loss.

    2. Disadvantages include the risk of venous air embolism and pneumocephalus and the potential for hemodynamic instability. Additional complications include sciatic nerve injury due to extreme flexion of the hip, massive swelling of the face and tongue due to extreme neck flexion and/or rotation, and midcervical quadriplegia (ostensibly caused by a combination of stretch or compression of the cord by extreme neck flexion and hypotension).

    3. The main contraindication to the use of the sitting position is presence of a documented right-to-left intracardiac or pulmonary shunt, which would facilitate systemic embolization of air.

C. Venous air embolism

    1. Venous air embolism (VAE) can occur any time that pressure within an open vessel is subatmospheric. Clinically significant VAE is unusual unless the surgical site is more than 20 cm above the heart. Hence, VAE is a particular problem during surgery in the seated position, but it also occurs, albeit less frequently, in patients operated in the lateral or prone position.

    2. When open vessels cannot collapse, which is the case with major venous sinuses as well as bridging and epidural veins, the risk of VAE increases substantially. Most studies indicate that the incidence of VAE during seated posterior fossa procedures is 40% to 45%. For seated cervical laminectomy or surgery in the prone or lateral positions, it is about 10% to 15%.

    3. Massive air embolism produces abrupt and catastrophic hemodynamic changes. Fortunately, this type of VAE is rare.

    4. More commonly, air entrainment occurs slowly over a longer period of time and may produce little or no respiratory or hemodynamic compromise.

       a. As air is cleared to the pulmonary circulation, pulmonary vascular resistance and pulmonary artery (PA) and right atrial pressures increase.

       b. This vascular obstruction increases dead-space ventilation, resulting in the decreasing end-tidal CO_2 ($ETCO_2$) and increasing $PaCO_2$ that are characteristic of VAE. In addition, nitrogen appears in exhaled gas.

      c. Due to the partially occluded pulmonary vasculature and to local release of vasoactive substances, hypoxemia develops.

      d. If unchecked, cardiac output decreases as a result of right heart failure and/or reduced left ventricular filling.

    5. Despite firmly held opinions and anecdotes, there is little evidence that the sitting position—at least when used in large centers doing numerous sitting cases—is less safe than alternative surgical positions. As such, it is difficult to argue that the sitting position should be abandoned purely because of the risk of VAE.

D. Paradoxic air embolism

    1. Any time air enters the venous circulation, there is a risk that it could pass via the pulmonary vascular bed or a patent foramen ovale to the arterial side and embolize to coronary or cerebral vessels. The incidence of clinically significant paradoxic air embolism (PAE) is unknown, and only a handful of cases have been reported (most without complications).

    2. Since about 25% of the population has a probe-patent foramen ovale (PFO) and the incidence of VAE is about 45%, approximately 10% to 12% of patients operated in the sitting position have a potential risk of PAE.

    3. Precordial echocardiography has been used preoperatively to identify patients at risk because of a PFO. While detection of a PFO indicates that a patient is at risk for PAE, failure to identify a PFO is not reassuring because precordial echo has a high false-negative rate. Hence, echo is not presently recommended as a routine part of the preoperative evaluation of such patients.

III. Anesthetic management

A. Premedication

    1. There is no contraindication to premedication of patients with small cranial nerve or cerebellar lesions. In the event of elevated ICP or symptomatic hydrocephalus, heavy premedication should be avoided.

B. General monitoring issues

    1. For most posterior fossa cases, routine operative monitoring, usually with addition of an intra-arterial catheter for blood pressure monitoring, will suffice.

    2. For sitting cases, two additional issues arise. First, blood pressure should be measured at the level of the head; since blood pressure as measured at the level of the heart will underestimate that perfusing the brain. Second, monitoring and prevention of VAE are major considerations.

C. **Monitoring for venous air embolism**
1. Monitoring may not provide advanced warning in the case of massive air embolism since hemo-dynamic changes are abrupt and catastrophic. Fortunately, this type of VAE is rare.
2. Clinically, several monitoring options are available. In general, Doppler and $ETCO_2$ monitoring are considered the acceptable minimum.
3. **Precordial Doppler**
    a. This device can detect 1 mL of air or less, which makes it more sensitive than any other monitor except transesophageal echocardiography (TEE). It is not quantitative, however, and knowing which of the various sounds it emits are indicative of air takes experience.
    b. The Doppler should be placed after the patient is in the operative position. The probe is usually positioned at the middle third of the sternum on the right side but, because the position of the right atrium will vary with patient position, proper placement must be confirmed. Hearing heart tones is not enough.
    c. To test for proper probe placement, 0.5 to 1.0 mL of air, CO_2, or circuit gas is injected through a right atrial catheter or peripheral intravenous line; injecting agitated saline is an acceptable alternative. The probe is properly placed if this maneuver produces characteristic Doppler sounds.
    d. Because of its extraordinary sensitivity, a properly positioned Doppler, combined with end-tidal gas monitoring, is an essential monitor for all sitting posterior fossa procedures.
4. **End-tidal gas monitoring**
    a. For reasons already stated, VAE is associated with a decreasing $ETCO_2$ and the presence of end-tidal nitrogen (ENT_2).
    b. End-tidal nitrogen monitoring, while theoretically quantitative, is less useful in practice because the ETN_2 concentration produced by even a large air embolus is small and just reaches the threshold of sensitivity of clinically available end-tidal gas monitors.
    c. $ETCO_2$ monitoring is of intermediate sensitivity but provides a qualitative estimate of the size of a VAE. In general, the larger the embolus, the greater the decrease in $ETCO_2$. A decrease in $ETCO_2$ is not specific for VAE, however, since a decrease in cardiac output from any cause will have the same effect.
    d. The $ETCO_2$ monitoring is particularly useful for corroborating evidence of VAE from the Doppler and judging the clinical and physiologic significance of the embolus.

5. **Central venous catheter**
   a. As a monitor for VAE, the central venous catheter (CVP) is insensitive and easily superseded by other devices. It has other utility, however.
   b. It can help with positioning of the Doppler (see above). Also, aspiration of air both confirms the diagnosis of VAE and serves as a treatment.
   c. To facilitate rapid aspiration of air, a multiorificed catheter is recommended. Since air tends to localize at the junction between the superior vena cava and the right atrium, greatest air retrieval occurs when the catheter orifices traverse this region.
   d. Catheter position can be confirmed in a number of ways. The catheter can be advanced until a right ventricular pressure trace is obtained and then withdrawn several centimeters. Alternatively, a chest x-ray can be obtained to confirm position. A popular and simple method involves using the electrocardiogram (ECG). In this case, the right arm lead is connected to the catheter by a fluid column of sodium bicarbonate or via the J wire used to place the catheter. The tip is advanced until a biphasic P wave appears, at which point the catheter is withdrawn a few centimeters.
   e. One should always attempt to place a CVP catheter in posterior fossa cases requiring the sitting position, but whether inability to do so should result in cancellation of the case is controversial.
6. **Pulmonary artery pressure**
   a. Because PA pressures rise with significant VAE, the catheter can be useful for both diagnosis and therapy.
   b. However, it is difficult to aspirate air from the distal port of a PA catheter and the middle port may not be in optimal location. Aspiration is more efficient with a CVP catheter.
   c. In addition, as a diagnostic tool, the PA catheter offers no advantage over CO_2 monitoring.
7. **Transesophageal echocardiography**
   a. Transesophageal echocardiography (TEE) is as sensitive as the Doppler and is also specific since air bubbles are directly visualized. It is the only monitor that can detect PAE.
   b. The problem is that TEE is expensive, requires special expertise, and demands near constant attention. For these reasons, it is not a routine monitor for VAE in most centers.

D. Prevention of venous air embolism

   1. Positive end-expiratory pressure

   a. Use of positive end-expiratory pressure (PEEP) to prevent VAE in the sitting position is controversial. High levels of PEEP (>10 cm H_2O) are needed to increase venous pressure at the head and studies are inconsistent as to whether PEEP decreases the incidence of VAE. It can also reduce venous return, cardiac output, and mean arterial blood pressure.

   b. Experimental data also indicate that discontinuation of PEEP promotes right-to-left shunting of air. Overall, PEEP is not recommended.

   2. Volume loading

   a. Although hypovolemia has been proposed as a predisposing factor to VAE, evidence for a prophylactic effect of volume loading either on the incidence of VAE or PAE is not strong enough to warrant routine use. Adequate hydration is the goal.

   3. Deliberate hypoventilation

   a. Recent work suggests that moderate hypoventilation might reduce the risk of VAE. As a consequence of higher cerebral blood flow and volume, it might also impair surgical exposure.

   b. Until the benefits of hypoventilation are confirmed, moderate hyperventilation remains the common practice.

E. Anesthetic technique

   1. There is no evidence that any particular anesthetic agent or technique is superior to another for posterior fossa surgery. Moreover, hemodynamic changes associated with assumption of the sitting position are minor regardless of the anesthetic technique.

   2. Use of nitrous oxide (N_2O) is controversial. Because of the risk of VAE and the ability of N_2O to expand air bubbles, some practitioners argue that N_2O should be avoided in sitting position cases. This is a debatable position, however, because (a) it has been shown that 50% N_2O does not increase the risk of VAE in sitting cases and (b) morbidity does not appear to be greater if N_2O is used provided it is discontinued the moment VAE is suspected. We subscribe to the latter reasoning; N_2O is used but discontinued when VAE occurs.

   3. The airway requires special attention. Often with posterior fossa cases, substantial neck flexion is required for optimal surgical exposure. Such flexion can advance the tip of the tube into a mainstem bronchus or cause kinking of the endotracheal tube in the posterior pharynx.

   a. Some clinicians use a wire-reinforced tube or prefer nasotracheal intubation. We use neither routinely but emphasize that careful assessment of tube patency and position is of utmost importance since access to the airway is quite limited subsequently.

   b. This assessment should be conducted once final patient positioning is complete but before skin incision has taken place. Palpation of the cuff above the sternal notch is useful in this regard.

   c. If there is evidence of partial tube obstruction (e.g., high airway pressures, slow upstroke on $ETCO_2$ trace), confirm that a suction catheter passes freely through the endotracheal tube and insist on head and neck repositioning if it does not.

4. In most cases, controlled moderate hyperventilation is desirable in order to improve surgical exposure and reduce retraction pressure on the brain. However, changes in respiration may be more sensitive to brain stem manipulation than hemodynamic changes. As such, use of spontaneous ventilation may be appropriate in rare circumstances.

   a. Because VAE can trigger a "gasp" that may in turn increase air entrainment, use of spontaneous ventilation in sitting cases is controversial and reserved for cases in which manipulation or ischemia of respiratory centers is likely. Moreover, the modest hypoventilation that occurs with spontaneous ventilation during general anesthesia may cause brain engorgement and make surgical exposure difficult.

F. Intraoperative considerations

  1. Cardiovascular reflexes

    a. Surgery on or near the brain stem (e.g., during acoustic neuroma surgery) can produce abrupt, often profound, cardiovascular responses that may signal potential damage to the brain stem.

    b. Stimulation of the floor of the fourth ventricle, medullary reticular formation, or trigeminal nerve results in hypertension, usually in association with bradycardia. Bradycardia also results from stimulation of the vagus nerve.

    c. If such changes occur, the surgeon should be alerted immediately so that he or she can avoid the manipulation that provokes the response.

      d. Masking such changes with pharmacologic treatment is undesirable unless they are recurrent and severe. Hypertensive responses are typically so abrupt and transient that by the time a drug is administered, the stimulus is gone and treatment unnecessary.

      e. Bradycardia can be both treated and prevented with glycopyrrolate or atropine, but the tachycardia produced by the former is less marked.

  2. Brain stem monitoring

      a. Cranial nerve injury is a significant risk of surgery in the area of the cerebellopontine angle and lower brain stem. Therefore, intraoperative stimulation and/or recording from cranial nerves V, VII, VIII, XI, and XII is often utilized.

      b. Monitoring techniques include somatosensory evoked potentials (SEPs), brain stem auditory evokes potentials (BAEPs), and the spontaneous and evoked electromyogram (EMG).

      c. This can be a challenge for the anesthesiologist since muscle relaxants complicate interpretation of the EMG and N_2O and high-dose inhalation anesthesia may interfere with SEPs. The BAEPs are robust and minimally influenced by anesthetics.

      d. Although direct intracranial stimulation of the facial nerve produces facial movement even in well-paralyzed patients, "spontaneous" (i.e., surgical manipulation–induced) EMG discharges are subtle. Hence, some electrophysiologists request that, with the exception of succinylcholine for intubation, no muscle relaxants be given. The clinical necessity for this "pure" state has not been documented, however, and some centers are satisfied with a continuous infusion of relaxant to maintain a constant level of modest twitch suppression.

  3. Treatment of VAE

      a. Except in rare cases of severe hemodynamic instability, changing the patient's position is seldom required and often inconvenient (the surgeon cannot identify a source of air entrainment if the wound faces the floor!). Other measures should be used first.

      b. Alert the surgeons; they should irrigate the field with saline.

      c. If N_2O is being used, discontinue it immediately.

      d. Aspirate the right atrial catheter.

      e. Provide cardiovascular support as needed.

      f. Modify the anesthetic technique as needed.

    g. Ask an assistant to compress both jugular veins lightly to minimize air entrainment.

    h. Change patient position if the above measures fail to prevent ongoing VAE.

G. Emergence from anesthesia

1. General objectives

    a. As with other types of intracranial neurosurgery, prompt, smooth emergence and avoidance of coughing, straining, or abrupt increases in blood pressure are desirable.

    b. The feasibility of extubation depends on the usual factors plus preexisting neurologic impairments, the nature and extent of the surgery, and the likelihood of brain stem edema or injury. Even if extubation is not planned, one should attempt to awaken the patient for postoperative neurologic evaluation.

2. Ventilation/airway abnormalities

    a. Because of disease- or surgery-induced dysfunction of cranial sensory or motor nerves, patients may have difficulty swallowing, vocalizing, or protecting the airway. In addition, damage to or edema of the respiratory centers from intraoperative manipulation can result in hypoventilation or erratic respiratory patterns. Thus, longer term ventilation and airway protection might be required in some patients.

    b. Severe tongue and facial edema can occur due to position-induced venous or lymphatic obstruction. The endotracheal tube should be left in place until the edema resolves.

    c. Pulmonary edema may result from large VAE. Although usually responsive to conservative measures such as supplemental O_2 and diuretics, continued postoperative ventilation may be appropriate until evaluation is completed.

3. Cardiovascular issues

    a. Hypertension is common after posterior fossa surgery and may contribute to edema formation and intracranial hemorrhage. Hence, one should be prepared to control postoperative hypertension.

4. Neurologic complications

    a. A variety of untoward neurologic outcomes can occur after posterior fossa surgery. These include altered level of consciousness, varying degrees of paresis, and specific cranial nerve deficits (e.g., visual disturbances, facial nerve paresis, impaired swallowing or phonation).

    b. Treatment is supportive, but evaluation of delayed emergence should proceed lest a treatable nonanesthetic cause go unrecognized.

5. Pneumocephalus

a. Air is retained in the cranial cavity after all craniotomies regardless of position. In the sitting position, CSF drains easily and a larger amount of air may be trapped when the wound is closed. In most cases, the air is reabsorbed uneventfully over several days and no treatment is necessary.

b. Tension pneumocephalus can occur when the brain reexpands and compresses the air. This situation is difficult to diagnose but should be suspected if emergence is delayed after an otherwise uneventful operation or if cardiovascular collapse or neurologic deterioration occurs postoperatively.

c. In such rare circumstances, surgical evacuation may be indicated.

Suggested Readings

Artu AA, Cucchiara RF, Messick JM. Cardiorespiratory and cranial nerve sequalae of surgical procedures involving the posterior fossa. *Anesthesiology* 1980;52:83.

Black S, Cucchiara RF. Tumor surgery. In: Cucchiara RF, Black S, Michenfelder JD, eds. *Clinical neuroanesthesia.* New York: Churchill Livingstone, 1998:343–365.

Black S, Ockert DB, Oliver WC, Cucchiara RF. Outcome following posterior fossa craniectomy in patients in the sitting or horizontal positions. *Anesthesiology* 1988;69:49.

Michenfelder JD. Central venous catheters in the management of air embolism: whether as well as where. *Anesthesiology* 1981;55:339.

Porter SS, Sanan A, Rengachary SS. Surgery and anesthesia of the posterior fossa. In: Albin MS, ed. *Textbook of neuroanesthesia.* New York: McGraw-Hill, 1997:971–1008.

Young ML. Posterior fossa: anesthetic considerations. In: Cottrell JE, Smith DS, eds. *Anesthesia and neurosurgery.* St. Louis: Mosby, 1994:339–363.

Anesthetic Management of Intracranial Aneurysms

Philippa Newfield

The anesthetic management of the surgical treatment of intracranial aneurysms is designed to:

●Facilitate the conduct of the operation and the patient's recovery.

●Minimize the risk of aneurysmal rupture, cerebral ischemia, neurologic deficit, and associated systemic morbidity to improve functional survival.

I. **Aneurysms**
   A. **Types**
      1. **Saccular aneurysms** (less than 2.5 cm in diameter) result from disintegration of the artery's elastic layer at the flow separator region from pounding of the arterial pulse wave.
      2. **Giant aneurysms** measure up to 10 cm in diameter and constitute 5% of all aneurysms.
      3. **Other types** include fusiform (associated with severe atherosclerosis or degenerative processes in childhood), dissecting (from a tear in the luminal endothelium that permits a blood column to dissect in between the endothelium and the media), traumatic (developing in the 2 to 3 weeks after severe head injury), and mycotic (infectious).
   B. **Location.** Ninety percent of aneurysms occur on the anterior circulation: most commonly the internal carotid–posterior communicating (more common in females), anterior communicating (more common in males), middle cerebral artery bifurcation. Ten percent occur on the posterior circulation, most commonly the basilar apex. The internal carotid artery bifurcation is commonly affected in children.
   C. **Epidemiology.** The annual incidence of aneurysmal subarachnoid hemorrhage (SAH) is approximately 10 per 100,000 persons. Aneurysms commonly present in the sixth decade. Smoking and hypertension are risk factors. Men outnumber women until age 50; women predominate thereafter. About 20% of patients will have more than one aneurysm. Aneurysmal SAH accounts for 10% of all cerebrovascular accidents.
   D. **Natural history.** One patient in six will die within minutes of an SAH. Of patients who survive to be admitted to the hospital, 25% will still die, and just over 50% will recover completely (Table 11-1). Without treatment, at least 50% of patients will rerupture within 6 months and then at a rate of 3% per year.
   E. **Prognostic factors.** Rate and volume of bleeding af-

Table 11-1. Cerebral aneurysms in North America: epidemiology

SAH patients/yr	28,000
Died immediately	10,000
Admitted to hospital	18,000
Died/disabled	9,000
Rebleeding	3,000
Vasospasm	3,000
Medical complications	1,000
Surgical complications	2,000
Functional survival	9,000

SAH, subarachnoid hemorrhage.

fect neurologic condition at hospital admission and determine outcome. Patients who remain conscious and complain only of severe headache after SAH do better than patients who are comatose on arrival. Old age, poor general health, evidence of clots in the brain substance or ventricles, and repeat hemorrhage all affect outcome adversely.

F. Genetics and associated diseases. Five to ten percent of patients with SAH will have one or more first-order relatives who also had a ruptured aneurysm. The inheritance is probably dominant with variable penetrance.

Conditions associated with intracranial aneurysms include polycystic kidney disease (5% of aneurysms series; 33% of polycystic kidney series), coarctation of the aorta (1% of aneurysm patients; 5% of coarctation patients, all of whom are hypertensive), sickle cell disease, drug abuse (cocaine: generalized vasoconstriction and hypertension; intravenous use: mycotic aneurysms), and hypertension (30% to 40% of SAH patients are hypertensive). Rarer associations are with fibromuscular dysplasia, Marfan's syndrome, tuberous sclerosis, Ehlers-Danlos syndrome, hereditary hemorrhagic telangiectasia, moyamoya disease, and pseudoxanthoma elasticum. Choriocarcinoma and cardiac myxomas are associated with multiple cerebral aneurysms.

II. Subarachnoid hemorrhage

A. Symptoms. Rupture of an intracranial aneurysm causes the sudden onset of an excruciating headache. After SAH, most patients complain of malaise and might be irritable, combative, and uncooperative.

Common misdiagnoses include flu, meningitis, cervical disc disease, migraine headaches, heart attacks, malingering, and intoxication. In the case of benign, nonaneurysmal headaches, there is a history of similar headaches under similar circumstances.

B. Signs. Impaired consciousness, nuchal rigidity (may be absent early after SAH), photophobia, ophthalmic hemorrhages (poor prognostic sign), focal neurologic deficits, seizures, nausea and vomiting, hypertension, fever (from subarachnoid blood), and fluid (hypovolemia) and electrolyte (hyponatremia) imbalance all occur after SAH.

C. Diagnosis
1. **History.** "Worst headache of my life."
2. **Physical examination.** Change in level of consciousness, focal neurologic deficit, fever, meningismus.
3. **Imaging.** Computed tomography (CT) scan for amount of subarachnoid, intracerebral, intraventricular blood; cerebral angiography for exact location and configuration of aneurysm and neck.

D. Grading
1. In 1956 Botterell introduced a system for the grading of patients after SAH to facilitate assessment of surgical risk, prediction of outcome after SAH, and evaluation of the patient's condition.
2. The five grades describe the patient's level of consciousness and degree of neurologic impairment as I to V, with each higher grade representing greater severity. Botterell's initial system was modified by Hunt and Hess to include a provision for the effect of serious systemic illness (Table 11-2a) and by the World Federation of Neurological Surgeons whose grading scale (Table 11-2b), based on the Glasgow Coma Scale, demonstrated that the preoperative level of consciousness correlated most directly with outcome.

III. Complications of subarachnoid hemorrhage
A. Rebleeding
1. Rebleeding is highest (4%) during the first 24 hours after SAH and subsequently decreases to 1.5% per day. The cumulative risk of rebleeding is 19% at 2 weeks and 50% at 6 months, and then decreases to 3% per year. The overall incidence of rebleeding is 11%, which represents 22% of the mortality from SAH.
2. Prognostic factors for rebleeding reflect a number of correlations:
   a. Impaired neurologic status indicates a large volume of blood in the subarachnoid space from a large tear at the time of the initial SAH.
   b. The shorter the interval from the initial hemorrhage, the higher the rebleeding rate will be.
   c. Females rebleed twice as frequently as males.
   d. Older patients and those in poor general medical condition are more prone to early rebleeding.

Table 11-2a.   Clinical grading after subarachnoid hemorrhage: Hunt and Hess modification

Grade 0	Unruptured aneurysm
Grade 1	Asymptomatic or minimal headache and slight nuchal rigidity
Grade 2	Moderate to severe headache, nuchal rigidity, no neurologic deficit other than cranial nerve palsy
Grade 3	Drowsiness, confusion, or mild focal deficit
Grade 4	Stupor, moderate to severe hemiparesis, possible early decerebrate rigidity, vegetative disturbances
Grade 5	Deep coma, decerebrate rigidity, moribund appearance

Note: Serious systemic diseases (hypertension, atherosclerotic heart disease, diabetes, chronic pulmonary disease, severe vasospasm seen on angiography) cause placement of the patient in the next less favorable category.
Source: Hunt WE, Hess EM. *J Neurosurg* 1968;28:14, with permission.

Table 11-2b.   World Federation of Neurological Surgeons grading scale

WFNS grade	GCS score	Motor deficit
I	15	Absent
II	14–13	Absent
III	14–13	Present
IV	12–7	Present or absent
V	6–3	Present or absent

WFNS, World Federation of Neurological Surgeons; GCS, Glasgow Coma Scale.
Source: Drake CG. *J Neurosurg* 1988;68:985, with permission.

    e. Systemic hypertension increases the risk of rebleeding.

3. Surgical obliteration of the aneurysm is the only definitive means of preventing rebleeding. Early operation (within 24 to 48 hours after SAH) is therefore favored because of its association with improved outcome, as demonstrated by the International Cooperative Study on the Timing of Aneurysm Surgery.

4. Treatment before operation includes:

      a. Prevention of hypertension and increases in transmural pressure [mean arterial pressure (MAP) minus intracranial pressure (ICP)].

      b. Short-acting antihypertensives (esmolol, labetalol) to control labile hypertension or transient spikes in blood pressure from therapeutic interventions.

      c. Maintenance of the patient's "normal" blood pressure as the lower acceptable limit to avoid initiation or exacerbation of vasospasm from a decrease in cerebral perfusion pressure (CPP).

      d. Narcotic analgesics and sedatives in titrated doses to reduce pain and anxiety.

      e. Avoidance of lumbar puncture and rapid ventricular drainage.

5. Although the use of ε-aminocaproic acid and other antifibrinolytic drugs halved the rebleeding rate in the initial 2 weeks after SAH, the incidence of vasospasm and hydrocephalus increased, resulting in no improvement in overall outcome. Many neurosurgeons have abandoned the use of antifibrinolytic drugs and gone to early surgery with definitive clipping of the aneurysm instead.

B. Vasospasm or delayed ischemic deficit

  1. Vasospasm is the reactive narrowing of the larger conducting arteries in the subarachnoid space that are surrounded by clot after SAH and affected by spasmogenic substances within the clot.

      a. Patients of all neurologic grades have a 50:50 chance of developing significant angiographic vasospasm. Symptoms of delayed ischemia will occur in 20% to 25% of patients, and 30% to 50% of patients will have evidence of infarction from vasospasm on CT. Death from vasospastic infarction will occur in 5% to 17% of patients.

      b. The incidence of vasospasm peaks between the fourth and ninth day after SAH and decreases over the next 2 to 3 weeks.

  2. Diagnosis of vasospasm is made by:

      a. Clinical signs of progressive impairment in level of consciousness or the appearance of new focal neurologic deficits more than 4 days after the initial SAH.

      b. Transcranial Doppler and angiography. A progressive increase in flow velocity reflects a reduction in vessel caliber. A peak flow velocity of 140 to 200 cm/second is indicative of moderate vasospasm; a peak flow velocity of more than 200 cm/second indicates severe vasospasm. Angiographically severe vasospasm is defined as a decrease of 50% or greater in arterial diameter.

3. **Treatment** of vasospasm involves pharmacologic and mechanical modalities.

  a. **Early surgery** permits the removal of fresh clot by irrigation and suction. The surgeon may instill tissue plasminogen activator directly into the subarachnoid space to dissolve the remaining clot. While this fibrinolytic drug can reduce vasospasm, it also might cause bleeding by dissolving normal clot. Thus, only patients at great risk of developing clinically significant vasospasm are candidates for this treatment.

  b. The use of the **calcium antagonist** nimodipine within 96 hours after SAH may reduce postaneurysmal cerebral infarction. Calcium antagonists tend to decrease blood pressure, so that patients might require hydration immediately before induction of anesthesia and careful attention to fluid balance intra- and postoperatively.

  c. **"Triple-H therapy,"** hypertensive hypervolemic hemodilution, will augment cerebral perfusion in autoregulation-impaired ischemic areas of the brain through increases in blood pressure, cardiac output, and intravascular volume. Relative hemodilution (hematocrit 32%) will promote blood flow through the cerebral microvasculature. The early institution of triple-H therapy is crucial to prevent the progression from mild ischemia to infarction.

    (1) Guides for optimal volume expansion include a central venous pressure (CVP) of 10 mm Hg and a pulmonary capillary wedge pressure (PCWP) of 12 to 16 mm Hg. The vagal and diuretic response to intravascular volume augmentation might necessitate the administration of atropine, 1 mg i.m. every 3 to 4 hours, and aqueous vasopressin (Pitressin), 5 units i.m., to reduce urine output to less than 200 mL/hour.

    (2) Vasopressor drugs, including dopamine, dobutamine, and phenylephrine, might also be required to increase blood pressure. If the aneurysm has not been secured, systolic pressure is maintained at 120 to 150 mm Hg. After the aneurysm is secured, systolic blood pressure may be increased to 160 to 200 mm Hg.

    (3) Complications of triple-H therapy include rebleeding, hemorrhagic infarction, cerebral edema, intracranial hypertension, myocardial infarction, pulmonary edema, coagulopathy, and dilutional hyponatremia.

   d. Transluminal angioplasty, the mechanical dilatation of a cerebral vessel at a segment of spastic narrowing by the use of an inflatable intravascular balloon, may effect improvement in level of consciousness and focal ischemic deficits. Early intervention is crucial to success.

IV. Central nervous system complications. The central nervous system (CNS) is directly affected by SAH and the resultant hematoma, vascular disruption, and edema. Subarachnoid hemorrhage interferes with cerebral autoregulation, the ability of the cerebral vasculature to maintain normal cerebral blood flow (CBF) in response to changes in cerebral perfusion pressure (MAP − ICP) from 50 to 150 mm Hg. Patients also experience a decrease in CBF and cerebral metabolic rate. The extent of impairment correlates with the patient's clinical grade.

 A. The response of the cerebral vasculature to changes in carbon dioxide tension ($PaCO_2$) is preserved after SAH. A decline in CO_2 reactivity usually does not occur without extensive disruption of cerebral homeostasis.

 B. Intracranial aneurysms themselves, particularly giant aneurysms, and the SAH-induced hematoma and edema all have the potential for causing **intracranial hypertension.**

 C. Hydrocephalus develops in 10% of patients from obstruction of cerebrospinal fluid (CSF) drainage pathways by intraventricular or intraparenchymal blood and development of arachnoidal adhesions that prevent reabsorption of CSF.

  1. Acute ventricular dilatation immediately after SAH, a cause of a spuriously poor neurologic grade, usually necessitates ventricular drainage to normalize ICP.

  2. Chronic hydrocephalus, which develops weeks after SAH, is an important cause of failure to improve in a patient who is initially comatose or of secondary slow decline in patients who were originally in good condition. Symptoms include impaired consciousness, dementia, gait disturbance, and incontinence. A CT scan is indicated a month after SAH to ascertain ventricular size.

 D. After SAH, the patient's clinical grade reflects the ICP. Grade I and II patients have normal ICP (but not necessarily normal elastance), whereas grade IV and V patients have intracranial hypertension.

V. Systemic sequelae of SAH

 A. Fluid and electrolyte balance

  1. Most (30% to 100%) patients develop a decrease in intravascular volume after SAH that correlates with clinical grade and the presence of intracranial hypertension.

  2. Hyponatremia occurs with the release of atrial natriuretic factor from the hypothalamus.

   3. Many patients (50% to 75%) develop hypokalemia and hypocalcemia and require replacement.
   4. Treatment includes hydration with normal or hypertonic (3%) saline to improve cerebral perfusion.
B. Cardiac sequelae
   1. Electrocardiogram (ECG) abnormalities occur in 50% to 100% of patients after SAH. The most common are T-wave inversion and ST segment depression. Other changes include U waves, QT interval prolongation, and Q waves.
   2. Rhythm disturbances, seen in 30% to 80% of patients, include premature ventricular complexes (most commonly), sinus bradycardia and tachycardia, atrioventricular dissociation, atrial extrasystole, atrial fibrillation, brady-/tachyarrhythmias, and ventricular tachycardia and fibrillation. The onset of arrhythmia is most frequently within the first 7 days after SAH. The peak occurrence is between the second and third day.
   3. The etiology has been attributed to injury to the posterior hypothalamus with release of norepinephrine and resultant subendocardial ischemic changes and electrolyte disturbances.
   4. The extent of myocardial dysfunction has correlated with the severity of the neurologic injury after SAH.
   5. Prophylactic adrenergic blockage has improved cardiac outcome in some patients.
   6. In determining whether to proceed with surgery on an emergent basis after SAH, the measurement of serial cardiac enzymes and the assessment of ventricular function by echocardiography might indicate the degree of ischemia.
   7. The use of a pulmonary artery catheter to monitor PCWP and cardiac output might facilitate management of both the patient's cardiac dysfunction and the response to triple-H therapy for the treatment of vasospasm.
   8. The presence of a severe arrhythmia (in 5% of patients who have arrhythmias) or significant cardiogenic pulmonary edema might necessitate the postponement of surgery until treatment has been instituted.
C. Respiratory system
   1. Pulmonary conditions including cardiogenic and neurogenic pulmonary edema, pneumonia, adult respiratory distress syndrome, and pulmonary emboli account for 50% of deaths from medical complications at 3 months after SAH, which themselves cause 23% of all deaths.
   2. The majority (60%) of patients become symptomatic from pulmonary edema between days 0 and

7 after SAH, with the greatest number of cases presenting on day 3. The incidence of pulmonary edema is greater in patients older than 30 years. Poor clinical grade at the time of admission also correlates with more respiratory dysfunction, suggesting neurogenic influences.

3. Treatment includes antibiotics, supportive care, and correction of intracranial (intracranial hypertension, cerebral edema, hydrocephalus) and fluid and electrolyte abnormalities.

D. **Other medical complications**

1. **Hepatic dysfunction** (hepatic failure and hepatitis) occurs in 25% of patients after SAH, correlates positively with poor clinical grade, and is frequently observed in patients who develop pulmonary edema after SAH.

2. **Renal dysfunction** is noted in 8% of patients after SAH, and it occurs more frequently in septic patients receiving antibiotics.

3. **Thrombocytopenia** occurs in 4% of patients after SAH and is associated with sepsis, severe neurologic deficits, and antibiotic use. Disseminated intravascular coagulation and leukocytosis have also been reported.

4. **Gastrointestinal bleeding** occurs in almost 5% of patients, and should be part of the differential diagnosis of any unexpected episode of hypotension and tachycardia.

VI. **Surgical intervention**

A. **Timing of surgery**

1. Early aneurysmal clip ligation in the first 24 to 48 hours after SAH has advantages: prevention of rebleeding, reduction in vasospasm from removal of blood from the subarachnoid space ("intracranial toilet"), and ability to treat vasospasm through volume expansion and deliberate hypertension with relative safety. Other advantages include reductions in medical complications, patient anxiety, and cost of hospitalization.

2. The International Study on the Timing of Aneurysm Surgery, published in 1990, defined predictors of mortality: decreased level of consciousness, older age, thicker subarachnoid clot on CT scan, elevated blood pressure, preexisting medical illness, and basilar location. While early (0 to 3 days after SAH) and late (11 to 14 days) surgery yielded similar overall morbidity and mortality in the study, the fact that results were better in the subset of North American patients who were alert and operated on early has made early surgical intervention a common practice.

a. **Preoperative evaluation** includes:

(1) Review of neurodiagnostic studies (mag-

netic resonance imaging, CT scan, angiogram).
(2) Neurologic examination.
(3) Notation of ward blood pressures and association between blood pressure decrease and neurologic deterioration.
(4) Assessment of fluid and electrolyte balance.
(5) Cardiac history and ECG with determination of need for echocardiogram, serum myoglobin, creatine kinase isoenzymes, myocardial nuclear scanning, and perioperative cardiovascular monitoring.
(6) Notation of current drug regimen.

b. **Premedication**
(1) Patients continue to receive calcium channel blocking drugs, anticonvulsants, steroids.
(2) Drugs to reduce gastric acidity (cimetidine, ranitidine) and speed gastric emptying (metoclopramide) are given before induction of anesthesia.
(3) Sedatives, hypnotics, anxiolytics, and narcotics are used sparingly to avoid respiratory depression and masking of neurologic deterioration.

Small doses of intravenous narcotic (morphine, 1 to 4 mg; fentanyl, 25 to 50 μg) and benzodiazepine (midazolam, 1 to 2 mg) may be administered by the anesthesiologist to good-grade patients.

Poor-grade patients do not receive premedication unless an endotracheal tube is in place, in which case they might require muscle relaxation, sedation, and blood pressure control.

c. **Monitoring during anesthesia** includes:
(1) Cardiac rate, rhythm, and ischemia via ECG with V_5 lead.
(2) Direct intraarterial blood pressure with pressure transducer at brain level to reflect cerebral perfusion.
(3) Central venous pressure via the antecubital, jugular, or subclavian route.
(4) Pulmonary capillary wedge pressure and cardiac output in patients who have cardiac compromise or severe vasospasm.
(5) Neuromuscular blockade.
(6) End-tidal CO_2, oxygen saturation via pulse oximeter.
(7) Intermittent arterial blood gases, glucose, electrolytes, osmolality, hematocrit.

(8) Brain temperature via tympanic or nasopharyngeal thermistor.

(9) Urinary output via indwelling catheter.

(10) Electrophysiologic monitors: electroencephalogram (EEG), brainstem auditory, somatosensory, and motor evoked potentials.

(11) Cerebral blood flow velocity via transcranial Doppler ultrasonography.

(12) Jugular bulb venous oxygen saturation.

d. The need for adequate intravenous access mandates the insertion of one or two large-bore intravenous catheters in addition to the CVP or pulmonary artery catheter before positioning for surgery, which may limit access to arteries and veins, and before interventions that will affect blood pressure, ICP, transmural pressure, and CBF.

VII. Anesthesia
A. Induction of anesthesia

1. The induction period is critical because rupture of the aneurysm at this juncture can be fatal. The incidence of rupture ranges from 0.5% to 2% and the mortality approaches 75%.

2. Smooth induction requires limitation of the hypertensive response to laryngoscopy and intubation, obliteration of coughing and straining on the endotracheal tube, and maintenance of adequate CPP while minimizing the change in transmural pressure.

3. Management of systemic blood pressure during induction varies with the patient's grade and ICP. The ICP of good-grade patients (grades 0, I, II) is usually normal: a decrease in blood pressure of 30% below normal values (or to a systolic blood pressure of 100 mm Hg) is not detrimental in the absence of evidence of cerebral ischemia.

   Poor-grade patients (grades IV and V) already have the potential for ischemia secondary to intracranial hypertension and impaired perfusion. Decreasing the blood pressure of these patients might exacerbate the cerebral ischemia. Measures are still necessary, however, to blunt the sympathetic response to laryngoscopy and intubation.

4. Good-grade patients do not require hyperventilation during induction ($PaCO_2$ 35 to 40 mm Hg) because they have normal intracranial elastance. The hyperventilation-induced reduction in CBF might also decrease ICP and increase transmural pressure (when the systemic pressure remains constant), risking aneurysmal rupture. Poor-grade patients who have intracranial hypertension will benefit from moderate hyperventilation to a $PaCO_2$ of 30 mm Hg during induction.

Table 11-3.   Induction of anesthesia: aneurysmal clip ligation

Optimal head position	
Deep level of anesthesia	
Sufentanil	0.5–1.0 µg/kg
Fentanyl	3.0–5.0 µg/kg
Thiopental	3.0–5.0 mg/kg
Propofol	1.0–2.0 mg/kg
Vecuronium	0.1 mg/kg
Low-dose isoflurane	
Controlled ventilation	100% O_2
Normal CO_2 (35–40 mm Hg)	
Before laryngoscopy	
Lidocaine	1.5 mg/kg
Thiopental	2.0–3.0 mg/kg
Propofol	0.5 mg/kg
Brief, gentle laryngoscopy	
Intubation	

5. The intravenous induction of anesthesia confers loss of consciousness while maintaining cardiovascular and intracerebral homeostasis during catechol-stimulating maneuvers (Table 11-3). Anesthesia is induced by the intravenous administration of thiopental (3 to 5 mg/kg), etomidate (0.1 to 0.3 mg/kg), or propofol (1 to 2 mg/kg), fentanyl (3 to 5 µg/kg) or sufentanil (0.5 to 1.0 µg/kg), lidocaine (1.5 mg/kg), and midazolam (0.1 to 0.2 mg/kg) and the patient is ventilated by mask with 100% oxygen.

6. If the patient does not have an increase in intracranial elastance, isoflurane, desflurane, or sevoflurane might be introduced before laryngoscopy to deepen the anesthesia.

7. Additional fentanyl (1 to 2 µg/kg), propofol (0.5 mg/kg), or lidocaine (1.5 mg/kg) is given before laryngoscopy and intubation to preserve hemodynamic and intracranial stability.

B. **Muscle relaxants**
1. **Vecuronium** (0.1 mg/kg), a nondepolarizing muscle relaxant of intermediate duration, increases neither the heart rate (and blood pressure) nor the ICP in the presence of a reduction in intracranial compliance.

2. **Succinylcholine** has increased ICP and caused ventricular fibrillation in patients after SAH. Susceptible patients include those who are comatose but nonparetic; have flaccid paralysis, spasticity, or clonus after head injury; or move their extremities in response to pain but not command.

For these patients, rocuronium (0.6 mg/kg), which does not adversely affect CBF or ICP, might be appropriate for rapid-sequence intubation.

C. **Cardioactive drugs**

1. Cardioactive drugs counteract the hypertensive response to laryngoscopy and intubation. Propranolol (1 to 2 mg), esmolol (0.5 mg/kg), and labetalol (2.5 to 5 mg) block the chronotropic and inotropic effects of sympathetic stimulation without affecting CBF or ICP.

2. **Sodium nitroprusside** (SNP), a direct-acting cerebral vasodilator, increases cerebral blood volume (CBV) and ICP. Although SNP, 100 μg i.v., can prevent the hypertensive response to laryngoscopy and intubation, it might be detrimental in patients who have a reduction in intracranial compliance. For them, prior hyperventilation and use of cerebral vasoconstricting drugs (e.g., barbiturates) might prevent the increase in ICP with SNP.

3. **Nitroglycerin** also increases CBV from the dilatation of capacitance vessels and increases CSF pressure.

4. **The calcium channel blocking drugs** nicardipine (0.01 to 0.02 mg/kg) and diltiazem (0.2 mg/kg or 10 mg) facilitate rapid control of intraoperative hypertension. Neither drug decreases local CBF or blood flow velocity.

5. For rapid-sequence induction in patients who have a full stomach, hypertension from laryngoscopy and intubation can be avoided by the addition of fentanyl (5 μg/kg), sufentanil (0.1 μg/kg), esmolol (0.5 mg/kg), or labetalol (0.2 to 0.4 mg/kg), or a supranormal dose of thiopental. Muscle relaxation is achieved by rocuronium (0.6 mg/kg).

D. **Intubation**

1. The difficult airway is secured by fiberoptic intubation before the induction of anesthesia. The combination of topical anesthesia (nebulized 4% lidocaine), translaryngeal injection (2.5 mL of 4% lidocaine) through the cricothyroid membrane, bilateral superior laryngeal nerve blocks (0.5 to 0.75 mL of 2% lidocaine), and incremental intravenous doses of fentanyl (25 μg) and midazolam (0.5 mg) will mitigate against hypertension and coughing.

2. Fiberoptic intubation can also be accomplished through the intubating mask or laryngeal mask airway. During this period of airway manipulation, it is essential to maintain oxygenation and ensure adequate anesthesia.

3. When neither intubation nor ventilation is possible, transtracheal jet ventilation is a temporizing measure during the performance of fiberoptic in-

tubation or, failing that, cricothyroidotomy or tracheotomy.

E. **Maintenance**

1. Intravenous and inhalational drugs are used alone or in combination to prevent aneurysmal rupture, optimize cerebral perfusion, protect against cerebral ischemia and edema, minimize brain retractor pressure through cerebral relaxation, manipulate blood pressure, and facilitate rapid emergence and timely neurologic assessment.

2. All inhalational anesthetics are cerebral vasodilators and have the potential for increasing ICP; and they all, with the exception of nitrous oxide, depress cerebral metabolism. Nitrous oxide is avoided, especially during the induction of anesthesia, in patients who have decreased intracranial compliance and is introduced only after giving cerebral vasoconstricting drugs and establishing hypocapnia.

3. Isoflurane increases CBF minimally, but it has increased ICP despite hypocapnia in patients who have space-occupying lesions. Isoflurane is therefore used in low concentrations or avoided altogether in patients known to have a decrease in intracranial compliance. The cerebral vascular effects of desflurane (4% to 6%) are similar to those of isoflurane. Sevoflurane is also a cerebral vasodilator, but it might not increase ICP when administered after the establishment of hypocapnia. The low blood gas solubility of desflurane and sevoflurane permits rapid emergence and prompt postoperative neurologic evaluation.

4. Narcotics are useful intraoperatively in conjunction with hyperventilation and vasoconstricting drugs. Fentanyl, sufentanil, and alfentanil improve cerebral relaxation during craniotomy in hyperventilated patients receiving isoflurane.

5. Narcotics may be administered with inhalational drugs or as an alternative. Either fentanyl (bolus: 25 to 50 μg i.v.; infusion: 1 to 2 μg/kg/hour) or sufentanil (bolus: 10 to 20 μg; infusion: 0.1 to 0.2 μg/kg/hour) may be combined with isoflurane (0.5% to 1%) or administered with an infusion of thiopental (1.0 to 1.5 mg/kg/hour) or propofol (40 to 60 μg/kg/minute) for the maintenance of anesthesia.

F. **Emergence**

1. Good-grade patients may be awakened in the operating room and their tracheas extubated at the end of the operation. The avoidance of coughing, straining, hypercarbia, and hypertension is essential.

2. The blood pressure of patients whose aneurysms have been wrapped rather than clipped or who have other untreated aneurysms is maintained

within 20% of their normal range (120 to 160 mm Hg systolic) to avoid rupture during emergence.

3. Poor preoperative status or a catastrophic intraoperative event (e.g., brain swelling, aneurysmal rupture, ligation of a feeding vessel) requires continued intubation, sedation, and postoperative ventilatory support.

4. When the patient fails to awaken or has a new neurologic deficit at the conclusion of the operation, the residual effects of sedatives, narcotics, muscle relaxants, and inhalational drugs should be reversed or dissipated, the $PaCO_2$ normalized, and other causes of depressed consciousness (e.g., hypoxia, hyponatremia) treated or ruled out. The persistence of diminished responsiveness or a new neurologic deficit for 2 hours after surgery requires a CT scan to diagnose the presence of hematoma, hydrocephalus, pneumocephalus, infarction, or edema. An angiogram might demonstrate a vascular occlusion.

VIII. Intraoperative management

A. Fluid administration

1. Intraoperative fluid administration is guided by the patient's maintenance requirements, blood loss, urine output, and CVP or PCWP.

2. Since patients have an SAH-induced decrease in circulating blood volume, they require hydration before the induction of anesthesia and the use of controlled hypotension to preserve cerebral perfusion.

3. Full restoration of the intravascular volume to a state of modest hypervolemia occurs after the aneurysm has been clipped to optimize CBF and prevent postoperative vasospasm.

4. All crystalloid administered is glucose-free because both focal and global ischemic deficits are exacerbated by hyperglycemia. Plasmalyte, Normo-Sol, and normal saline are better than Ringer's lactate, which is hypoosmolar to plasma and can exacerbate cerebral edema if the blood–brain barrier is disrupted.

5. The use of blood and blood products is indicated to maintain the hematocrit at 30% to 35%. Five percent albumin may confer rheologic advantage, but more than 500 mL of hetastarch might interfere with hemostasis and cause intracranial bleeding.

B. Cerebral volume reduction

1. The volume of the intracranial contents is reduced and brain relaxation improved to facilitate the surgical approach to the aneurysm after the opening of the dura. The maneuvers are timed to prevent aneurysmal rupture from an increase in transmural pressure secondary to the decrease in ICP induced by hyperventilation, administration

of mannitol (0.25 to 1.0 g/kg i.v.), an osmotic diuretic, and drainage of CSF.

2. Moderate hyperventilation to a $PaCO_2$ of 30 to 35 mm Hg is maintained until the dura is incised and intracranial compliance is normal at which time the $PaCO_2$ is reduced to 25 to 30 mm Hg to decrease CBF, CBV, and brain bulk. With a preoperative increase in intracranial elastance, the $PaCO_2$ is reduced to 25 to 30 mm Hg during induction. Higher $PaCO_2$ values are necessary in patients who have vasospasm and during the period of induced hypotension.

3. Mannitol's onset of action is within 10 to 15 minutes. The administration should be timed to avoid any decrease in CBV and ICP, with an attendant rise in transmural pressure and the chance of aneurysmal rupture, before the dura is opened. Furosemide (0.25 to 1.0 mg/kg) potentiates the action of mannitol and diminishes the dose. Fluid and electrolyte balance is monitored closely after the administration of these diuretics.

4. Cerebrospinal fluid may be drained through a lumbar subarachnoid catheter inserted after induction of anesthesia, a ventricular catheter, or intraoperative drainage of the basal cisterns. Leakage of CSF is avoided while the cranium is still closed to prevent a decrease in ICP and the concomitant rise in transmural pressure. If the ICP is elevated preoperatively, the subarachnoid puncture before craniotomy with escape of CSF might also lead to tonsillar herniation.

C. **Temporary proximal occlusion**

1. Lowering the blood pressure during microscopic dissection of the aneurysm has been advocated in the past to reduce the risk of rupture by decreasing aneurysmal wall tension and augmenting the malleability of the aneurysmal neck. Controlled hypotension also decreases bleeding.

2. Controlled hypotension can compromise regional CBF in patients whose autoregulation is impaired after SAH; since these patients have a higher incidence of cerebral ischemia, infarction, and postoperative neurologic deficit, neurosurgeons prefer to avoid the use of induced hypotension. An exception might be to gain control of the parent vessel if the sac ruptures during surgical manipulation.

3. Temporary proximal occlusion of the parent vessel is now favored by neurosurgeons to reduce the risk of rupture during aneurysmal manipulation. The application of temporary clips produces "local hypotension" and reduction of transmural pressure without the problems caused by systemic hypotension.

4. The risks of distal ischemia and infarction, cerebral edema, and damage to the parent vessel are directly related to the duration of the temporary occlusion and the integrity of the collateral circulation. The chance of developing a new neurologic deficit after temporary proximal occlusion is exacerbated by older age, poor preoperative neurologic status, and aneurysms involving distributions of the basilar and middle cerebral arteries.

5. The duration of temporary occlusion should be limited to less than 20 minutes since most studies have shown a higher incidence of neurologic deficits and infarction postoperatively when the duration exceeds 20 minutes.

6. To enhance collateral circulation during temporary proximal occlusion, the patient's blood pressure is maintained in the high normal range. This may require dopamine or phenylephrine, although patients who have coronary artery disease might be at risk for the development of cardiac ischemia.

7. Drugs administered to extend the duration of occlusion include mannitol, vitamin E, dexamethasone, and sodium thiopental.

D. Cerebral protection (see Chapter 4)

E. Intraoperative aneurysmal rupture

1. Rupture of the aneurysm during induction of anesthesia and operation (7% before dissection, 48% during dissection, 45% during clip ligation) markedly increases mortality and morbidity.

2. Diagnosis of rupture during or after induction is based on an abrupt increase in blood pressure with or without bradycardia. The ICP might increase as well. The transcranial Doppler may demonstrate the rupture and the efficacy of management.

3. Therapy is designed to maintain cerebral perfusion, control ICP, and reduce bleeding through lowering of systemic pressure with thiopental or SNP.

4. Intraoperative rupture of the aneurysm requires rapid surgical control. The MAP may be reduced to 40 to 50 mm Hg to facilitate clip ligation of the aneurysmal neck or temporary proximal and distal occlusion of the parent vessel. Once the parent vessel is occluded, the blood pressure is increased to enhance collateral circulation. This might be preferable to the use of induced hypotension, especially with hypovolemia. Alternatively, the ipsilateral carotid artery may be manually compressed for up to 3 minutes to produce a bloodless field.

5. The intravascular volume is repleted with whole blood, blood products, crystalloid, or colloid.

6. Although barbiturates have been advocated for

protection against focal ischemia, their efficacy has not been demonstrated in this clinical situation, and their effects might be detrimental in hypovolemic patients.

IX. Hypothermic circulatory arrest for giant and vertebrobasilar aneurysms

- **A. Giant cerebral aneurysms** are greater than 2.5 cm in diameter, lack an anatomic neck, and have perforating vessels traversing the aneurysmal wall. They occur in 2% of patients who have aneurysms and cause signs and symptoms of a mass lesion, headache, visual disturbance, and cranial nerve palsies.

- **B. Surgical treatment** of giant aneurysms, associated with significant perioperative morbidity and mortality, includes the use of proximal and distal temporary occlusion to collapse the aneurysm and empty the aneurysmal sac during circulatory arrest under profound hypothermia. Circulatory arrest affords good visualization, a bloodless field, and easy aneurysmal manipulation and clip placement.

- **C.** The morbidity from femoral vein–femoral artery bypass is lower than that from open chest bypass with median sternotomy and ventricular venting. Electrical activity of the heart is terminated with potassium chloride, 40 to 80 mEq, to the pump or with cardioversion at 100 to 250 W/second to avoid ischemic injury. The most serious complication is postoperative intracranial hemorrhage.

- **D. Cerebral protection** during circulatory arrest is afforded by decreasing the cerebral metabolic oxygen consumption. Barbiturates reduce the active component (maintenance of neuronal activity) of the cerebral metabolic rate and may be administered before cooling and arrest as a single dose of 30 to 40 mg/kg over 30 minutes or as a continuous infusion. When EEG monitoring is used to indicate burst suppression, the patient receives an initial loading dose of 3 to 5 mg/kg i.v. and then a continuous infusion of 0.1 to 0.5 mg/kg/minute for the duration of cardiopulmonary bypass. The EEG becomes isoelectric below 18°C, even without pharmacologic suppression. At this point the infusion rate that had previously maintained burst suppression is continued.

- **E. Hypothermia** reduces the active and basal (maintenance of cellular integrity) components of metabolic oxygen consumption, and confers cerebral protection during anoxic conditions. The tolerable period of circulatory arrest doubles for every 8°C temperature reduction. At 15°C to 18°C clinical circulatory arrest has been used safely for up to 60 minutes.

  - **1.** Brain temperature may be measured directly, but it correlates closely with esophageal, tympanic membrane, and nasopharyngeal thermistors, but not with rectal or bladder temperatures.

2. Hypothermia increases blood viscosity with sludging of red blood cells. The deliberate lowering of the hematocrit through phlebotomy and simultaneous volume repletion with crystalloid will avoid this complication while preserving platelet-rich autologous blood for transfusion during rewarming.

3. Hypothermia, by interfering with glucose utilization and metabolism, might cause hyperglycemia, which might in turn exacerbate neuronal damage during ischemia. Frequent monitoring of serum glucose, maintenance of acid–base balance, and treatment of hyperglycemia with insulin are crucial.

F. **Preoperative evaluation** before hypothermic circulatory arrest includes attention to coexisting cardiac, pulmonary, hematologic, and neurologic disorders that might modify the approach or exclude the technique altogether.

G. **Monitors** in addition to those recommended for aneurysmal clip ligation include EEG to indicate burst suppression, somatosensory evoked potentials to measure sensory conduction to the cortex, brainstem auditory evoked potentials, and transesophageal echocardiography to assess ventricular function.

H. The major **postoperative complications** associated with hypothermic circulatory arrest are coagulopathy and intracranial hemorrhage. To reduce the risk:

1. The surgeon dissects the aneurysm and achieves hemostasis before the initiation of hypothermic circulatory arrest.

2. Heparinization is evaluated with the activated clotting time (ACT) and maintained between 400 and 450 seconds.

3. Heparinization is reversed with protamine after rewarming until the ACT is 100 to 150 seconds.

4. Previously phlebotomized blood is transfused.

5. Additional blood products, fresh frozen plasma, cryoprecipitate, and platelets are given as needed.

6. Hemostasis is achieved before dural closure.

I. **Cardiovascular sequelae** of hypothermia and bypass including arrhythmias are treated. Patients might require inotropes during warming and into the postoperative period. Extubation of the trachea and neurologic assessment are performed within 12 to 24 hours.

Suggested Readings

Ausman JI, Malik GM, Tomecek FJ, et al. Hypothermic circulatory arrest and the management of giant and large cerebral aneurysms. *Surg Neurol* 1993; 40:289–298.

Gianotta SL, Oppenheimer JH, Levy ML, Zelvian V. Management

of intraoperative rupture of aneurysms without hypotension. *Neurosurgery* 1991;28:531–536.

Kassell NF, Torner JC, Haley EC, et al. The International Cooperative Study on the timing of aneurysm surgery. 1. Overall management results. *J Neurosurg* 1990;73:18–36.

Kassell NF, Torner JC, Jane JA, et al. The International Cooperative Study on the timing of aneurysm surgery. 2. Surgical results. *J Neurosurg* 1990; 73:37–47.

Newfield P, Hamid RKA, Lam AM. Anesthetic management— intracranial aneurysms and A-V malformations. In: Albin M, ed. *Textbook of neuroanesthesia with neurosurgical and neuroscience perspectives.* New York: McGraw-Hill, 1997:859–900.

Solenski NJ, Haley EC Jr., Kassell NF, et al. Medical complications of aneurysmal subarachnoid hemorrhage: a report of the multicenter cooperative aneurysm study. *Crit Care Med* 1995; 23:1007–1117.

Solomon RA, Fink ME, Lennihan L. Early aneurysm surgery and prophylactic hypervolemic hypertensive therapy for the treatment of aneurysmal subarachnoid hemorrhage. *Neurosurgery* 1988;23: 699–704.

Ischemic Cerebrovascular Disease

Ian A. Herrick and Adrian W. Gelb

Patients presenting for carotid endarterectomy (CEA) are often elderly, have advanced cerebrovascular disease, and frequently have significant coexisting diseases involving other organ systems. Anesthetic management of these patients requires both an understanding of the physiologic stress imposed by the surgical procedure (disruption of the major cerebral hemispheric blood supply) and an appreciation of the physiologic constraints imposed by the coexisting diseases.

I. **Guidelines for performing CEA**
   A. Several prospective, randomized studies have reported superior outcome for medically stable patients with symptomatic, high-grade carotid stenoses (70% to 99%) after CEA combined with best medical therapy compared to medical treatment alone.
   B. Based on these studies, guidelines for performing CEA have been formulated by both the American Heart Association and the Canadian Neurosurgical Society (Table 12-1).

II. **Physiologic considerations**
   A. **Cerebral blood flow and metabolism**
      1. The brain is highly active metabolically but is essentially devoid of oxygen and glucose reserves, making it dependent on the continuous delivery of oxygen and glucose by the cerebral circulation.
      2. Cerebral blood flow (CBF) is provided by the internal carotid arteries (approximately 80%) and the vertebral arteries (approximately 20%), which anastomose at the base of the brain to form the circle of Willis.
      3. Patients with advanced occlusive cerebrovascular disease may be dependent on other collateral channels to maintain adequate CBF.
      4. Normally CBF is autoregulated to match the brain's metabolic requirements and maintain normal neuronal function.
   B. **Cerebral perfusion**
      1. Cerebral blood flow is related to cerebral perfusion pressure (CPP) and cerebrovascular resistance (CVR) according to the equation $CBF = CPP/CVR$.
      2. Factors affecting CBF
         (a) Cerebral perfusion pressure equals mean arterial blood pressure (MAP) minus intra-

Table 12-1.   Surgery guidelines for carotid endarterectomy

- Appropriate candidate for CEA
    Symptomatic 70%–99% stenosis with
        TIA(s) or nondisabling stroke
        Surgically accessible stenosis
        Stable medical and neurologic condition
- Uncertain candidate for CEA[a]
    Symptomatic <70% stenosis with[b]
        TIA(s) or nondisabling stroke
        Surgically accessible stenosis
        Stable medical and neurologic condition
    Asymptomatic >60% stenosis with
        Surgically accessible stenosis
        Stable medical condition
- Inappropriate candidate for CEA
    Asymptomatic ≤60% stenosis
    Symptomatic or asymptomatic with
        Intracranial stenoses more severe than the extracranial
        stenosis
        Uncontrolled diabetes mellitus, hypertension, congestive
        heart failure, or unstable angina pectoris
        A major neurologic deficit or decreased level of con-
        sciousness

The percentage stenosis should be defined by cerebral angiography and the NASCET method. The surgeon's rate of surgical complications (stroke or death) should be less than 6% for CEA in cases of symptomatic stenoses (appropriate or uncertain candidates), and less than 3% in cases of asymptomatic stenoses (uncertain candidates).
TIA, transient ischemic attack; CEA, carotid endarterectomy; NASCET, North American Symptomatic Carotid Endarterectomy Trial.
[a] Guidelines uncertain = insufficient evidence to support a definitive recommendation.
[b] Guideline for symptomatic <70% stenosis expected to be clarified this year with publication of NASCET results for this group of patients.
Adapted from Findlay JM, et al. Guidelines for the use of carotid endarterectomy: current recommendations from the Canadian Neurosurgical Society. *Can Med Assoc J* 1997;157:653.

cranial pressure (ICP) or central venous pressure (CVP), whichever is greater.
   (b)   Cerebrovascular resistance is a function of blood viscosity and the diameter of the cerebral resistance vessels.
   3.   Optimization of CBF during CEA is hampered by the fact that the only factors readily amenable to intraoperative manipulation are arterial blood pressure and arterial carbon dioxide tension ($PaCO_2$), which impact on CPP and CVR, respectively.
C.   Carbon dioxide tension
   1.   Within the range of $PaCO_2$ from 20 to 80 mm Hg, CBF changes by 1 to 2 mL/100 g/minute for every 1 mm Hg change in $PaCO_2$.

    2. The most common approach to ventilatory management during CEA is maintenance of normocapnia (i.e., a $PaCO_2$ that produces a normal pH in the absence of coexisting metabolic acidosis).

D. Blood pressure

    1. Cerebral blood flow remains remarkably constant within the range of MAP from 50 to 150 mm Hg. Beyond this range, the limit of vasomotor activity is exceeded and CBF becomes directly dependent on changes in CPP.

    2. In patients with preexisting chronic hypertension, both the upper and lower limits of autoregulation are shifted to higher pressures.

    3. In patients with cerebrovascular disease, and during carotid cross-clamping, the CBF response to changes in $PaCO_2$ is impaired. Under these conditions, improvement in CBF is likely to be largely dependent on increases in CPP, emphasizing the relatively greater importance of blood pressure control during CEA surgery.

    4. During CEA, blood pressure should be maintained within the normal preoperative range. Mild increases in systolic blood pressure of up to 20% above normal at the time of cross-clamping are acceptable but hypotension and severe hypertension should be avoided.

III. Preanesthetic assessment

A. The patient's state of health should be assessed based on history, pertinent physical examination, and chart review.

B. Coexisting diseases should be assessed and optimized. Common coexisting diseases include coronary artery disease, arterial hypertension, peripheral vascular disease, chronic obstructive pulmonary disease, diabetes mellitus, and renal insufficiency.

C. For patients with diabetes, perioperative blood glucose should be carefully managed to avoid both hypo- and hyperglycemia. Current evidence suggests that hyperglycemia adversely affects outcome after temporary focal or global cerebral ischemia.

D. Cardiac complications are a major source of mortality after CEA. Preoperative factors reported to correlate with increased perioperative cardiac morbidity include poorly controlled hypertension, congestive heart failure, and recent myocardial infarction.

E. Cerebral angiograms should also be reviewed to identify patients at increased risk due to the presence of significant contralateral carotid disease or poor collateral circulation.

F. A risk stratification scheme for perioperative complications has been proposed for patients undergoing CEA (Table 12-2).

IV. Anesthetic management

    Carotid endarterectomy can be performed safely under general anesthesia or regional anesthesia (including local

**Table 12-2.   Preoperative risk stratification
for patients undergoing carotid endarterectomy**

Risk group	Characteristics	Total morbidity and mortality (%)
1	Neurologically stable, no major medical or angiographic risk	1
2	Neurologically stable, significant angiographic risk, no major medical risk	2
3	Neurologically stable, major medical risk, ± major angiographic risk	7
4	Neurologically unstable, ± major medical or angiographic risk	10

Type of risk	Risk Factors
Medical risk	Angina Myocardial infarction (<6 mo) Congestive heart failure Severe hypertension (>180/110 mm Hg) Chronic obstructive pulmonary disease Age >70 yr Severe obesity
Neurologic risk	Progressing deficit New deficit (<24 h) Frequent daily TIA(s) Multiple cerebral infarcts
Angiographic risk	Contralateral ICA occlusion ICA siphon stenosis Proximal or distal plaque extension High carotid bifurcation Presence of soft thrombus

TIA, transient ischemic attack; ICA, internal carotid artery.
Adapted from Sundt TM Jr, Sandok BA, Whisnant JP. Carotid endarterectomy. Complications and preoperative assessment of risk. *Mayo Clinic Proc* 1975;50:301–306. Reproduced with permission from Herrick IA, Gelb AW. Occlusive cerebrovascular disease: anesthetic considerations. In: Cottrell JE, Smith DS, eds. *Anesthesia and neurosurgery,* 3rd ed. St Louis: Mosby, 1994:484.

anesthetic infiltration). Experienced centers report similar morbidity and mortality, and available evidence is insufficient to establish the superiority of either technique definitively.

A. Regional anesthesia
   1. Superficial and deep cervical plexus blocks are the most common regional anesthetic technique for CEA.
      a. A superficial cervical plexus block is performed by injecting local anesthetic subcu-

taneously along the posterior border of the sternocleidomastoid muscle where the cutaneous branches of the plexus fan out to innervate the skin of the lateral neck.

b. A deep cervical plexus block is a paravertebral block of the C_2 to C_4 nerve roots. This technique involves injecting local anesthetic at the vertebral foramina (transverse processes) of the C_2, C_3, and C_4 vertebrae to block neck muscles, fascia, and the greater occipital nerve.

c. The techniques are described in detail in many regional anesthesia textbooks and should be reviewed before performing the blocks.

2. Intraoperative monitors include:
   a. Intraarterial cannula for blood pressure measurements.
   b. Continuous electrocardiogram (ECG).
   c. Pulse oximetry.
   d. Capnography sampled via nasal prongs for monitoring respiratory rate.

3. Supplemental oxygen should be provided with a mask or nasal prongs positioned to avoid the site of surgery.

4. Carefully titrated sedation using small, repeated, intravenous doses of fentanyl (10 to 25 μg) and/or midazolam (0.5 to 2 mg) should ensure a comfortable and cooperative patient during the operation. Propofol is a reasonable alternative administered as intermittent intravenous bolus doses (0.3 to 0.5 mg/kg) or as a low-dose continuous infusion (0.3 to 1.0 mg/kg/hour).

5. Equipment should be immediately available to convert to a general anesthetic if intraoperative conditions warrant.

6. Advantages of regional anesthesia include:
   a. Superior neurologic monitoring associated with an awake patient.
   b. Potential to minimize interventions such as shunt insertion based on symptoms at cross-clamping.
   c. Less expensive.
   d. Reports of more rapid recovery and shorter hospitalization.

7. Disadvantages of regional anesthesia include:
   a. Requires an operating room staff committed to working with patients under regional anesthesia, which requires patience, gentle technique, and reinforcement of block as needed.
   b. Lack of airway and ventilatory control.
   c. Potential need to deal with complications in an awake patient: stroke or transient cere-

bral ischemia, cross-clamp intolerance, seizure, airway obstruction, hypoventilation, confusion, agitation, angina.

d. Complications associated with cervical plexus blocks: local anesthetic toxicity, inadvertent injection into subarachnoid space or vertebral artery, phrenic or recurrent laryngeal nerve block.

B. General anesthesia

1. General anesthesia represents the most common anesthetic technique for CEA.
2. Intraoperative monitors include:
   a. Intraarterial cannula for blood pressure measurements.
   b. Continuous ECG.
   c. Pulse oximetry.
   d. Capnography.
   e. Central venous or pulmonary artery pressure monitoring is optional. A central venous catheter facilitates the management of intraoperative fluid administration and provides central access for drug administration or resuscitation. A pulmonary artery catheter can be used in patients with high-risk cardiovascular disease (e.g., unstable angina, poor left ventricular function, recent myocardial infarction, etc.). Care should be exercised to avoid carotid puncture when placing these lines.
3. The key consideration during induction of anesthesia is the maintenance of stable hemodynamic conditions during intubation, positioning, and draping.
4. Thiopental, midazolam, propofol, and etomidate are all appropriate induction drugs and should be supplemented with opioid.
5. Tracheal intubation is facilitated with any of the nondepolarizing neuromuscular blocking drugs. Succinylcholine is a reasonable alternative. However, its use is contraindicated in patients who have had a recent paretic cerebral infarct.
6. General anesthesia is usually maintained with a combination of volatile anesthetic (typically isoflurane, desflurane, or sevoflurane) and opioid. Neuromuscular blockade is maintained throughout the procedure. Propofol infusion is a reasonable alternative.
7. The administration of nitrous oxide is controversial due to reports of potential adverse effects on cerebral metabolism. However, its use remains popular.
8. Blood pressure is maintained at preoperative levels. Small bolus doses of vasopressor (e.g., phenylephrine, 40 to 60 μg; or ephedrine, 5 to

7.5 mg) can be administered to support blood pressure if necessary. Infusions of phenylephrine are used at some hospitals to maintain or increase blood pressure, especially during cross-clamping. However, evidence suggests that this practice may be associated with an increased risk of myocardial ischemia.

9. Ventilation is adjusted to maintain normocapnia.

10. Advantages of general anesthesia include:
    a. Potentially more comfortable for patients and operating room staff.
    b. Facilitates intraoperative control of ventilation, airway, and sympathetic responses.
    c. Facilitates management of complications (e.g., cross-clamp intolerance and transient cerebral ischemia) through the use of induced hypertension or pharmacologic suppression of electroencephalographic activity.
    d. Reduces the need for expedience in performing surgery since patient tolerance is not a factor.
    e. General anesthesia may provide some cerebral protection.

11. Disadvantages of general anesthesia include:
    a. Need for an alternate method for monitoring cerebral function.
    b. In the absence of a completely reliable cerebral function monitor, it is possible that some remediable complications will not be detected prior to irreversible neuronal injury (e.g., cross-clamp intolerance, kink in carotid shunt, etc.).
    c. Prolonged emergence might confuse postoperative evaluation.
    d. More expensive.

C. **Carotid cross-clamping**
   1. Prior to cross-clamping, heparin (75 to 100 U/kg) is administered intravenously.
   2. Carotid cross-clamping is often associated with an increase in blood pressure (up to approximately 20% above preoperative levels). Excessive increases may reflect cerebral ischemia. This should be considered before the increase in blood pressure is controlled pharmacologically.
   3. **Neurologic monitoring**
      a. The purpose of neurologic monitoring is to identify patients at risk for adverse neurologic outcome due to the development of cerebral ischemia, particularly during carotid cross-clamping.
      b. An awake patient represents the least expensive and most sensitive neurologic function monitor during CEA.

    c. Since an awake patient is not available during general anesthesia, a variety of other techniques have been investigated for monitoring neurologic function. Electroencephalography, carotid stump pressure measurements, transcranial Doppler, and CBF measurements are used most commonly, either individually or in combination (i.e., electroencephalography and transcranial Doppler).

    d. Each of these techniques can identify significant reductions in cerebral perfusion. However, controversy continues to surround the reliability of each technique or combination to predict outcome accurately.

    e. Interventions available in response to evidence of cerebral ischemia include:

        (1) Increasing CPP by administering systemic vasopressor drugs (e.g., phenylephrine).

        (2) Reducing the risk of ischemia by pharmacologically suppressing cerebral metabolic requirements (e.g., thiopental, etomidate, propofol, etc.).

        (3) Restoring internal carotid artery blood flow by placing a carotid shunt.

D. Emergence

  1. Emergence should be designed to avoid excessive coughing or straining and surges in systemic blood pressure, which might strain the fresh arteriotomy.

  2. Heparin is usually partially reversed at the time of wound closure.

  3. Many surgeons prefer patients to be awake and their tracheas extubated at the conclusion of the procedure to facilitate neurologic examination in the early postoperative period.

V. Postanesthetic management

  A. The intraarterial cannula is maintained during the initial postoperative period to permit continuous blood pressure monitoring.

  B. All patients receive supplemental oxygen and the adequacy of oxygenation is monitored by pulse oximetry. Bilateral CEA is associated with abolition of the ventilatory and cardiovascular responses to hypoxemia. Provision of supplemental oxygen and close monitoring of ventilatory status are particularly important in these patients.

  C. Postoperative hemodynamic instability is common (>40%) after CEA and is postulated to be related to carotid baroreceptor dysfunction.

    1. CEA performed using a carotid sinus nerve sparing technique is associated with a higher incidence of postoperative hypotension. This is most likely due to increased exposure of the carotid sinus after removal of the atheromatous plaque. Associated with a marked decrease in systemic vascular resistance, hypotension can be prevented or treated with local anesthetic blockade of the carotid sinus nerve, intravenous fluid administration, or, if necessary, the administration of vasopressor drugs such as phenylephrine.

2. Hypertension after CEA is less well understood and has been reported to be more common in patients with preoperative hypertension and in patients who undergo CEA in which the carotid sinus is denervated. Mild increases in postoperative blood pressure are acceptable (up to 20% of preoperative normotensive levels), but marked increases are treated with antihypertensive drugs.

3. Other causes of hemodynamic instability after CEA include myocardial ischemia/infarction, arrhythmias such as atrial fibrillation, hypoxia, hypercarbia, pneumothorax, pain, confusion, and distention of the urinary bladder.

D. In most hospitals, patients are discharged from the postanesthetic care unit to an environment where intensive neurologic and cardiovascular monitoring is available (e.g., intensive care unit or neurosurgical observation unit).

VI. Complications

Major postoperative complications after CEA include stroke, myocardial infarction, and hyperperfusion syndrome.

A. Stroke

1. Approximately two thirds of strokes associated with CEA occur in the postoperative period. Most of these appear to be related to surgical factors resulting in carotid occlusion (e.g., thrombosis, intimal flap) or emboli originating at the surgical site.

2. Intraoperative strokes represent approximately one third of strokes that occur in the perioperative period. The majority of intraoperative strokes occur at the time of carotid cross-clamping and are technical (i.e., shunt malfunction) or embolic, rather than hemodynamic, in origin.

3. Intraoperative neurophysiologic function monitoring is directed to the identification of a relatively small group of patients who develop hemodynamically induced ischemia, which is potentially reversible with early recognition and intervention.

4. It is likely that, beyond using current anesthetic and monitoring techniques and meticulously manipulating hemodynamic and ventilatory parameters, the anesthesiologist has little ability,

at present, to further affect stroke outcome during CEA.

B. Myocardial infarction

1. Myocardial infarction represents the major cause of mortality after CEA. The incidence of fatal postoperative myocardial infarction is 0.5% to 4%, and the proportion of total perioperative mortality (within 30 days of operation) attributed to cardiac causes is estimated to be at least 40%.

2. Based on the high incidence of coronary artery disease among patients undergoing CEA, routine coronary angiography has been advocated. However, little evidence supports the premise that routine preoperative coronary angiography improves cardiac outcome after CEA. It seems more reasonable to assume that all patients presenting for CEA have atherosclerotic disease involving the coronary arteries and gage perioperative risk in relation to the patient's functional status.

3. High-risk patients such as those with unstable angina, recent myocardial infarction, or recent heart failure may be considered more appropriate candidates for CEA staged or combined with a coronary artery bypass graft (CABG) procedure.

4. Existing evidence is insufficient to formulate firm recommendations regarding the staging of CEA with CABG surgery. The risk of stroke is similar if CEA precedes or is combined with CABG. This risk is lower than when CABG is performed before CEA. However, the incidence of myocardial infarction and death is greater when CEA precedes CABG. Pending results from well-designed prospective studies, recommendations from the Canadian Neurosurgical Society suggest that CEA should precede CABG if possible. When the patient's cardiac condition is too unstable to permit a prior CEA, combined surgery should be considered.

C. Death

1. Stroke and myocardial infarction represent the major causes of perioperative mortality associated with CEA.

2. Operative risk is affected by patient selection, the experience of the surgeon, and the institution where the surgery is performed.

3. Based on these considerations, the American Heart Association Stroke Council has recommended that the combined risk for death or stroke associated with CEA should not exceed 3% for asymptomatic patients, 5% for symptomatic (transient cerebral ischemia) patients, 7% for patients who have suffered a previous

stroke, and 10% for patients undergoing reoperation for recurrent carotid stenosis.

D. Hyperperfusion syndrome

1. An increase in CBF occurs frequently after CEA. Typically the magnitude of this increase is relatively small (<35%). However, in severe cases, increases in CBF can exceed 200% of preoperative levels and can be associated with increased morbidity and mortality.

2. Clinical features of this hyperperfusion syndrome include headache (usually unilateral), face and eye pain, cerebral edema, seizures, and intracerebral hemorrhage.

3. Patients at greatest risk include those with reduced preoperative hemispheric CBF due to bilateral high-grade carotid stenoses, unilateral high-grade carotid stenosis with poor collateral cross-flow, or unilateral carotid occlusion with contralateral high-grade stenosis.

4. The syndrome is thought to result from restoration of perfusion to an area of the brain that has lost its ability to autoregulate due to chronically decreased CBF. Restoration of CBF leads to a state of hyperperfusion that persists until autoregulation is reestablished, usually over a period of days.

5. Patients at risk for this syndrome should be monitored closely in the perioperative period and blood pressure should be meticulously controlled.

E. Other complications

Other complications associated with CEA include hematoma formation and cranial nerve palsies. Hematoma formation can lead to airway compromise due to mass effect, which might require opening the wound acutely to reestablish the airway for emergent reoperation. Cranial nerve palsies are typically temporary and might manifest as vocal cord paralysis and/or altered gag reflex.

VII. Summary

This chapter has focused on the anesthetic management of patients undergoing CEA. Physiologic concepts that form the basis for current recommendations regarding the choice of anesthetic technique, drugs, monitoring, and hemodynamic and ventilatory management have been discussed. Enormous progress has occurred in the past decade validating the efficacy of CEA and defining indications for the procedure. Despite advances in surgical and anesthetic techniques, morbidity and mortality associated with CEA remain substantial. Further improvement in outcome after CEA will require advances in the development of effective interventions to prevent and/or treat cerebral ischemia (especially embolic events) and myocardial ischemia in the perioperative period.

SUGGESTED READINGS

Beebe HG, et al. Assessing risk associated with carotid endarterectomy. *Stroke* 1989;20:314.

Cheng MA, Theard MA, Tempelhoff R. Anesthesia for carotid endarterectomy: a survey. *J Neurosurg Anesth* 1997;9:211.

Drader KS, Herrick IA. Carotid endarterectomy: monitoring and its effect on outcome. *Anesthesiol Clin North Am* 1997;15(3):613.

Findlay JM, et al. Guidelines for the use of carotid endarterectomy: current recommendations from the Canadian Neurosurgical Society. *Can Med Assoc* 1997;J 157:653.

Herrick IA, Gelb AW. Occlusive cerebrovascular disease: anesthetic considerations. In: Cottrell JE, Smith DS, eds. *Anesthesia and neurosurgery,* 4th ed. St. Louis: Mosby, 1999 (in press).

Moore WS, et al. Guidelines for carotid endarterectomy. A multidisciplinary consensus statement from the ad hoc committee, American Heart Association. *Stroke* 1995;26:188.

Sundt TM Jr, Sandok BA, Whisnant JP. Carotid endarterectomy. Complications and preoperative assessment of risk. *Mayo Clinic Proc* 1975;50:301.

Neuroendocrine Procedures

M. Jane Matjasko

I. **Anatomy**
   A. **Intracranial mass.** Many tumors are microadenomas and require routine induction and maintenance of anesthesia. Some tumors are very large and require attention to blood pressure (BP), airway dynamics, and other factors affecting intracranial pressure (ICP) during induction.
   B. **Pituitary gland and stalk** are very close to the optic chiasm, intracranial carotid arteries, and cavernous sinuses.
   C. **Pituitary adenomas** may be intrasellar, not intracranial, but may extend laterally into the cavernous sinuses.
      1. **Cavernous sinus** contains the intrasphenoid carotid artery and cranial nerves III, IV, V_1, V_2, and VI.
      2. **Magnetic resonance imaging (MRI)** appearance and extension of tumor are important for planning anesthetic management and neurophysiologic monitoring.
   D. **Pituitary tumors** can extend out of the sella into the intracranial space and involve the optic chism and carotid arteries.
II. **Endocrine physiology–anterior pituitary**
   A. **Hypothalamus** secretes hormone-releasing factor (RF), which is transported to the median eminence of the hypothalamus by axonal flow. Releasing factor is transported via the hypothalamo-hypophyseal portal system to the anterior pituitary. Hormones are secreted into the systemic circulation in response to a variety of stimuli. Target organs respond to stimuli and send negative feedback to the pituitary and the hypothalamus to turn off the secretion of RF and stop release of the hormone.
   B. **Anterior pituitary hormones** [adrenocorticotropic hormone (ACTH), growth hormone (GH), prolactin (PRL), thyroid-stimulating hormone (TSH), luteinizing hormone (LH), melanocyte-stimulating hormone (MSH), and follicle-stimulating hormone (FSH)] have all been known to be produced by microadenomas; ACTH, GH, and PRL are the most common. All have inhibiting and releasing factors; all can be accurately measured in blood using radioimmunoassay techniques.
   C. **Cushing's disease** is due to an ACTH-secreting pituitary tumor.
      1. **Cushing's syndrome** is due to ACTH-dependent

(ACTH administration, ectopic ACTH syndrome) or ACTH-independent (adrenal adenoma, carcinoma, or exogenous cortisol administration) excess secretion of cortisol.

2. **Ectopic ACTH** is due to primary oat cell carcinoma of the lung.
   a. Tumor produces ACTH- and corticotropin-releasing factor (CRF)–like peptides
   b. Plasma cortisol >50 μg/dL
   c. Explosive hypercortisolism
      (1) **Hypertension**
      (2) **Glucose intolerance**
      (3) **Hyperaldosteronism** (hypokalemic alkalosis)
      (4) **Marked pigmentation**

3. **Cushing's disease**
   a. **Truncal obesity**, posterior cervical fat pads, osteoporosis.
   b. **Hypertension**, glucose intolerance.
   c. **Adrenal hyperplasia.** In the past many patients had bilateral adrenalectomy to treat what was thought to be a primary adrenal condition. Patients who have Nelson's syndrome might come to surgery to remove a primary pituitary tumor.
   d. **Corticotropin-releasing factor** is stimulated by acetylcholine and serotonin and inhibited by norepinephrine.
   e. **Cortisol secretion** is 16 μg/day, 75% of which is bound to transcortin protein.
   f. **Normal diurnal variation:** 4 to 8 a.m. 25 μg/dL; 4 to 8 p.m. <10 μg/dL.
   g. **Diagnosis.** Loss of diurnal variation; ACTH increased; MRI evidence of sellar adenoma.

D. **Acromegaly.** A GH-producing tumor leading to:
   1. **Signs and symptoms**
      a. Bone and soft tissue enlargement
      b. Hypertension
      c. Glucose intolerance
      d. Visual loss if tumor large and involving chiasm
      e. Hoarseness (soft tissue stretching Xth cranial nerve)
      f. Dyspnea (narrow glottis due to soft tissue overgrowth)
      g. Cardiomyopathy (lymphocytic infiltration), which is common cause of death if untreated
      h. Carpal tunnel (soft tissue) and cervical compression
      i. Lumbar spinal stenosis (bony overgrowth)
   2. **GH** random blood level 2 to 5 ng/mL in normals.
   3. **Hypoglycemia** is most potent stimulus to secretion; somatostatin inhibits the release of GH.
   4. **Diagnosis.** Random GH >10 ng/mL; somatomedin C elevation (produced in liver only in re-

sponse to GH stimulation); high levels are only due to acromegaly.

5. **Acromegaly and airway**
   a. Hypertrophy of mandible, nasal turbinates, soft palate, tonsils, epiglottis, arytenoids, tongue, lips, nose.
   b. Glottis might be narrow.
   c. Vocal cord paralysis might be present.
   d. Most often routine intubation successful but be prepared with extra long blade and smaller endotracheal tubes.
   e. Anticipate difficult mask fit; potential post-extubation stridor.
   f. Rarely will awake fiberoptic intubation be necessary.
   g. Patients frequently have an ear–nose–throat consultation prior to surgery; report of indirect laryngoscopy is obtained from that consultation to allow anticipation of airway difficulty.

E. **Prolactin-secreting tumors** may be larger in men than women who seek medical attention earlier because of infertility. Other symptoms include amenorrhea, galactorrhea, anovulation, decreased libido, gynecomastia, osteoporosis.
   1. **Prolactin secretion** is primarily regulated by an inhibitory factor (dopamine). Prolactin-releasing factors are thyroid-releasing hormone (TRH), serotonin, and the stress of anesthesia and surgery. Prolactin secretion is increased with pituitary stalk section, phenothiazines, and α-methyldopa.
   2. **Normal prolactin** level is 15 to 25 ng/mL.
   3. **Diagnosis.** Prolactin > 25 ng/mL. When PRL > 200 ng/mL, 80% have adenomas even if neuroradiologic procedures do not demonstrate adenoma. When PRL > 2,000 ng/mL, cavernous sinus invasion is likely. This may warrant extra intravenous access and electroencephalogram/evoked potential (EEG/EP) monitoring.
   4. **Amenorrhea.** Prolactin > 30 ng/mL
      Loss of libido. Prolactin > 300 ng/mL
      Menopause. Prolactin ↑ ; estrogen ↓

F. **Nonfunctioning pituitary tumors** include adenomas, craniopharyngiomas, meningiomas, or aneurysms. These tend to be large and involve perisellar structures.

III. **Endocrine physiology–posterior pituitary**
A. **Antidiuretic hormone (ADH)**
   1. Produced in the supraoptic and paraventricular nuclei of the hypothalamus.
   2. Stored in the median eminence of the hypothalamus.
   3. Transported with carrier protein, neurophysin, along hypothalamic hypophyseal tract to posterior pituitary.

4. Released into the systemic circulation after appropriate stimulus (decreased blood volume → greatest ADH release and concurrent vasoconstriction; increased serum osmolality; pain; opiates).

5. Secretion inhibited by decreased serum osmolality, alcohol ingestion, increased blood volume, phenytoin.

B. Antidiuretic hormone attaches to an adenyl cyclase receptor on the medullary interstitial surface of the collecting duct epithelium. This causes an increase in cyclic AMP, which increases the permeability of the collecting duct to water and water is reabsorbed. In the absence of ADH, pure water is lost.

C. Diabetes insipidus (DI) can be present preoperatively. It can occur intraoperatively and may be temporary or permanent in the postoperative period.

1. **Signs and symptoms** include polyuria (3 to 15 L/day), polydypsia, serum hyperosmolality (>320 mosmol/kg), dilute urine (specific gravity 1.001 to 1.005, osmolality 50 to 150 mosmol/kg)

2. **If any salt-containing fluids are administered**, patient will develop severe hypernatremia and hyperosmolality.

3. **If glucose-containing fluids are administered**, patient will develop hyperglycemia and osmotic diuresis.

4. **Calculate total body water deficit** in 70-kg patient.

   Normal serum sodium (Na^+) = 140 mEq/L
   Total body water = 60% total body weight = 42 L
   Normal body sodium = 42 L × 140 mEq/L = 5880 mEq Na^+
   Patient's serum sodium = 160 mEq/L
   Patient's body water = 5880 mEq/160 mEq/L = 36.7 L
   Water deficit = 42 L − 36.7 L = 5.3 L

5. **Drug therapy** indicated in patients who cannot drink the volumes necessary and in the anesthetized or NPO patient:

   a. **1-Deamino-8-D-arginine   vasopressin (DDAVP) intranasal** q12h; also can be given intravenously.

   b. **Lysine vasopressin** 5 to 10 U s.c. q4h.

   c. **Other drugs**: vasopressin tannate-in-oil used more rarely; effect lasts up to 36 hours after single dose.

IV. Perioperative management

A. Pituitary tumor signs and symptoms include:

1. Headache (bitemporal or bifrontal).

2. Visual symptoms (classically bitemporal hemianopsia but depends on relationship of stalk to optic chiasm).

3. Ophthalmoplegia (III, IV, VI) and facial paralysis (VII).
4. Corneal anesthesia (V) related to cavernous sinus invasion or compression.
5. Seizures related to temporal lobe extension—rare.
6. Hypothalamic symptoms (abnormal temperature regulation, thirst, appetite changes—all rare).
7. Diabetes insipidus.
8. Endocrinopathies [syndrome of multiple endocrine neoplasia which may include parathyroid dysfunction with hypercalcemia and TSH, ACTH, LH, FSH-producing adenomas].

B. **Panhypopituitarism** is a clinical diagnosis confirmed by assay of specific hormones.
   1. The majority of patients with microadenomas are clinically normal and do not demonstrate any signs of panhypopituitarism.
   2. Nonetheless, in some institutions it is customary to administer hydrocortisone 50 to 100 mg i.v. prior to induction and 10 mg/hour by infusion until the patient's postoperative course indicates that the drug is no longer necessary.
   3. Thyroid replacement may be administered orally, as levothyroxine sodium (Synthroid); very rarely as intravenous.
   4. Diabetes insipidus is treated with DDAVP and appropriate fluids. If panhypopituitarism has been diagnosed preoperatively, the patient might be receiving replacement steroids and DDAVP.

C. **Intraoperative management**
   1. **Usual monitoring** appropriate for physiologic status of patient.
      a. Consider EEG/EP monitoring if cavernous sinus or perisellar involvement is marked.
      b. In some institutions pituitary surgery is performed in a head-elevated position. Venous air embolism (VAE) might occur, so that end-tidal gas monitoring is recommended. If VAE occurs, the head can be lowered rapidly to treat. The need for central venous access is determined by the size and location of the tumor and/or by the patient's medical condition.
      c. Visual evoked responses are not measured in most institutions and are not indicated in microadenoma patients.
   2. **Anesthetic technique** is selected to permit early postoperative assessment of vision, ocular movements, pupil size, and motor strength.
   3. **Careful monitoring** of fluid intake and output.
   4. **Antibiotic prophylaxis** (typically cefazolin 1 gm, i.v. q6–8h).
   5. **Topical cocaine and injected lidocaine** with epinephrine: if both are used, severe hypertension might occur.

D. **Postoperative management**
1. **Careful fluid/electrolyte management**. Treatment of DI, SIADH, or cerebral salt wasting.
2. **Steroid maintenance and tapering**. Cushing's disease patients may have prolonged adrenal insufficiency and require steroids for several months.
3. **Acromegalics and Cushing's disease** patients have excess body water and will diurese postoperatively.
4. **Patients with previous adrenalectomies** (Nelson's syndrome) require mineralocorticoid replacement such as Florinef (fludrocortisone acetate 0.1 to 0.2 mg/day p.o.).
5. **Deep vein thrombosis** and pulmonary emboli are not uncommon.

V. **Pituitary apoplexy**
A. **Syndrome** related to the sudden enlargement of a pituitary tumor due to hemorrhage or necrosis.
B. **Symptoms and signs** include acute loss of consciousness, hypertension, meningismus, eye pain, blindness, ophthalmoplegia, panhypopituitarism.
C. **Diagnosis is made on clinical grounds** and with radiologic evidence of a pituitary tumor.
D. **Treatment is urgent:** surgical decompression of the optic system, systemic steroid replacement, and other hormone replacement as necessary. Some recommend bromocriptine therapy in lieu of surgery.

VI. **Treatment of pituitary tumors**
A. **Radiation therapy** is rarely used now because of the high incidence of panhypopituitarism and the long lag time for clinical effect.
B. **Medical therapy**
1. **ACTH (Cushing's disease).** Since there is no effective medical therapy, surgery is most desirable.
2. **Growth hormone (acromegaly).** Octreotide, a somatostatin inhibitor, is an expensive ($7,800 annually) agent that requires multiple daily subcutaneous injections. Octreotide reduces headaches and improves cardiomyopathy, and can be used to treat less than optimal surgical results. Surgery is preferred.
3. **Prolactin.** Bromocriptine or similar drugs such as pergolide are the first-line treatment.
   a. They reduce tumor size and PRL levels.
   b. They restore fertility. The risks of pregnancy with a pituitary tumor include enlargement during pregnancy, necessitating surgery. Perhaps tumor removal should precede pregnancy.
   c. If patients are intolerant of the drug's side effects (nausea, dizziness, orthostatic hypotension), surgery is indicated.
   d. Medical therapy must be continued long

term to indefinitely when surgery is not performed.
C. **Surgical therapy**
1. **Transsphenoidal.** Transnasal, transsphenoidal approach to floor of sella.
   a. **Advantages.** Less damage to frontal lobes and olfactory apparatus, no external scar, direct visualization of microadenomas, minimal damage to normal pituitary, lower incidence of temporary and (rarely) permanent DI, less blood loss, and shorter hospitalization.
   b. **Disadvantages.** Potential for CSF leak, meningitis, no direct visualization of the optic apparatus, inaccessibility of large tumors, blood loss more difficult to control; may require packing of cavernous sinus and compression of cranial nerves and carotid artery, which could lead to neurologic deficit.
2. **Transfrontal: bifrontal or unilateral craniotomy**
   a. **Advantages.** Can access suprasellar tumor extension, can visualize optic system and other perisellar structures.
   b. **Disadvantages.** Higher morbidity than transsphenoidal; temporary and permanent DI more likely.

SUGGESTED READINGS

Ciric I, Ragin A, Baumgartner C, Pierce D. Complications of transsphenoidal surgery: results of a national survey, review of the literature, and personal experience. *Neurosurgery* 1997;40:225.

Harrigan MR. Cerebral salt wasting: a review. *Neurosurgery* 1996;38:152.

Matjasko MJ. Anesthetic considerations in patients with neuroendocrine disease. In: Cottrell JE, Smith DS, eds. *Anesthesia and neurosurgery*, 3rd ed. St. Louis: Mosby, 1994:604–623.

O'Brien T, O'Riordan DS, Gharib H, Scheithauer BW, Ebersold MJ, van Heerden JA. Results of treatment of pituitary disease in multiple endocrine neoplasia, type 1. *Neurosurgery* 1996;39:273.

Epileptic Patients and Epilepsy Surgery

Pirjo Helen Manninen

I. Epileptic patient
A. Definitions
1. **Epileptic seizures** are the clinical manifestations (signs and symptoms) of excessive and/or hypersynchronous abnormal activity of neurons in the cerebral cortex. This activity is usually self-limited. The features of the seizure reflect the functions of the cortical areas from which the abnormal activity originates and to which it spreads. Epileptic seizures have electrophysiologic correlates that are recorded on a scalp electroencephalogram (EEG).
2. **Epilepsy** is a chronic disorder caused by a variety of pathologic processes in the brain and is characterized by epileptic seizures. Incidence of epilepsy is from 0.5% to 2% of the total population, with 25% to 30% of persons with epilepsy having more than one seizure a month.

B. Classification of epileptic seizures
1. **Partial seizures** have an onset that is localized or focal within the brain.
   a. **Simple partial:** There is no alteration in consciousness during these seizures. They are further classified according to symptoms: motor, sensory, autonomic, and psychic. **Auras** are the sensory, autonomic, or psychic symptoms that precede a progression to impaired consciousness or motor seizure.
   b. **Complex partial:** Seizures spread into multiple areas of the brain and alter consciousness; they are also called **psychomotor** or **temporal lobe** seizures. A simple partial seizure can progress to become complex.
   c. **Convulsive:** These seizures have a partial onset but then spread to involve most areas of the brain and brain stem. They are not easily distinguishable from generalized seizures.
2. We speak of **generalized seizures** when the EEG shows simultaneous involvement of both cerebral hemispheres and consciousness is impaired.
   a. Inhibitory or nonconvulsive, such as atonic or absence seizures (petit mal).
   b. Excitatory or convulsive, which produce myoclonic, tonic, or clonic seizures.
3. **Unclassified seizures**

C. **Mechanisms of epilepsy** are diverse and include abnormalities in the regulation of neural circuits and the balance of neural excitation and inhibition. Factors that influence the appearance of epilepsy can be genetic, environmental, or physiologic.

D. **Associated medical problems**
   1. Psychiatric disorders.
   2. Rare syndromes: tuberous sclerosis, neurofibromatosis, multiple endocrine adenomatosis.
   3. History of trauma.
   4. Sleep deprivation.

E. **Treatment of epilepsy**
   1. **Medical therapy**
      a. A variety of antiepileptic drugs are used including phenytoin, phenobarbital, primidone, carbamazepine, clonazepam, valproic acid, and diazepam.
      b. Treatment can consist of single medication or multiple drug therapy.
      c. The choice is dependent on considerations of the pharmacokinetics, clinical toxicity, efficacy, and type of epilepsy.
   2. **Adverse effects of antiepileptic drugs** are dose-dependent and are usually associated with long-term therapy.
      a. Many drugs have neurologic side effects such as sedation, confusion, learning impairment, ataxia, and gastrointestinal problems such as nausea and vomiting.
      b. Most anticonvulsants are metabolized by the liver. Thus, long-term usage may cause liver enzyme induction, which increases the rate of metabolism of other drugs, particularly anesthetic agents.
      c. Long-term therapy with phenytoin causes gingival hyperplasia with poor dentition and, potentially, difficult airway management.
      d. Carbamazepine can depress the hemopoietic system and, in rare cases, causes cardiac toxicity.
      e. Valproic acid might occasionally result in thrombocytopenia and platelet dysfunction.
   3. **Surgical treatment.** Epilepsy becomes intractable to medical therapy in 5% to 15% of patients. Approximately 13% of patients who have intractable epilepsy are candidates for surgical resection of the epileptogenic focus.

F. **Status epilepticus**
   1. Status epilepticus is defined as epileptic seizures that are so frequently repeated or so long in duration as to create a fixed and lasting epileptic condition, either convulsive or nonconvulsive. This is considered a neurologic emergency.
   2. **Treatment.** To prevent brain damage, seizures must be stopped as quickly as possible.

a. Secure the airway, provide oxygen, and maintain circulation.

b. Protect patient from traumatic injury secondary to involuntary motor movements.

c. If hypogylcemia is present or cannot be ruled out, 50% glucose 50 mL i.v. and thiamine 100 mg i.v. should be given.

d. There are different approaches, but the initial drug choices usually include phenobarbital, phenytoin, and benzodiazepines; an example would be diazepam 0.2 mg/kg i.v., or lorazepam 0.1 mg/kg i.v., followed by phenytoin 15 to 20 mg/kg given slowly at no more than 50 mg/min.

e. Seizures that continue to be refractory might require barbiturate coma, titrated to EEG effect.

f. Other anesthetic agents that have been used include etomidate, ketamine, propofol, halothane, enflurane, and isoflurane.

G. **Pro- and anticonvulsant effects of anesthetic agents.** Numerous reports describe how anesthetic agents can paradoxically exhibit convulsant and anticonvulsant properties with different doses, under different physiologic situations, and with different species.

1. The inhalation agents halothane and isoflurane are both effective anticonvulsants. However, enflurane activates epileptiform activity on EEG and has produced seizures in patients with and without epilepsy. Nitrous oxide does not have any anticonvulsant properties, nor does it produce seizure activity on EEG. Desflurane and sevoflurane are not epileptogenic during deep anesthesia or under hypocapnic conditions.

2. Barbiturates are anticonvulsants, but when given in a small dose, thiopental and methohexital will activate the epileptiform activity from a seizure focus on EEG monitoring. Etomidate and ketamine can activate the epileptogenic focus and have also been used to treat status epilepticus. Benzodiazepines are effective anticonvulsants. Propofol is an anticonvulsant but there are controversial reports of clinical seizure activity following its use.

3. Droperidol has no effect on the EEG.

4. Opioids, e.g., fentanyl and alfentanil, can activate the epileptiform activity in patients with epilepsy.

5. Local anesthetic agents are anticonvulsant in low doses but at higher serum levels can produce central nervous system excitation.

H. **Interaction of anesthetic drugs with antiepileptic agents**

1. The requirements for muscle relaxants, opioids,

and barbiturates are increased in patients taking most long-term anticonvulsants, particularly phenytoin and phenobarbital, due to the enhanced hepatic microsomal enzyme activity, which accelerates hepatic biotransformation.

2. Interactions with endogenous neurotransmitters and changes in the number of receptors, including opioid, may occur.

I. **Anesthetic management of an epileptic patient for nonepilepsy surgery**
   1. **Preoperative assessment**
      a. General assessment and preparation.
      b. Specific concerns with an epileptic patient.
         (1) Medical problems associated with epilepsy.
         (2) Complications from anticonvulsant therapy.
         (3) Continuation of anticonvulsant therapy.
   2. **Anesthetic management and monitoring** depend on the needs of the patient and the procedure.
      a. Agents that potentiate seizure activity should not be used.
      b. There might be an increase in the requirement of anesthetic agents.
      c. Consideration should be given to the administration of additional doses of antiepileptic drugs during prolonged procedures.
      d. Hyperventilation might potentiate seizure activity and should be avoided unless necessary for surgery.
      e. Seizures can occur postoperatively as blood levels of antiepileptic drugs can be significantly affected by the anesthetic and by changes in body physiology during surgery.

II. **Epilepsy surgery**
   A. **Procedure**
      1. Surgery for partial seizure disorders involves the resection of a specific epileptogenic focus that may show sclerosis or gliosis. This is frequently accomplished by some form of a temporal lobectomy.
      2. Generalized seizures are treated by interruption of the seizure circuits by a corpus callosoctomy or a hemispherectomy.
      3. A surgical cure, i.e., a patient remaining seizure-free or with a significant reduction in seizure frequency, occurs in 50% to 80% of patients.
      4. Cognitive improvement also results as the doses of anticonvulsive drugs are reduced or eliminated.
   B. **Patient suitability for epilepsy surgery.** A complete evaluation is needed to assess whether the patient is a candidate for epilepsy surgery.
      1. **Noninvasive evaluation** includes medical his-

tory; assessment of the frequency, severity, and type of seizures; physical examination; and psychosocial and neuropsychiatric testing. Surface electrode monitoring of EEG activity may also include video-camera monitoring of seizures.

2. **Radiologic imaging** may supplement EEG data. Computed tomography and magnetic resonance imaging can help identify areas of sclerosis or low-grade intracranial neoplasms.

3. **Functional imaging** is done with positron emission tomography, single-photon emission computed tomography, and other methods that detect cerebral blood flow (CBF). These are helpful in localizing the seizure focus and in evaluating the metabolic effects of seizure focus resection.

4. **Thiopental testing** may be performed to assist in EEG localization of the seizure focus. The technique is performed by producing a gradual increase in the blood level of thiopental during EEG recording. This will cause an increase in beta activity in normally functioning neural tissue, but not in the seizure focus.

5. a. **Invasive evaluation** is accomplished by the insertion of intracranial electrodes. Epidural electrodes are inserted through multiple burr holes; subdural grids or strip electrodes are inserted through a full craniotomy. Stereotactic techniques can also be used. These electrodes are inserted several weeks prior to definitive surgery in order to monitor the patient for many days. The patient's behavior and EEG are continuously recorded and displayed on a television monitor in specialized units.

b. **Placement of intracranial electrodes or grids** is usually performed under general anesthesia. The anesthetic plan should take into consideration the concerns of a patient with epilepsy and the precautions that apply to any craniotomy. Routine noninvasive monitoring is required with the addition of intraarterial blood pressure measurement as indicated. The anesthetic agents used are not specific as there is no EEG recording. Electrode plates or large grids are quite bulky and might require brain shrinkage with the use of mannitol and hyperventilation. These patients might develop postoperative problems with brain edema and require urgent removal of the grid due to the development of intracranial hypertension.

C. **Intraoperative localization \of epileptogenic focus**

1. **Electrocorticography (ECoG)** is performed during surgery after opening of the dura by the

placement of electrodes directly on the cortex over the area predetermined to be epileptogenic as well as on adjacent cortex. Additional recordings can be performed with microelectrodes placed into the cortex or depth electrodes into the amygdala and hippocampal gyrus.

2. **Stimulation of epileptogenic focus** is possible pharmacologically if insufficient information to define the seizure focus adequately is obtained during routine ECoG. Agents used in adults include a small dose of methohexital (10 to 50 mg), thiopental (25 to 50 mg), propofol (10 to 20 mg), or etomidate (2 to 4 mg). If the patient is under general anesthesia, other agents can be used such as alfentanil (20 to 50 μg/kg) and enflurane with or without hypocarbia.

3. **Delineation of eloquent areas** of brain function, such as speech, memory, and sensory and motor function, is performed by direct electrical stimulation of the cortex. This allows these areas to be preserved during resection of the seizure focus. Only motor testing can be done when the patient is under general anesthesia.

D. **Preoperative preparation for epilepsy surgery.** Communication among all members of the team, including neurologist, surgeon, and anesthesiologist, is vital to the successful management of the patient throughout the perioperative period.

1. Routine and specific epilepsy assessment is carried out.

2. Appropriate preparation of the patient for the chosen technique of anesthesia is carried out.

3. The administration of anticonvulsant agents prior to surgery is done in consultation with the neurologist and surgeon.

4. Premedication for the purpose of sedation is rarely required as these patients are usually well informed; and all agents that might influence EEG, such as benzodiazepines, should be avoided.

E. **Techniques of anesthesia.** Historically, epilepsy surgery was performed with the patient awake for at least some part of the procedure. These procedures are now performed with the use of either neurolept anesthesia or general anesthesia. The decision is usually made by the surgeon but also depends on the location of the seizure focus, the need for testing of eloquent function, and the ability of the patient to withstand an awake procedure.

1. **Conscious sedation/neurolept**

a. **The reasons** for having an awake patient are:

(1) Better ECoG localization of the seizure focus without the influence of general anesthetic agents.

(2) Direct electrical stimulation of the cerebral cortex to delineate eloquent areas of

brain function in order to preserve them during surgical resection.

    (3) Continuous clinical neurologic monitoring of the patient throughout the procedure.

b. The challenge is to have the patient comfortable enough to remain immobile through a long procedure, but sufficiently alert and cooperative to comply with testing. The analgesic and sedative drugs employed must have minimal interference with ECoG and stimulation testing.

c. Specific preoperative preparation

    (1) The patient is prepared psychologically and informed about the complexities and demands of an awake craniotomy.

    (2) The establishment of good rapport by the anesthesiologist with the patient is absolutely essential.

    (3) The anesthesiologist should be aware of any signs or symptoms that the patient might have at the onset of a seizure.

    (4) Reassurance of the patient should begin here.

d. Preparation of the operating room. An awake craniotomy adds additional stress to the patient and the entire team. All preparations should be complete before the patient arrives in the room so that the patient can receive everyone's full attention.

    (1) Anesthetic agents and equipment for conscious sedation, induction of general anesthesia, and for the treatment of complications.

    (2) Routine monitoring equipment.

    (3) Positioning of patient: extra pillows, soft mattress, soft head rest or fixed head frame.

    (4) Room environment: normal room temperature, quiet, reassuring

e. Patient management

    (1) Positioning is usually in the lateral decubitus, which is most comfortable for the patient.

        (a) Pillows should be placed behind patient's back, between the legs, and under the arms.

        (b) Extra blankets are initially needed, but they should be placed so as to be easily removable as patients frequently get very warm during the procedure.

        (c) Patients should be positioned in such a way as to have some freedom of movement of extremities.

(d) The patient's head should be placed on a pillow of appropriate size and shape. Alternatively, the surgeon's preference might be to have the patient in a rigid head pin fixation. Pins are inserted with the use of local anesthesia.

(e) The placement of surgical drapes should allow for maximum visibility of the patient's face by the anesthesiologist and for the patient to see the anesthesiologist continuously.

(2) **Scalp block** is performed by the surgeon before the patient comes into the operating room or after positioning.

(a) Long-acting local anesthetic agents, such as bupivacaine with the addition of epinephrine, are used because these are long procedures.

(b) Lidocaine, which has a faster onset, may be added and also used to infiltrate areas that are still painful during the procedure, such as dura.

(c) The maximum dose for bupivacaine is 3 mg/kg and for lidocaine 5 to 7 mg/kg.

(d) The scalp block is probably the most painful part of the procedure. Sedation may be started before this is done.

(3) **Monitors**

(a) Electrocardiogram, noninvasive blood pressure cuff, pulse oximeter, and end-tidal CO_2 via nasal prongs that are used to deliver supplemental oxygen. Invasive monitoring is not routinely required.

(b) The intravenous catheter should be placed in the arm not involved in seizure activity.

(c) Fluids are kept to a minimum and thus a urinary catheter is not routinely needed.

(d) Dextrose-containing fluids should be avoided.

(4) **Anesthetic agents**

(a) The techniques of drug administration and dosage requirements vary greatly and should be titrated to each patient.

(b) The drugs may be administered by intermittent boluses, by continuous infusions, or by a combination.

(c) The anesthetic agents usually include a combination of an opioid, a major tranquilizer, and propofol. Traditionally, intermittent boluses of fentanyl (0.5 to 1.0 µg/kg) and droperidol (0.015 to 0.1 mg/kg) were used. Other opioids, e.g., sufentanil, alfentanil, and remifentanil, have also been used.

(d) Propofol infusion (25 to 100 µg/kg/minute) is easily titratable to the requirements of the patient but has to be discontinued at least 20 minutes prior to ECoG recording.

(e) Patient-controlled analgesia with propofol has also been used effectively.

(f) Antiemetic agents (dimenhydrinate, prochlorperazine, metoclopramide, droperidol) are useful and some may also provide additional sedation without affecting the ECoG.

(g) All drugs should be discontinued prior to ECoG recording and testing.

(5) **Nonpharmacologic measures** are very useful to help the patient through the procedure. These include frequent reassurance, allowing the patient to move intermittently, warning the patient in advance about loud noise (drilling bone) and painful areas, ice chips, a cold cloth to face, and just holding the patient's hand.

f. **Intraoperative complications**

(1) **Pain/discomfort.** There are certain times when patients might feel pain or discomfort; they should be warned about these, e.g., the scalp block. Pain and/or discomfort might also be experienced during the bone work if dural vessels come in contact with instruments, and during the manipulation of the dura mater and major vessels within brain tissue. The loud noises of drills and rongeurs can be frightening, if not painful.

(2) **Nausea/vomiting.** Many factors can influence the high incidence of nausea and vomiting, such as anxiety, medications, and surgical stimulation, especially the stripping of dura and manipulation of the temporal lobe or meningeal vessels.

(3) **Seizures** can occur at any time.

(a) Short, mild seizures might not require any treatment. Seizures that are convulsive or generalized need to be treated.

(b) The patient should be protected from injury.

(c) Ensure patent airway, adequate oxygenation, and circulatory stability.

(d) Prior to ECoG recording, seizures can be treated with a small dose of thiopental (25 to 50 mg) or propofol (10 to 20 mg).

(e) After all recordings are completed, benzodiazepines may be used.

(f) If repeated treatments are required, the patient may become very drowsy and need airway support.

(4) **Induction of anesthesia.** If a patient becomes uncooperative or complications such as continuous seizures or hemorrhage develop, the induction of general anesthesia might be required. To do this safely one needs to have a plan of action. Airway assessment will determine the best approach.

(a) Frequently, routine oral intubation with patient on his side is possible. With adequate assistance, the anesthesiologist is positioned at the head of the patient with the surgeon protecting the sterile brain field. After preoxygenation, anesthesia is induced with a small dose of thiopental or propofol (with or without opioid) and a short-acting muscle relaxant (succinylcholine).

(b) If any difficulty in securing the airway is anticipated, an awake intubation with local anesthesia should be performed. This may be with direct or fiberoptic laryngoscopy, and intubation may be either orally or nasally.

(c) The laryngeal mask airway may be another alternative.

(5) Other complications that are less common include excessive blood loss and a tight brain.

g. **Closure.** During closure the patient may be sedated with other agents that were not used prior to this, such as benzodiazepines. Frequently, patients will require nothing as they are tired and will fall asleep.

   h. **Recovery** of the patient should be in an intensive care unit or specialized observation unit. Postoperative complications are the same as for any patient following a craniotomy. Seizures might still occur and may require treatment.

2. **General anesthesia**
   a. **The reason** for choosing general anesthesia is the preference of the surgeon and/or the inability of the patient to tolerate an awake craniotomy.
   b. **The challenge** is to provide good conditions for EEG/ECoG and for motor testing, ensuring that the influence of the anesthetic agents be kept at a minimum, but also avoiding long periods of potential awareness on the part of the patient.
   c. **Specific preoperative preparation** is to inform patients of the possibility that awareness might occur at the time of ECoG recording and testing, but reassuring them that this will be brief and painless.
   d. **Preparation** of the operating room, anesthetic equipment and agents, and for positioning are as for any craniotomy. In addition to routine monitors, intraarterial and urinary catheters are frequently used.
   e. **Anesthetic management**
      (1) **Specific concerns** include the effects of long-term anticonvulsant therapy with the increased dosage requirements of opioids and neuromuscular blocking agents.
      (2) **Nitrous oxide.** If the patient has had a recent craniotomy or burr holes for electrode placement, intracranial air might still be present. Nitrous oxide should be avoided to prevent complications from an expanding pneumocephalus.
      (3) **Anesthetic agents**
         (a) Should be short acting with minimal influence on EEG/ECoG and non-seizure-producing activity.
         (b) A balanced technique is best with opioids, muscle relaxant, nitrous oxide, and low concentrations of inhalation agent.
         (c) Total intravenous anesthesia with propofol may also be used.
         (d) Inhalation agents and propofol must be eliminated at least 20 minutes prior to ECoG recordings. Nitrous oxide might also have to be eliminated.
         (e) The addition of droperidol may

help decrease the chance of awareness.

    (4) Motor testing is possible during general anesthesia by discontinuing all inhalation agents and propofol, and reversing or allowing the muscle paralysis to wear off. This testing demands very careful planning and care of the patient. Additional opioids or lidocaine might decrease the chance of the patient's coughing.

  f. Complications
    (1) The complications of any craniotomy
    (2) The possibility of awareness
    (3) Movement from seizures if the patient is not adequately paralyzed

  g. Recovery is the same as for awake patients.

F. Pediatric surgery. The considerations for pediatric surgery for epilepsy are similar to those for the adult, except that most children will not be able to tolerate an awake craniotomy. Therefore, most procedures are under general anesthesia. An older child might be able to cooperate. Coexisting conditions with multiple organ system involvement or significant psychological and behavior problems might be present. Parents may be very closely involved in the patient's management and will require consideration as well.

G. Cerebral hemispherectomy and corpus callosotomy. Treatment of generalized seizures that are diffuse might require the resection of substantial portions of the entire cerebral hemisphere or section of the corpus callosum. These procedures are usually done under general anesthesia as they involve a large craniotomy and most of the patients are children. The major concerns of these lengthy procedures are the possibility of extensive blood loss and air emboli as the surgical site is close to major vessels and sinuses.

SUGGESTED READINGS

Eldredge EA, Soriano SG, Rockoff MA. Surgical treatment of epilepsy in children: neuroanesthesia. *Neurosurg Clin North Am* 1995;6:505.

Engel J Jr. *Seizures and epilepsy.* Philadelphia: FA Davis Co, 1989.

Kofke WA, Tempelhoff R, Dasheiff RM. Anesthetic implications of epilepsy, status epilepticus, and epilepsy surgery. *J Neurosurg Anesthesiol* 1997;9:349.

Manninen PH, Contreras J. Anesthetic considerations for craniotomy in awake patients. *Int Anesthesiol Clin* 1986;24:157.

Modica PA, Tempelhoff R, White PF. Pro- and anticonvulsant effects of anesthetics, Parts 1 and 2. *Anesth Analg* 1990;70:303, 70:433.

15

Disruption of the Blood–Brain Barrier

Paolo Bolognese

The central nervous system (CNS) is provided with a specialized environment that is watery in composition, chemically precise, and sheltered from the blood by the blood–brain barrier (BBB). The extracellular (EC) compartment of the CNS has two fluids:

- Interstitial fluid (ISF)
- Cerebrospinal fluid (CSF)

I. **The Blood–Brain Barrier.** The BBB is a structure guarding the passage of plasma constituents into the EC compartment of the brain. It is formed by two main structures: the capillary endothelium and the perivascular astrocytes.
   A. **The capillary endothelium.** In most areas of the brain, the cells of the capillary endothelium differ from those found in other tissues of the body.
      1. The distinctive features of the cerebral capillary endothelium are:
         a. The absence of **fenestrations**.
         b. The presence of **tight junctions** (zonulae occludentes).
         c. The low (thin) cellular profile of **plasmalemmal pits and vesicles**.
         d. The high (thick) cellular profile of **mitochondria**.
      2. The tight junctions of the cerebral endothelium impose an obligatory restraint on the movement of substances between blood and brain based on molecular size.
      3. The cerebral endothelium is unquestionably impermeable to large or polar molecules. It is, however, highly permeable to most lipid-soluble substances and exhibits variable permeability to ions, small nonelectrolytes, and urea.
      4. When **hyperosmotic agents** such as urea or mannitol are injected intraarterially, there is a shrinkage of cerebral endothelial cells and a "reversible opening" of the tight junctions.
   B. **The foot processes of the perivascular astrocytes** are spread beyond the capillary tubule and are closely applied to its basement membrane, forming a complete cuff around the circumference of the vessel.
      1. Astrocytes contain high concentrations of important enzymes involved with water and sodium (Na^+) transport and energy production.

2. Astrocytic foot processes appear to have a capacity for making rapid and sensitive adjustments in the microchemical environment of the EC compartment.

II. **Specialized ependyma of circumventricular organs**. In a few circumscribed areas of the brain, the cells of the capillary endothelium are not joined by tight junctions. The vessels are fenestrated or "open" like those in other organs of the body. Each of these areas borders the cerebral ventricles, and all are involved with specific secretory activities that presumably require a direct contact with the plasma. They include:
   A. The four choroid plexuses.
   B. The median eminence.
   C. The neural lobe of the hypophysis.
   D. The organum vasculosum lamina terminalis.
   E. The subfornical organ.
   F. The subcommissural organ.
   G. The pineal gland.
   H. The area postrema.

III. **Internal milieu**. An essential function of the BBB is to provide a specialized environment for nervous tissue. Within limits, the chemical composition of the brain EC fluid is carefully regulated, and a variety of substances, especially those that are large, polar, or lipid-insoluble, are almost totally excluded from the brain. In this manner, the CNS is protected from toxic or potentially toxic substances, and the CSF is maintained as a protein-poor product of the plasma. The cells of the CNS are metabolically active. The milieu that surrounds them is responsible for a number of functions:
   A. Providing a large and continuous supply of substrates, despite transient and often wide variations in the plasma concentrations of these substances (e.g., glucose).
   B. Maintaining a chemically precise environment that is suitable for the electrophysiologic needs of nervous tissue.
   C. Removing products of metabolism and disease.

IV. **Brain extracellular compartment**. The EC spaces of the brain form a series of narrow, interconnecting channels that are anatomically continuous with the cerebral ventricles and subarachnoid space.
   A. The macroscopic CSF cavities consist of two main compartments:
      1. **An internal compartment**, formed by the three cerebral ventricles, the aqueduct of Sylvius, the fourth (cerebellar) ventricle, and the central canal of the spinal cord.
      2. **An external compartment** formed by the cisterns, fissures, and sulci of the subarachnoid space.
   B. Each cavity is continuous with the next through one or more well-defined openings, and the pathway terminates at the level of the dural sinuses where

expansions of the subarachnoid space, the arachnoid villi, protrude into the venous circulation.

C. In humans, the total volume of the CSF cavities is approximately 140 mL. The subarachnoid space, which is by far the larger of the two main compartments, contains approximately 118 to 120 mL of fluid, of which 30 mL belongs to the spinal subarachnoid space.

D. The volume of the cerebral ventricles is given as 20 to 23 mL, with each lateral ventricle accounting for approximately 7.5 mL. It is estimated that the total brain EC compartment (interstitial and CSF spaces) represents 10% to 15% of total brain.

V. **Lymphatic-like function of brain EC fluid**. The CSF formation rate in humans is approximately 0.37 ± 0.1 mL/minute, or 500 mL/day. The CSF volume is renewed every 8 hours.

A. **CSF is formed** by two mechanisms:
1. Secretion of the choroid plexuses.
2. Lymphatic-like drainage of brain interstitial fluid (ISF).

B. The **production of brain ISF** appears to involve the following steps:
1. Ultrafiltration and active transport by the cerebral endothelium.
2. Formation of water of metabolism by the cellular elements of the brain.
3. Addition of metabolic wastes.

C. The **movement of brain ISF** occurs by bulk flow through the narrow intercellular clefts of the neuropil and appears to be influenced by the hydrostatic pressure gradient between ISF and CSF.

D. The **CSF flows** in bulk from the cerebral ventricles into the subarachnoid space from which it is absorbed across the arachnoid villi and perineural lymphatics.

E. The following factors contribute to the circulatory movement of CSF:
1. The continuous outpouring of newly formed ventricular fluid.
2. The ventricular pulsations, representing the combined effects of respiratory variations and pulsations emanating from cerebral arteries and choroid plexuses.
3. The pressure gradient across the arachnoid villi.

VI. **Traditional classification of cerebral edema**. Cerebral edema may be defined as an increase in brain water content of sufficient magnitude to produce clinical symptoms.

A. It is current practice to classify the cerebral edemas into two main types:
1. Vasogenic edema, caused by increased permeability of the BBB.
2. Cytotoxic edema, characterized by an abnormal

uptake of water by the cellular elements of the brain.

B. While useful, this classification equates cellular swelling with "edema" and fails to include a number of important types, such as periventricular edema occurring with hydrocephalus and parenchymal edema occurring with water intoxication, plasma hypoosmolarity, and inappropriate secretion of antidiuretic hormone.

VII. **A comprehensive approach to the classification of cerebral edema**. Like other organs in the body, the brain has three anatomic compartments that can accumulate fluid in excessive amounts: the vascular compartment, composed of arteries, capillaries, and veins; the cellular compartment, composed of cells and their subcellular extensions; and the EC compartment, composed of the ISF and the CSF spaces. Many diseases produce mixed types.

A. **Increased vascular volume.** Volumetric expansion of the cerebrovascular bed can occur as a consequence of two mechanisms:

1. **Arterial dilatation.** Under normal conditions, the cerebral circulation responds rapidly and precisely to the metabolic needs of the brain. Pathologic processes can alter metabolic needs or directly disturb arterial tone and caliber.

2. **Venous obstruction.** Obstruction of the cerebral veins or dural sinuses can occur with a wide variety of disorders including bacterial meningitis, subdural abscess, parasagittal tumors, head trauma, radical neck dissection, head and neck tumors, strangulation, superior vena cava syndrome, and right heart failure.

B. **Cellular swelling.** The excessive uptake by cells of fluid or other abnormal substances can lead to varying degrees of brain swelling. Two general types of cellular swelling are:

1. **Cytotoxic edema.** This is a disturbance of cellular osmoregulation that results in the abnormal uptake of fluid within the cytoplasm of cells. The primary mechanism appears to be a disturbance of the energy dependent Na^+-K^+ pump of the cell membrane which serves to exclude Na^+, and hence water, from the intracellular compartment. The most common clinical disorder to cause cytotoxic brain swelling is cerebral ischemia.

2. **Metabolic storage.** The intracellular uptake of abnormal metabolites is common to a rare group of inherited disorders known collectively as the storage diseases. These include the intracellular storage of mucopolysaccharides (Hurler's disease), GM_2 ganglioside (Tay-Sachs disease), and sphingomyelin (Niemann-Pick disease).

C. **Extracellular edema.** Extracellular or "wet" brain edema includes four general types:

1. **Vasogenic.** This is the most common type of EC edema. The spread of vasogenic edema follows the normal pathways of ISF bulk flow, preferentially through the white matter. Its driving force is the mean arterial pressure. The magnitude of edema formation depends on a number of other variables including the severity of BBB dysfunction, the size of the lesion, and the duration of barrier opening. It occurs as a consequence of increased permeability of brain capillaries. The mechanisms of increased brain capillary permeability include:

    a. **Structural injury of the cerebral endothelium** leading to opening of tight junctions, increased pinocytosis, or disruption of cells.

    b. **Metabolic impairment** of endothelial transport systems.

    c. **Neovascularization** by vessels lacking BBB characteristics.

2. **Osmotic edema.** Formation of this type of edema depends on the establishment of an unfavorable osmotic gradient between the plasma and the brain EC fluid. For osmotic edema to develop, the BBB must be intact. Osmotic edema might occur in association with a number of hypoosmolar conditions including the improper administration of intravenous fluids, compulsive drinking by psychiatric patients, inappropriate secretion of antidiuretic hormone, pseudotumor cerebri, and excessive hemodialysis of uremic patients.

3. **Compressive edema.** Compressive edema can be caused by any mass lesion that obstructs the bulk flow of brain ISF. This type of edema is a common complication of benign tumors that do not alter BBB permeability (e.g., meningioma), but probably occurs to some extent with all large intracranial masses.

4. **Hydrocephalic edema.** The edema of hydrocephalus, more than any other type of cerebral edema, resembles lymphedema in the general body tissues. With few exceptions, both result from obstruction of the drainage channels, which leads to distention of the cavities proximal to the block with retrograde flooding of the EC compartment. In acute hydrocephalus, the earliest finding involving the brain parenchyma is periventricular edema. The formation of hydrocephalic edema probably involves two mechanisms:

    a. **Stasis of brain ISF**, occurring as a consequence of the reduced gradient for bulk flow into the cerebral ventricles.

    b. Reflux of CSF into the periventricular tissues, occurring as a consequence of increased intraventricular pressure.

VIII. Treatment of cerebral edema

  A. Surgical excision. Surgical excision of mass lesions (e.g., tumors, abscesses, subdural hematoma) is effective in the treatment of compressive edema and the vasogenic component that attends neovascularization or increased capillary permeability. In addition to removing leaky capillaries, surgical excision reduces the release of potentially toxic substances, such as free radicals and prostaglandins, and usually improves local cerebral perfusion by reducing mass effect.

  B. Head elevation. It is standard clinical practice to elevate the head of patients with cerebral edema in order to facilitate cerebrovenous drainage and reduce ICP. However, there is evidence that the cerebral perfusion pressure is maximal in the horizontal position and that elevation of the head above the heart reduces the hydrostatic force of the systemic arterial circulation.

  C. Hyperventilation. Since cerebral vessels are exquisitely sensitive to changes in CO_2 tension, hyperventilation is an effective means for reducing ICP. This vasoconstricts cerebral arteries and arterioles, and leads to a commensurate reduction of cerebral blood flow and volume. This effect continues until CSF pH returns to a near-normal range. Prolonged or excessive hyperventilation can lead to diffuse cerebral hypoxia and the accumulation of lactic acid within the parenchymal tissues.

  D. Osmotherapy. The use of hypertonic drugs (osmotherapy) is an effective means for producing a rapid reduction of brain water content. The clinical benefits of hypertonic drugs derive from their ability to withdraw water from tissues osmotically and not to their diuretic effect, although the duration of action of osmotherapy can be prolonged by the use of loop diuretics (e.g., furosemide, ethacrynic acid) that preferentially excrete water as compared to solute.

    Contrary to popular belief, hypertonic drugs have little direct effect on edematous tissues and do not remove edema fluid per se. Although hypertonic drugs have only a limited direct effect on edema fluid, they have been shown to reduce blood viscosity and tend to increase local cerebral blood flow (CBF). If autoregulation is intact, such changes can potentially lead to some vasoconstriction with a reduction of "filtration edema" or to an increased efflux of fluid as a consequence of enhanced drug action.

E. Steroids. To date, the most clearly established benefits of glucocorticoids concern their ability to influence perifocal edema surrounding mass lesions.

1. A dramatic response to steroids is seen in patients with vasogenically induced causes such as Addison's disease, intoxications, and allergic reactions.

2. The administration of glucocorticoids appears to be relatively ineffective when cerebral autoregulation is impaired.

3. Steroid therapy is rarely of benefit in the treatment of acute hemorrhagic conditions (e.g., intracerebral hematoma) and not helpful in the management of patients with severe closed head injuries.

4. The mechanisms by which steroids influence vasogenic edema are as follows:

   a. **Stabilization of the cerebral endothelium** leading to a decrease of plasma filtration.

   b. **Increase in lysosomal activity** of cerebral capillaries.

   c. **Inhibition of the release of potentially toxic substances** such as free radicals, fatty acids, and prostaglandins.

   d. **Electrolyte shifts** favoring transcapillary efflux of fluid.

   e. **Increase in local and global cerebral glucose utilization** leading to improved neuronal function.

F. Antiinflammatory agents. Because of the many recognized complications of steroid therapy, increasing attention has been focused on the potential use of nonsteroidal antiinflammatory drugs (e.g., indomethacin, probenecid, ibuprofen) in the treatment of vasogenic edema. The mechanism of action of nonsteroidal antiinflammatory drugs has not been fully elucidated but appears to be related to a direct inhibition of the arachidonic acid–prostaglandin cascade.

G. Antihypertensive drugs. Since the formation and spread of vasogenic edema are directly related to the systemic arterial pressure, it is desirable to reduce any untoward elevations of blood pressure.

H. CSF Drainage. Cerebrospinal fluid shunting is effective in resolving periventricular edema associated with hydrocephalus and is sometimes required in the treatment of patients with refractory pseudotumor cerebri.

I. Barbiturate coma. The therapeutic benefits of barbiturate coma are difficult to assess because the treatment is often a choice of last resort and is used in conjunction with many other modalities. However, barbiturates have been shown to reduce the metabolic needs of the brain, and their apparent usefulness in management of vasogenic edema might be related to the ability to control systemic arterial pressure and hence to reduce the filtration of fluid across leaky capillaries. Objections to barbiturate coma include:

1. **Reduction or elimination of neurologic responses** that are often crucial in assessing the patient's progress.
2. **The procedure requires continuous physiologic monitoring** (e.g., intracranial pressure, blood gases, central venous pressure, arterial pressure) and assisted ventilation in a critical care unit.

J. **Operative decompression**. The creation of a cranial opening (external decompression) with or without the resection of brain tissue (internal decompression) is a time-honored way to combat massive brain swelling. It is desirable to perform a generous subtemporal decompression and open the dura. If the brain is devitalized, necrotic tissue should be removed, and resection of the temporal lobe tip might relieve compression of the brain stem.

SUGGESTED READINGS

Chestnut RM. The management of severe traumatic brain injury. *Emerg Med Clin North Am* 1997;15(3):581–604.

Jafar JJ, Johns LM, Mullan SF. The effect of mannitol on cerebral blood flow. *J Neurosurg* 1986;64:754–760.

Milhorat TH. *Cerebrospinal fluid and the brain edemas.* New York: Neuroscience Society of New York, 1987.

Selmaj K. Pathophysiology of the blood brain barrier. *Springer Semin Immunopathol* 1996;18(1):57–73.

Spinal Cord: Injury and Procedures

Gary R. Stier, Joseph P. Giffin, Daniel J. Cole, and Elie Fried

I. General considerations

A. Spinal anatomy and physiology

1. **Structure**
   a. The vertebral column is composed of seven cervical (C), twelve thoracic (T), five lumbar (L), five sacral (fused), and four coccygeal (fused) bones. Individual vertebrae are composed of a ventral vertebral body and a dorsal bony neural arch composed of a pedicle on either side of the vertebral body, each supporting a lamina, which combine posteriorly to form a spinous process. The vertebral foramen is formed by the posterior vertebral body, pedicles, and lamina. The neural laminar arches bear lateral transverse processes and superior and inferior articular facets.
   b. The vertebral column is stabilized by ligaments (from posterior to anterior): supraspinous, interspinal, ligamentum flavum, posterior longitudinal, and anterior longitudinal ligaments. The ligaments provide flexibility and limit excessive movement that could damage the cord.
   c. The spinal cord begins at the foramen magnum and terminates at the conus medullaris (L_2 in adults). Below the termination of the spinal cord, the lumbar and sacral roots form the cauda equina. The anterior portion of the cord gives rise to the motor nerves. Nerves that originate posteriorly are sensory in function.

2. **Blood supply**
   a. **Anterior spinal artery.** A single vessel formed by the two vertebral arteries supplies the anterior 75% of the cord.

b. **Posterior spinal arteries.** Two vessels orig-inating from the posterior inferior cerebellar arteries supply the posterior 25% of the cord.

c. **Radicular arteries.** Originate from branches of the vertebral, deep cervical, in-tercostal, and lumbar arteries. They anasto-mose with the anterior and posterior spinal arteries. The artery of Adamkiewicz (arteria radicularis magna), the major radicular ar-tery, is most commonly located in the lower thoracic or upper lumbar region and provides most of the blood supply to the lower cord.

3. **Regulation of blood flow.** Autoregulation main-tains spinal cord blood flow by altering vascular resistance in response to changes in mean arte-rial pressure (MAP).

a. Normal autoregulation exists for a MAP be-tween 50 and 150 mm Hg.

b. Failure of autoregulation at a MAP of less than 50 mm Hg leads to ischemia.

c. At a MAP of greater than 150 mm Hg, the increased flow leads to tissue edema and dis-ruption.

d. The autoregulatory range of individuals with chronic hypertension is shifted to the right (higher range of MAP).

e. Alterations in $PaCO_2$ and PaO_2 disrupt auto-regulation in the spinal cord much as they do in the brain.

II. Spinal cord injury

A. **Introduction.** There are 10,000 new cases per year of spinal cord injury (SCI) in the United States. Early mortality is around 50% with less than 10% of survi-vors experiencing a neurologic improvement. Accord-ingly, the perioperative care of patients during the acute phase of injury is of extreme importance. Peri-operative strategies that prevent an injury, limit the extension of an existing injury, or salvage even a few dermatomal levels can have a significant influence on morbidity, mortality, long-term disability, quality of life, and health care costs.

There is an equal distribution of SCI among incom-plete quadriplegia, complete quadriplegia, incomplete paraplegia, and complete paraplegia. Common causes of SCI include motor vehicle accidents, falls, violence, and sports. Most injuries occur at the midcervical or thoracolumbar region and are often associated with concomitant injuries. Surgical treatment for SCI is aimed at immobilization, medical stabilization, spinal alignment, operative decompression, and spinal stabilization. This section focuses on the perioperative care of the patient with or at risk for acute SCI. Specific issues pertaining to an intermediate or chronic phase of injury are also discussed.

B. Pathogenic correlates of spinal cord injury

1. **Primary SCI**, caused by the mechanical forces of the trauma, results in direct neuronal disruption and destruction, petechial hemorrhages, and hematomyelia. Histologic changes consist of hemorrhage and protein extravasation into the central gray matter, which spread to adjacent white matter. The traumatized areas then undergo cavitating necrosis and ultimately glial scar formation. Spinal cord edema is maximal at 3 days and may persist for 2 weeks. Rarely does physical transection of the spinal cord occur.

2. **Secondary SCI** is due to activation of biochemical, enzymatic, and microvascular processes in proportion to the severity of the initial lesion. Damage is caused by progressive hemorrhagic necrosis, edema, and inflammation. These processes lead to vascular stasis, decreased spinal blood flow, ischemia, and cell death.

C. Anatomical correlates of spinal cord injury (see Table 16-1). Flexion injuries cause anterior subluxation or fracture-dislocations of the vertebral bodies. Hyperextension is associated with transverse fractures of the vertebra, disruption of the anterior longitudinal ligaments, and posterior dislocations. Vertical compression produces burst fractures and ligamentous rupture. Rotational injuries might result in fractures of the vertebral peduncles and facets.

D. Clinical correlates of spinal cord injury. Spinal cord injury can result in complete (total loss of sensory and motor function distal to the injury) or incomplete (presence of any nonreflex function distal to the

Table 16-1. Spinal injury, clinical finding, and indicated treatment

Spinal Injury	Clinical Finding	Treatment
Atlantooccipital dislocation	Usually unstable; commonly fatal	Reduction, immobilization, fusion
Atlantoaxial injury:		
Isolated atlas fracture	Usually stable/no neurologic injury	Philadelphia collar
Isolated odontoid fracture	Usually neurologically intact	Immobilization
Displaced fracture C_{1-2}	Commonly fatal or quadriplegic	Immobilization and reduction
Posterior subluxation C_{1-2}	Usually neurologically intact	Immobilization
Axis pedical fracture	May be neurologically intact	Immobilization
Hyperflexion dislocation C_3–T_1	Any subluxation is unstable	If neurologic deficit, decompression
Dislocated facets	Neurologically variable	Traction and surgery
Flexion-rotation injuries	Neurologically variable	Surgical reduction and fusion if anterior subluxation and jumped facet
Compression fractures C_3–T_1:		
Wedge compression/burst fractures	Frequent neurologic damage	Surgical decompression
Teardrop fractures (vertebra dislocated anteriorly with inferior vertebral fracture)	Usually unstable	Posterior fusion
Hyperextension injuries C_3–T_1:	Geriatric patients with spondylosis producing central cord syndrome	Immobilization; if significant spinal canal narrowing, decompression
Thoracic spine injuries	Incomplete neurologic injury most common	Realignment and stabilization
Thoracolumbar injuries	Neurologic deficits complex	Decompression and fusion
Lumbar injuries	Incomplete neurologic injury	Realignment and decompression
Penetrating injuries	Neurologic deficit variable	Decompression/foreign body removal

Table 16-2.   Incomplete spinal cord injury syndromes

Syndrome	Clinical Findings
Anterior cord syndrome	Motor, sensory, temperature, and pain lost; vibration/position intact.
Central cord syndrome	Motor impairment of upper more than lower extremities.
Posterior cord syndrome	Loss of fine, vibratory, and position sensation; preserved motor function.
Brown-Séquard (hemicord) syndrome	Ipsilateral paralysis; loss of proprioception, touch, and vibration; contralateral loss of pain and temperature.
Conus medullaris syndrome	Areflexic bladder, bowel, and lower extremities; sacral reflexes might be preserved; reduced rectal tone and perirectal sensation.
Cauda equina syndrome	Sensory loss with flaccid weakness. Sacral reflexes abnormal or absent.

injury; see Table 16-2) loss of neurologic function. Complete spinal cord injuries have less than a 10% chance of complete return of normal neurologic function. Incomplete SCI has a 59% to 75% chance of recovering lost function. The range of cardiac and respiratory dysfunction, dependent on the site of acute

Table 16-3.   Level of spinal cord injury and pulmonary/cardiac function[a]

Level of SCI	Pulmonary Function		Cardiovascular Function	
	Ventilatory Function	Cough	Sympathetic Function	Cardiovascular Reserve
$C_{1,2}$	0	0	Minimal	Minimal
$C_{3,4}$	0	0	Minimal	Minimal
$C_{5,6}$	+	+	Minimal	Minimal
C_7	+--++	+-++	Minimal	+
High thoracic	++	++	+-++	++
Low thoracic	++-+++	++-+++	++-+++	++-+++
Lumbar	+++	+++	+++	+++
Sacral	+++	+++	+++	+++

SCI, spinal cord injury.
[a]Scale is 0 (no function) to +++ (normal).

SCI, is detailed in Table 16-3. Medical problems include:

Cardiovascular
- Spinal shock
- Bradycardia
- ↓ Myocardial contractility
- Deep venous thrombosis
- Hypothermia

Respiratory
- Respiratory impairment
- Poor cough
- Viscous mucus

Gastrointestinal
- Atony
- Prone to aspiration

Genitourinary
- Bladder distension
- Infection

Electrolytes
- Hypercalcemia
- Hyperphosphatemia
- Hyponatremia
- Hyperkalemia

The effects that SCIs have on the cardiovascular system depend on the level of injury (see Table 16-3). For levels of SCI below T_6, the major problem involves varying degrees of hypotension resulting from the functional sympathectomy. With complete SCI above C_6, more significant cardiovascular abnormalities are encountered including bradycardia, hypotension, ventricular dysfunction, and dysrhythmias.

1. **Spinal shock,** seen with physiologic or anatomic transection of the spinal cord above C_6, results from a total loss of impulses from higher centers as an immediate consequence of injury.
    a. This syndrome of loss of sensory and motor function and autonomic dysfunction lasts from days to weeks and is prolonged by serious infection.
    b. Spinal shock is characterized by flaccid paralysis, loss of reflexes below the level of the lesion, paralytic ileus, and loss of visceral and somatic sensation, vascular tone, and vasopressor reflex. The lack of sympathetic outflow can cause vasodilatation, pooling of blood in peripheral vascular beds, postural hypotension, and bradycardia.
        (1) **Bradycardia,** universal with complete cervical SCI, results from a functional sympathectomy with interruption of cardiac accelerator nerves (T_{1-4}) and unopposed vagal innervation. Bradycardia usually resolves over a 3- to 5-week period. More profound degrees of bradycardia, as well as cardiac arrest, might occur during stimulation of the patient (e.g., turning the patient, tracheal suctioning). Familiarity with the factors precipitating bradycardia will lead to preventive interventions (sedation, anti-

cholinergics, 100% oxygen prior to suctioning, and limiting the time allowed for suctioning). Although these episodes are effectively treated with atropine in most cases, a temporary pacemaker might be required.

(2) **Hypotension** occurs because the loss of sympathetic tone causes peripheral vasodilatation. Early intervention to maintain diastolic blood pressure above 70 mm Hg is necessary to preserve neurologic function as autoregulation is impaired. The heart rate is useful in differentiating between neurogenic shock, associated with bradycardia, and hemorrhagic shock, which causes tachycardia. Hypovolemia from coexisting hemorrhagic shock in patients with spinal shock is treated with prompt blood replacement and administration of isotonic crystalloid. The total volume of fluid administered is limited as pulmonary edema and cardiac decompensation can occur, especially in the setting of high SCI.

(a) If hypotension persists despite adequate fluid administration, vasopressor therapy should be instituted. The vasopressor should have β-agonist properties (e.g., dopamine or dobutamine). Supplementation with an α agonist such as phenylephrine might be necessary. However, care is indicated when choosing a more potent α-agonist, such as norepinephrine, which may substantially increase cardiac afterload, impair cardiac output, and precipitate frank left ventricular failure.

(b) Invasive central hemodynamic monitoring is recommended in high SCI as an aid in guiding clinical management of hypotension. A pulmonary artery occlusion pressure of 15 to 18 mm Hg appears to optimize spinal cord perfusion. In patients who have suffered multiple trauma, hypotension and bradycardia secondary to spinal shock might conceal hemorrhagic shock. Operative intervention for spinal injury is postponed until the patient's hemodynamic status has been optimized.

2. **Disturbances of cardiac rhythm** are commonly observed in SCI and include bradycardia, primary asystole, supraventricular dysrhythmias (atrial fibrillation, reentry supraventricular tachycardia), and ventricular dysrhythmias. An acute autonomic imbalance resulting from a disruption of sympathetic pathways in the cervical cord is causative. The arrhythmia usually resolves within 14 days after injury.

3. **Left ventricular impairment** has been noted in complete cervical SCI and is also attributed to the functional sympathectomy with resulting autonomic imbalance.

4. **Autonomic hyperreflexia** occurs in 85% of patients with spinal cord transections above T_6. This clinical constellation is secondary to autonomic vascular reflexes, which usually begin to appear about 1 to 3 weeks after injury.
   a. Afferent impulses originating from cutaneous, proprioceptive, and visceral stimuli (bladder or bowel distention, childbirth, manipulations of the urinary tract, or surgical stimulation) are transmitted to the isolated spinal cord. They, in turn, elicit a massive sympathetic response from the adrenal medulla and sympathetic nervous system, which is no longer modulated by the normal inhibitory impulses from the brain stem and hypothalamus. Vasoconstriction occurs below the lesion. Reflex activity of carotid and aortic baroreceptors produces vasodilatation above the lesion, which is often accompanied by bradycardia, ventricular dysrhythmias, and even complete heart block.
   b. Common symptoms include hypertension, bradycardia, hyperreflexia, muscle rigidity and spasticity, diaphoresis, pallor, flushing above the lesion, and headache. Horner's syndrome, pupillary changes, anxiety, and nausea occur less frequently. Systolic pressures in excess of 260 mm Hg and diastolic pressures of 220 mm Hg have been reported.
   c. Adverse sequelae include myocardial ischemia, intracranial hemorrhage, pulmonary edema, seizures, coma, and death.
   d. Treatment involves cessation of the offending stimulus and change to the upright position. Pharmacologic intervention includes direct-

acting vasodilators (e.g., sodium nitroprusside), beta blockers (e.g., esmolol), combination alpha and beta blockers (e.g., labetalol),
calcium channel blocking agents, or ganglionic blocking agents. As the attacks are often
paroxysmal, drugs of rapid onset and short
duration are preferred.

E.   Acute care of the patient with spinal cord injury.
Preservation of spinal cord function involves maintaining oxygen delivery, stabilizing the spine, decreasing spinal cord edema, and decreasing secondary
biochemical processes that worsen neurologic injury.
The initial care of the patient with a SCI can be considered in the following areas:

   1.   External splinting and immobilization. Immobilization of the spine is done in the field by placing the patient on a spine board with sandbags
on either side of the head to prevent rotation.

   2.   Medical management. Identification of associated injuries is crucial. These include:

   *Cervical Spine   Thoracic Spine
      Injury   Injury*
   • Head   • Myocardial
   • Airway   • Pulmonary
   • Esophagus   • Ribs
   Lumbar Spine Injury   • Major vascular
   • Abdominal
   • Pelvic

   a.   Airway
      (1)   Spinal cord injury presents several prob-
lems in airway management. Many ma-
neuvers used for intubation can cause
displacement and worsening of the injury, especially at the level of the cervical spine (C-spine). For this reason, all
patients with head trauma, multiple
trauma, or decreased level of consciousness should be considered as having a
spinal injury until proven otherwise ra-

diographically (see Fig. 16-1 for a decision algorithm in airway management for suspected C-spine injury).

(2) Patients with a normal level of consciousness, an intact "gag reflex," and a patent airway may be managed conservatively with supplemental oxygen. These patients should be observed closely to detect progressive loss of ventilatory ability as a result of developing diaphragmatic or intercostal paralysis.

(3) Blind nasal intubation is commonly recommended. The benefit of this technique is minimal head movement. Potential disadvantages include an extended period of time to perform and trauma to the nasal passage. Nasotracheal intubation is contraindicated in the presence of a basilar skull fracture or extensive facial trauma.

(4) Fiberoptic intubation is appropriate in non-emergent situations where the airway is free of blood and stomach contents.

(5) A catheter passed through a needle inserted into the cricothyroid membrane ("retrograde intubation") and directed out the nose or mouth may also serve as a guide for intubation.

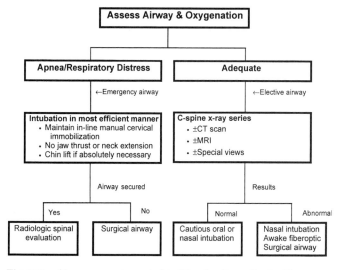

Fig. 16-1. Airway management algorithm for the patient with suspected cervical spine injury.

(6) Flexion and extension of the neck during maintenance of the airway and intubation might lead to catastrophic exacerbation of the spinal injury. Therefore, in-line manual stabilization should be utilized when traditional laryngoscopy proves necessary. This is accomplished by having an assistant hold the sides of the neck and the mastoid process, preventing any movement of the neck. The airway can be opened with a "jaw thrust" technique while the head is maintained in a neutral position (lack of flexion and extension).

(7) Because of gastric atony and paralytic ileus, SCI patients are considered to have "full stomachs" and are at increased risk for aspiration. Therefore, airway adjuncts like the laryngeal airway mask, while helpful in maintaining oxygenation in a situation where intubation has proven difficult, should not be relied on as a long-term solution. Cricoid pressure is administered with minimum pressure to avoid inadvertent further injury to the cord. Since neck displacement of up to 9 mm can occur with the application of cricoid pressure, the risk of causing or exacerbating C-spine injury should be judged against the risk of pulmonary aspiration.

(8) While excessive movement of the spine is to be avoided, hypoxia secondary to a failure to intubate has a worse prognosis and intubation should be accomplished as expeditiously as possible. Cricothyroidotomy is an appropriate choice when faced with an anatomically abnormal airway in an emergent situation.

(9) A brief examination after intubation of the trachea will reveal any further deterioration in the patient's neurologic condition related to manipulation of the airway or positioning.

b. Pulmonary system. Spinal cord injury can have a profound effect on the respiratory system, depending on the level and degree of injury, because of paralysis of the abdominal, intercostal, diaphragmatic, and accessory muscles. Problems include respiratory failure, recurrent lobar atelectasis, hypoventilation, ventilation-perfusion mismatching, pulmonary edema (neurogenic, cardiogenic), bacterial pneumonia, aspiration pneumonitis, and coexisting blunt chest trauma.

(1) Respiratory failure is present in nearly all patients with SCI above C_7. The resultant abnormality in respiratory mechanics leads to a reduction in lung volume (tidal volume, expiratory reserve volume, functional residual capacity), impairment of respiratory function [decreased forced vital capacity, FEV_1, (forced expiratory volume in one second) peak forces, peak flows], and retention of pulmonary secretions with progressive hypoxemia and CO_2 retention. In addition, patients might have abdominal distention secondary to gastric atony, which further impairs pulmonary function. Even patients whose weakness does not extend above the abdominal muscles are at risk of abnormal respiratory function because of their inability to clear secretions.

(2) Patients require frequent assessment of respiratory function as significant declines in pulmonary reserve can occur before overt clinical signs of respiratory failure are seen. It is particularly important to perform serial measurements of vital capacity (VC) and negative inspiratory force. When the VC decreases to less than 50% of predicted, more frequent serial determinations of VC must be made (i.e., every 6 hours). When the VC decreases to less than 1 L, especially if the patient is dyspneic and hypoxemic, endotracheal intubation should be performed.

(3) The aim of mechanical ventilation in this scenario is to incorporate spontaneous patient effort into the respiratory dynamic so as to maintain diaphragmatic muscle mass. The combination of synchronized intermittent mandatory ventilation with pressure support will achieve this goal.

   (a) Positive end-expiratory pressure is added, beginning with 5 cm H_2O, to recruit collapsed alveoli and prevent further atelectasis. Choosing larger mechanical tidal volumes (e.g., 10 to 15 mL/kg) might also enhance alveolar recruitment.

   (b) Weaning from mechanical ventilation after cervical SCI is facilitated by the respiratory muscles' development of spasticity (in about 3 weeks). This stabilizes the chest wall sufficiently to cause improvement in lung volume and in overall ventilatory ability. The vital capacity doubles in volume within 5 weeks of injury in patients with injuries at the $C_{4,5}$ level. Respiratory dynamics in the supine position improve due to the more cephalad position of the diaphragm. This position is therefore used when weaning.

(4) Lobar atelectasis, common in SCI above C_7, requires aggressive pulmonary therapy emphasizing the prevention, recognition, and treatment of secretion retention. This regimen, instituted at the time of hospitalization, includes frequent nasotracheal suctioning, frequent repositioning or rotational beds, chest percussion, bronchodilator therapy, deep breathing exercises, incentive spirometry, and assisted coughing. Even with the most aggressive pulmonary care and management, retained secretions result in repeated lobar collapse during the first 2 weeks of hospitalization. Therapeutic bronchoscopy is frequently required.

(5) Pulmonary edema is observed in patients with acute SCI. Neurogenic causes include intracranial hypertension with high cervical cord injury and increases in extravascular lung water secondary to autonomic dysfunction with sympathetic discharge at the time of injury. Cardiogenic pulmonary edema might also occur because of reduced myocardial inotropy and overzealous fluid administration. Meticulous fluid management guided by central monitoring is essential in limiting pulmonary complications.

(6) Pneumonia is observed in 70% of cervical and high thoracic spinal cord injuries. Pneumonia might result from aspiration of gastric contents at the time of the initial injury or occur later due to bacterial infection.

(7) Chest trauma resulting in hemothorax, pulmonary contusions,

pneumothorax, and rib fractures might be present in patients with SCI. These injuries might necessitate prolonged mechanical ventilation with difficulty in weaning and delay operative intervention to stabilize the spine.

c. **Cardiovascular support.** For the first few minutes after SCI there is a brief and substantial autonomic discharge from direct compression of sympathetic nerves. This results in severe hypertension and arrhythmias and can cause left ventricular failure, myocardial infarction, and pulmonary capillary leak. This transient phase is usually not evident by the time the patient arrives in the hospital when hypotension from spinal shock and traumatic hypovolemia is commonly seen.

d. **Gastrointestinal.** During the acute stages of SCI, the gastrointestinal tract loses autonomic neural input and becomes atonic. Intestinal ileus (especially after thoracic and lumbar SCI) and gastric atony might cause gastric distention and place the patient at risk for aspiration. Moreover, the dilatation might cause upward pressure on the diaphragm, adversely affecting ventilation. Insertion of a nasogastric tube will limit distention and reduce the risk of regurgitation.

(1) As hypochloremic metabolic alkalosis may occur with excessive gastric suctioning, careful monitoring of fluid and electrolyte balance must be provided.

(2) Gastritis and gastric ulceration and hemorrhage can occur after SCI, especially in patients requiring mechanical ventilation, or as a result of administration of corticosteroids. Preventive techniques include monitoring of gastric pH and the use of antacids or H_2 blockers.

(3) Other diseases occurring in critically ill patients after SCI include pancreatitis, acalculous cholecystitis, and gastric perforation (especially in those on high-dose steroids).

(4) Patients with acute SCI characteristically are catabolic. Early nutritional supplementation is advised.

e. **Genitourinary.** During the acute stages of SCI, the bladder is flaccid. Insertion of an indwelling urinary catheter is often necessary. Adequate hydration is likely if urinary volume is greater than 0.5 mL/kg/hour in the absence of renal dysfunction.

(1)   Bladder flaccidity is followed by bladder spasticity. The abnormalities with bladder emptying predispose the patient to recurrent urinary tract infections, bladder stones, nephrocalcinosis, and recurrent urosepsis.

(2)   Although an indwelling drainage catheter is required during the initial 2 to 3 weeks after injury to prevent urinary retention and reflex vagal responses, intermittent straight catheterization of the bladder should be instituted as soon as feasible.

(3)   Acute renal failure is uncommon but can occur as a result of hypotension, dehydration, sepsis, or associated trauma.

f.   **Temperature control.** The body temperatures of patients with injuries above C_7 tend to approach that of the environment (poikilothermia) due to the inability to conserve heat in cold environments through vasoconstriction and the inability to sweat in hot ambient conditions. Consequently, these patients are prone to hypothermia if the ambient temperature is lower than normal body temperature. While hypothermia can provide some degree of spinal cord protection, it can also increase the incidence of arrhythmias and prolong the effects of anesthesia. Delayed awakening can be problematic as it interferes with prompt neurologic examination.

g.   **Deep venous thrombosis**. Deep venous thrombosis (DVT) and pulmonary embolism (PE) occur in 12% to 24% and 10% to 13% of SCI patients, respectively. Three fourths of PE occur in the first month after SCI but rarely after 3 months. Pulmonary embolism occurs more often with thoracic injuries and complete SCI. The high incidence of DVT necessitates some form of prophylaxis, including a combination of mechanical compression devices and subcutaneous heparin, low molecular weight heparin, or coumadin. Percutaneous placement of an inferior vena caval filter should be considered if anticoagulation is contraindicated.

3.   **Neurologic examination.** The examination determines areas in need of radiologic evaluation and establishes a baseline for subsequent assessment. The following neurologic examination can be performed quickly and efficiently. A more thorough examination can be performed if indicated:

a. **Consciousness.** Is the patient alert, oriented, and responsive?

b. **Motor system.** Function and strength of the major muscle groups are graded with reference to the normal segmental innervation. If possible, cerebellar function can be assessed by having the patient touch finger to nose.

c. **Sensory system.** Includes an assessment of proprioception and the patient's response to light touch and pinprick. Perirectal sensation and the presence of the bulbocavernosus reflex or the anal-cutaneous reflex are important indicators of the preservation of distal function (sacral sparing), which may mean a more favorable prognosis. A rectal exam is performed to assess voluntary contraction of the anal sphincter. The most caudad level with normal motor and sensory function is designated as the level of injury (see Table 16-4).

d. **Cranial nerves.** The specific nerves evaluated depend on the level of injury, associated injury, and the patient's level of consciousness. The responses most often evaluated include the pupillary reflex, ocular movement,

Table 16-4.   Muscle group with corresponding level of innervation

Injury Level	Sensory Deficit	Affected Muscle Group
C_4	Acromioclavicular joint	Diaphragm
C_5	Antecubital fossa (lateral)	Shoulder rotators and abductors, elbow flexors
C_6	Thumb	Supinators, pronators, wrist extensors
C_7	Middle finger	Elbow extensors, wrist flexors
C_8	Little finger	Finger flexors, distal phalanx
T_1	Antecubital fossa (medial)	Intrinsic hand muscles
L_2	Upper anterior thigh	Hip flexors
L_3	Medial femoral condyle	Knee extensors
L_4	Medial malleolus	Ankle dorsiflexors
L_5	Dorsum of foot	Toe extensors
S_1	Lateral heel	Plantar flexors
S_{2-5}	Popliteal fossa, ischial tuberosity, perianal area	Sphincter ani, bulbocavernosus reflex

tongue movement, and function of the trigeminal and facial nerves.

  e. Reflexes. Commonly tested reflexes include the biceps, triceps, patellar, achilles, abdominal, cremasteric, and Babinski.

4. Radiologic evaluation

  a. Assessment begins with a plain x-ray film. For C-spine injuries, a useful method of analysis of the plain film is:

   (1) *Adequacy* and quality of the occipital-cervical junction, C_{1-7}, and the C_7–T_1 junction.

   (2) *Alignment* of the anterior edge of the vertebral body, the posterior edge of the vertebral body, the spinolaminar junction, and the tips of the spinous process (Fig. 16-2).

   (3) *Bones.* Look for fractures of the vertebral body, pedicle, lamina, and spinous process.

   (4) *Cartilage.* Analyze the disk space and the facet joints.

   (5) *Soft* tissue space. Observe for edema and other abnormalities.

  b. As many as 15% to 20% of patients with a C-spine injury will not have an abnormality on the plain film. A more comprehensive radiologic evaluation may be indicated.

   (1) Computerized tomography (CT) is helpful to:

    (a) Define bony and soft tissue abnormalities.

    (b) Evaluate the lower C-spine.

    (c) Measure spinal canal and neuroforaminal diameter.

    (d) Provide detailed anatomy of the facet joints.

    (e) Detect hematoma formation.

    (f) Determine compression of the spinal canal and spinal stability.

    (g) Detect a unilateral jumped facet or bone fragments in the canal or root foramen.

    (h) Confirm complete reduction of a dislocation.

    (i) Demonstrate hyperdense acute blood or retropulsed vertebral body fragments.

   (2) Magnetic resonance imaging (MRI) is helpful for:

    (a) Determining the degree of injury to

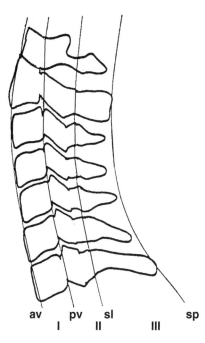

Fig. 16-2. The lateral cervical spine. Spinal column stability after traumatic injury is often based on a system that divides the spine into four longitudinal lines from anterior to posterior, starting with the anterior edge of the vertebral body (av), the posterior edge of the vertebral body (pv), the spinolaminar junction (sl), and the tips of the spinous process (sp). Each line provides the border for three columns (I, II, and III). Disruption of two or more of these columns is indicative of spinal instability.

the soft tissue contents of the spinal cord.

(b) Identifying ligamentous injury, nerve root compression, and spinal cord pathologic signals.

(c) Predicting functional neurologic outcome in the subacute stage of SCI.

(d) Visualizing the epidural and subarachnoid spaces.

(e) Detecting elevation of the anterior or posterior longitudinal ligaments.

5.   Neuroprotective strategies
a.   Spinal alignment

(1) Studies have shown that movement of the injured segment leads to exacerbation of the initial injury. Thus, an important neuroprotective strategy is to relieve cord compression and ischemia and prevent further neurologic compromise by immediate and effective immobilization of the spine with tongs or halo traction devices. Failure to accomplish this may lead to loss of residual neurologic function or even ascension of the patient's neurologic level of injury.

(2) Patients who have unstable injuries are placed in traction to align and immobilize the spine, decompress neural structures, and prevent further injury. Diminished pressure on the cord improves microvascular circulation which might reduce spinal cord edema. If there is no bony instability, traction is not usually needed for patients with penetrating injuries.

(3) Thoracic and lumbar fractures and dislocations may initially be stabilized by restricting the patient to bed rest and turning in a log roll fashion to keep the spine rigid. Subluxations in these regions usually are stabilized by surgical intervention.

b.   Surgical reduction and stabilization might be necessary for dislocations that cannot be reduced by traction and/or manipulation because of the nature of the injury. **Surgical decompression** within the first 2 hours of injury may increase the chances of recovery. The decision as to the timing of surgery depends on:

(1) An assessment of the underlying injury.

(2) Failure of medical, manipulative, and bracing procedures to achieve adequate alignment.

(3) The benefit of early decompression or stabilization of the spine.

(4) The presence of progressive neurologic deficits and/or refractory pain.

(5) The severity of any coexisting illnesses, infections, or trauma.

(6) The possibility of earlier patient mobilization by early surgical intervention.

c.   Physiologic therapy

(1) Cooling has been shown to be effective in the treatment of SCI. Limitations of the clinical studies are small cohorts

and no controls. The high mortality is also of concern. The effect of modest hypothermia on spinal recovery after trauma is currently being evaluated.

(2) Hypertension is advocated by some to improve perfusion in the posttraumatic patient who has evidence of impaired autoregulation and hypoperfusion of the spinal cord. Definitive human data are not available. The MAP is maintained in the normal to high-normal range by volume replacement (non-dextrose-containing crystalloid and/or colloid) if hemorrhagic shock predominates or by inotropes and pressors if neurologic shock is the cause of hypotension. More aggressive hypertension conveys the risk of intramedullary hemorrhage and edema.

(3) Glucose-containing solutions are avoided. Studies in experimental models have shown that even minimally increased blood glucose levels worsen neurologic outcome.

d. **Pharmacologic therapy**

(1) **Methylprednisolone**, in an initial dose of 30 mg/kg, is followed by an infusion of 5.4 mg/kg/hour for 23 hours. This is of benefit only if given within 8 hours of the initial injury. The National Acute Spinal Cord Injury III study, published in 1997, showed that if methylprednisolone is given within 3 hours of SCI, the steroid infusion need only be continued for 24 hours, whereas if therapy is initiated between 3 and 8 hours of injury, 48 hours of steroid infusion should be administered. There has been no increase in the incidence of septic complications with steroids.

(2) **Mannitol**, 0.25 to 1.0 g/kg, may be used to treat cord edema. The ensuing osmotic diuresis necessitates close attention to the patient's intravascular volume.

F. **Anesthetic management of acute spinal cord injury**

1. **Preoperative evaluation.** The SCI patient frequently has multiple medical complications that may impact the anesthetic plan.

a. Indicated studies include complete blood count, serum electrolytes, blood urea nitrogen, creatinine, glucose, liver function tests, and a urinalysis. A preoperative electrocardiogram (ECG), arterial blood gas, chest x-ray, and pulmonary function tests may also be indicated.

b. **Airway evaluation.** Examination of the airway must include the oropharynx with a Mallampati classification and range of motion of the neck with particular attention to any limitation due to pain or neurologic symptoms. If movement elicits any abnormality the offending position is avoided. Airway problems are most frequently encountered in patients with atlantoaxial subluxations, traumatic C-spine injuries in combination with facial trauma, severe kyphoscoliosis or spinal deformities, and spinal stabilization devices. When the patient is in a halo brace or other cervical fixation device, plans for either an awake tracheal intubation or another technique of securing the airway should be made.

c. **Neurologic evaluation** is performed preoperatively and any preexisting neurologic deficits are documented. Regional anesthesia is chosen only after careful evaluation and review of all preexisting deficits.

d. **Pulmonary evaluation** must take into consideration the level of SCI. For instance, patients with C-spine injury have restrictive pulmonary defects and marked reductions in lung volumes which predispose them to hypoxemia. Injuries of the cervical and high thoracic spine also engender difficulties with clearance of secretions, which might predispose patients to hypoxemia and hypercarbia.

e. **Cardiac evaluation** is essential to elicit evidence of cardiovascular dysfunction due to acute SCI or preexisting abnormalities. In addition, assessment of the degree of orthostatic hypotension and the risk of autonomic hyperreflexia should be made.

2. **Monitoring.** Decisions regarding the utilization of advanced monitoring are based on the level of injury and neurologic deficit, the complexity and length of the surgical procedure, and any preexisting underlying medical diseases.

a. **Neurophysiologic** monitoring is often indicated either for patients who have no neurologic injuries but are at high risk due to the instability of their spinal abnormalities or for patients with incomplete neurologic injuries who are undergoing spinal stabilization surgery. Neurophysiologic monitoring might consist of an intraoperative wake-up test, somatosensory evoked potential (SSEP) monitoring, or motor evoked potential monitoring. Somatosensory evoked potentials monitor the posterior columns of the spinal cord, whereas motor evoked potentials monitor the anterior portion of the spinal cord. For a more comprehensive description of spinal cord monitoring, see Chapter 3.

b. Intracranial pressure monitoring might be indicated for patients who also have head injuries.

c. Routine monitors (ECG, pulse oximetry, capnography, non-invasive blood pressure, temperature) are employed for every procedure. A urinary catheter is used to monitor the patient's volume status.

d. In patients with spinal shock, the institution of direct blood pressure monitoring is indicated, ideally before induction. The arterial line is also useful for blood gas measurements and other laboratory determinations that might be necessary intraoperatively.

e. Early use of pulmonary artery catheters during spinal shock is appropriate. Measurement of intracardiac pressures [central venous pressure (CVP), pulmonary capillary wedge pressure (PCWP), left ventricular end diastolic pressure (LVEDP)], in conjunction with cardiac output (CO) and blood pressure (BP) is necessary to differentiate hypovolemia from low systemic vascular resistance (SVR). The information obtained is helpful in determining the appropriate form of management (fluid versus vasopressors), as well as monitoring the response to therapy.

(1) Patients with low SVR may be treated with titrated infusions of a direct-acting alpha agonist, as above.

(2) Patients who are hypovolemic can receive fluid boluses of 250 to 500 mL. A Starling curve, identifying the optimal fluid filling pressure, can be derived from the changes in intracardiac pressures (CVP, PCWP, LVEDP), CO, and BP in response to the fluids:

3. Anesthetic technique

a. Securing the airway without causing or exacerbating SCI is the principal concern.

(1) **An awake intubation.** The advantage is that the patient acts as a monitor to avoid worsening of the spinal cord condition. In addition, a neurologic evaluation can document the absence of any new changes. An awake intubation also avoids the use of succinylcholine and the attendant risk of hyperkalemia.

(2) **A *blind* nasal endotracheal intubation** is often recommended as one of the best means to avoid spinal manipulation during intubation. This approach is contraindicated if there is facial trauma or a basilar skull fracture. Topical application of 0.2% phenylephrine hydrochloride in 4% lidocaine is essential to shrink nasal tissues and limit bleeding. Anesthesia of the tongue can be achieved using 2% lidocaine ointment or local anesthetic sprays. Vocal cord and laryngeal anesthesia is provided with the combination of transtracheal injection of 4% lidocaine via a percutaneous puncture of the cricothyroid membrane, and superior laryngeal nerve blocks with bilateral injection of 2 mL of 1% lidocaine into the thyro-hyoid membrane just above the lateral wings of the thyroid cartilage. An alternative technique could include 4% nebulized xylocaine with the patient receiving no more than 4 to 5 mg/kg. Toxicity calculations must include all topical and injected local anesthetics.

(3) **Fiberoptic endotracheal intubation** may be used in a nonemergent situation after local anesthesia of the airway as detailed above. If using the oral route, a bite block or large oral airway with a central passageway for the fiberoptic scope is essential. In addition, oral intubation often mandates use of mild sedation for patient acceptance. Blood, debris, and vomitus in the airway mitigate against fiberoptic intubation.

(4) **Direct laryngoscopy** may be appropriate if the previous methods do not seem feasible. Neutrality of the neck must be maintained to prevent further SCI. Extension or flexion during intubation can cause displacement and worsening of the original SCI. Inline manual cervical immobilization appears to be the safest method to minimize spinal column motion.

(5) In situations where severe facial trauma or neck instability exists, or if the airway is lost, a **surgical airway** via cricothyrotomy or tracheotomy might be indicated. The method chosen for intubation depends on perceived airway difficulties, coexisting disease and trauma, or other factors including facial trauma and soft tissue swelling.

b. **Induction**

(1) The sympathetic function of spinal injury patients is unpredictable and, as they are frequently hypovolemic, the induction should proceed slowly in an elective situation. When the patient has a full stomach, a rapid sequence induction is indicated after volume replacement.

   (a) Ketamine (1 to 2 mg/kg) will provide a more stable hemodynamic profile during induction. It has the added advantage of amplifying the electrophysiologic monitor's signal amplitude but its use is not generally recommended in the presence of intracranial hypertension.

   (b) Etomidate provides cardiovascular stability during induction.

(2) During induction of general anesthesia, maintenance of a spinal cord perfusion pressure of at least 50 mm Hg (ideally 70 to 90 mm Hg) is essential. If the patient is in the early phase of spinal shock with a high cord injury, the patient is at risk of developing bradycardia or asystole. Accordingly, some have advocated the use of a prophylactic anticholinergic to avoid this complication.

(3) Excessive fluctuations of cardiovascular parameters should be treated with direct-acting agonists and antagonists. These drugs should preferably be short acting and delivered via intravenous infusion. Sympathetic agonists and antagonists that release catecholamines indirectly are avoided.

c. **Muscle relaxants.** The SCI patient whose injury involves skeletal muscles develops a supersensitivity to depolarizing muscle relaxants. With muscle denervation, the number of postsynaptic acetylcholine receptors increases greatly and amplifies any small neuromuscular signal that may be present. When depolarized by succinylcholine, pores on the neuromuscular junction open maximally allowing massive egress of stored intracellular potassium. The occurrence of succinylcholine-induced ventricular fibrillation secondary to acute hyperkalemic response has been reported.

Since the time course for the development of the extrajunctional receptors is not clear (but may be as short as 24 hours), succinylcholine is best avoided even in recently injured patients. It is also important to realize that the magnitude of potassium release is more a function of the amount of muscle mass affected than the dose of depolarizing drug given. Even small doses of succinylcholine have triggered significant hyperkalemia. The administration of succinylcholine should be avoided in patients with SCI.

d. **Positioning.** Spinal surgery is most often performed in the **prone** position. Patients can be anesthetized on the bed or stretcher and then log-rolled onto the operating table. Important goals include maintaining the head and neck in a neutral position; providing adequate padding to the chest, abdomen, head, and extremities; and avoiding excessive neck flexion or extension. Special attention should be given to the endotracheal tube as significant movement or obstruction can occur with positional changes. In addition, sudden changes of position are avoided because they may have significant hemodynamic consequences due to the lack of adequate compensatory vasoconstrictor and cardiac reflexes to maintain venous return and cardiac output.

The head is positioned so that its weight is supported by bony prominences and there is no pressure on the eyes, ears, or nose. Head position can be adjusted slightly every 15 minutes or so throughout the procedure to ensure adequate perfusion under the weight-bearing area.

When an awake intubation is employed, the use of nerve blocks instead of sedatives will enable the patients to position themselves. This allows a neurologic exam to be performed after positioning and helps ensure that the operative position does not aggravate the injury. Information gleaned from the preoperative neurologic exam (range of motion, motions that worsen symptoms) will also help to prevent positioning from exacerbating the neurologic injury.

e. **Maintenance.** The choice of anesthetic technique is guided by the patient's underlying condition. When neurologic monitors are utilized, the anesthetic technique should maintain optimal spinal cord blood flow, and avoid drugs (e.g., volatile anesthetics) that suppress the monitored responses or cause fluctuations in the anesthetic depth, which can confuse interpretation of the evoked responses.

In general, drug regimens that utilize opiate infusions serve this purpose. While regional techniques may be considered, the incidence of coexisting injury, as well as the frequently compromised hemodynamic and respiratory status, virtually guarantees that general anesthesia will be preferable.

There is some evidence that hypocapnia decreases SCI due to ischemia. However, hypocapnia might also decrease perfusion. Normocapnia is recommended.

4. **Fluid management**. Fluid administration is based on estimated preoperative fluid deficits, intraoperative blood and fluid losses, and a knowledge of the effect of the level of SCI on cardiac and pulmonary function. Meticulous fluid management is essential since patients with high thoracic and cervical spine injuries have an increased propensity for developing pulmonary edema. In addition, cervical spine injury can cause cardiac dysfunction with decreased inotropy and chronotropy (due to reduced sympathetic neural input to the heart). Whether to use crystalloid or colloid for volume resuscitation is of less importance than the need to avoid glucose-containing solutions, which are known to exacerbate SCI.

5. **Temperature regulation.** SCI patients have impaired thermoregulation below the level of injury. Prophylactic measures to prevent intraoperative hypothermia should be aggressively instituted. These include a warm ambient environment, warm intravenous fluids, standard warming mattresses, humidification of the respiratory circuit, and forced hot-air blankets. Keep in mind, however, that hyperthermia worsens neurologic injury.

6. **Postoperative care.** Even patients who had adequate respiratory function before surgery might require a weaning period postoperatively before

extubation due to the residual effects of the anesthetics. Because of the potential difficulty in rein-
tubating the trachea of the spinal injury patient,
one should be extremely conservative in determining the appropriate time for extubation.
Critical care weaning parameters are used in
place of routine extubation criteria after most operative procedures. Once the trachea is extubated, the patient is monitored for several hours
to ensure that the respiratory status does not de-
teriorate.

Extubation criteria include:
a. **Blood gases:**
   (1) pH >7.3
   (2) PaO2 >60 mm Hg
   (3) PaCO2 <50 mm Hg
   (4) Alveolar- arterial oxygen difference
       <350 mm Hg ($FIO_2 = 100\%$)
   (5) Arterial to alveolar ratio >0.75
b. **Pulmonary functions:**
   (1) Maximal inspiratory pressure < -20 cm
       H_2O
   (2) Vital capacity >15 mL/kg
   (3) Respiratory rate <25/minute
   (4) Dead space–to–tidal volume ratio <0.6
c. **Other:**
   (1) Patient is conscious and oriented
   (2) Stable cardiac function
   (3) Optimal intravascular fluid volume and
       electrolyte status
   (4) Absence of infection
   (5) Unlabored breathing

G. **Chronic spinal cord injury.** As improved emergent
medical care increases the survival of patients with
high-level spinal injuries, one is more likely to encounter patients with chronic SCIs undergoing surgical procedures for spinal and other indications. Many
of the issues raised regarding acute spinal injuries
apply equally to patients with chronic injury. There
are, in addition, a number of medical problems (Table
16-5).

1. **Preoperative.** Respiratory complications are the
   most common cause of morbidity in spinal injury
   patients. Pneumonia is second only to anoxia at
   the time of injury as a cause of death. Any fever
   with a leukocytosis or physical or radiographic
   evidence of pneumonitis should be treated aggressively.

Table 16-5. Summary of medical problems in the patient with chronic spinal cord injury

System	Abnormality	Relevant comment
Cardiovascular	• Autonomic hyperreflexia • → Blood volume • Orthostatic hypotension	Susceptible to hypertensive crisis if SCI level above T$_7$. Positional changes and intrathoracic pressure might cause hypotension.
Respiratory	• Muscle weakness • → Respiratory drive • → Cough	SCI patient susceptible to postoperative pneumonia and might be difficult to wean from mechanical ventilation.
Muscular	• Proliferation of acetylcholine receptors • Spasticity	Hyperkalemia from succinylcholine.
Genitourinary	• Recurrent urinary tract infections • Altered bladder emptying	Might lead to renal insufficiency, pyelonephritis, sepsis, or amyloidosis.
Gastrointestinal	• Gastroparesis • Ileus	Susceptible to aspiration.
Immunologic	• Urinary tract infection • Pneumonia • Decubitus ulcers	Watch for subtle signs of infection and sepsis. Questionable risk of seeding an infection from invasive monitoring.
Skin	• Decubitus ulcers	Prevention.
Hematologic	• Anemia • Risk of DVT	DVT prophylaxis.
Bone	• → Bone density	Osteoporosis, hypercalcemia, heterotopic ossification, and muscle calcification.
Nervous system	• Chronic pain	Perioperative pain can be difficult to manage.

SCI, spinal cord injury; DVT, deep venous thrombosis.

Patients with chronic injury are more prone to episodes of hypertension secondary to autonomic hyperreflexia, especially with lesions above T_7. Muscle spasms also occur because of hyperactive spinal reflexes without the modulating effect of cortical, brain stem, and cerebellar centers. This "mass reflex" might require the therapeutic use of skeletal muscle relaxants in the awake patient.

2. Intraoperative

a. Regional anesthesia may offer some advantage for patients who still have instability of the cervical spine, or whose initial repair limits their cervical range of motion. Should general anesthesia prove necessary for this subset of patients, all precautions for airway manipulation should be employed.

b. General anesthesia and regional anesthesia are equally effective in preventing autonomic hyperreflexia. Techniques based on the use of oxygen/nitrous oxide/narcotics seem to be less efficacious in this regard. When deciding on the appropriateness of a regional technique, one should consider the site of injury as well as the site of surgery. The patient's underlying hemodynamic status should also be taken into account. Regardless of the technique, direct-acting vasodilators (e.g., nitroprusside), α-adrenergic blockers (e.g., phentolamine), antiarrhythmics (e.g., lidocaine, esmolol), atropine, and other antihypertensives (e.g., labetalol) should be readily available.

c. Chronic SCI puts all patients at risk for a hyperkalemic response to depolarizing muscle relaxants. Decreasing the dose does not reliably attenuate the response. Therefore, succinylcholine is to be avoided.

Since the receptors at the neuromuscular junction of denervated muscle are upregulated, basing the dose of nondepolarizing muscle relaxants on twitch response from a denervated limb will lead to a relative overdose of muscle relaxant. This should be considered when giving the initial dose, when reversing the relaxation at the end of the procedure, and when judging readiness for extubation.

d. Urinary retention and urinary tract infections are a persistent problem. A distended bladder can trigger the hypertensive response of autonomic hyperreflexia. Therefore, in addition to routine monitors, these patients should have a urinary catheter inserted for most procedures.

3. **Postoperative.** The postoperative management, including when to extubate the trachea, should be guided primarily by the requirements of the surgical procedure and the patient's underlying medical condition.

III. **Spinal cord tumors**. Spinal tumors can be primary or metastatic in origin. The medical problems associated with the patient will be determined by the location of the spinal lesion and by the location of the primary tumor in metastatic lesions. Depending on the length of time since the onset of the spinal lesion and its associated symptoms, these patients might present with many of the same complications found in patients with traumatic injury to the cord.

A. **Preoperative management**

1. Upper cord lesions are the most damaging physiologically. Respiratory impairment secondary to loss of intercostal muscle and/or diaphragmatic activity is common and a blood gas measurement is indicated to determine the patient's baseline respiratory status. In addition, the decreased ability to clear secretions may frequently result in pneumonitis, which may require further intervention. Such infections might not always be associated with elevated temperature, nor will elevated temperature always point to an infection, as temperature regulation is frequently impaired.

2. Cardiovascular tone might be diminished with resulting hypotension, as occurs in patients with acute SCI. One must differentiate neurogenic hypotension from the hypotension resulting from dehydration and malnutrition, commonly associated with cancer patients. Such dehydration might be exacerbated in patients who have undergone diagnostic radiographic tests that in-

volved the use of contrast dyes, as these usually act as diuretics.

3. In addition to the basic chemistries, preoperative blood determinations should include liver function tests to identify the presence, if any, of metastasis to the liver. The possibility of pituitary and adrenal insufficiency should also be considered as these are frequent sites of metastatic lesions.

4. Premedication should be kept to a minimum, as it is useful to be able to reassess neurologic function immediately prior to surgery. In particular, sedatives are avoided in situations where the respiratory status is already impaired.

B. Intraoperative management

1. The choice of monitors, beyond the routine, will be dictated by the planned procedure and the location of the lesion. Patients who exhibit signs of spinal shock will be managed more effectively with the cardiovascular information provided by a pulmonary artery catheter and an arterial line. Those patients at risk for autonomic hyperrflexia may also require the "beat-to-beat" blood pressure monitoring provided by an arterial line.

2. The positioning of these patients for the procedures frequently places the surgical site above the level of the heart. This increases the risk for pulmonary air embolism. A monitor for the detection of air embolism (e.g., precordial Doppler, transesophageal echocardiography, pulmonary artery pressure), as well as an appropriately positioned CVP line to aspirate air, should be incorporated into the anesthetic plan.

3. The risk of hyperkalemia with the use of succinylcholine is increased as it was for the patient with

spinal injury. The use of nondepolarizing relaxants is recommended to ensure a quiet surgical field. However, because of upregulation of receptors in the neuromuscular junction secondary to denervation, care should be taken to select an appropriate site for the monitoring of twitch suppression via the nerve stimulator.

4. Maintenance of anesthesia can be accomplished with any general anesthetic technique. However, in procedures where the use of SSEPs is anticipated, agents that suppress the monitored potentials are avoided. In such circumstances a nitrous oxide/narcotic technique is more appropriate. Frequent changes of anesthetic depth are avoided as they will interfere with SSEP interpretation.

C. **Postoperative management.** The decision regarding early extubation of these patients is made on a case-by-case basis. Early extubation in a fully awake patient facilitates postoperative neurologic examination. The appropriateness of early extubation will depend on baseline respiratory function, location and size of the tumor, and duration and degree of difficulty of surgical dissection. Patients who were operated for high-level lesions require close monitoring for as long as 48 to 72 hours postoperatively. During this time, edema at the surgical site can cause renewed compression of the spinal cord and lead to progressive respiratory compromise and loss of protective gag reflexes. Reintubation, when necessary, should be done early in the course of respiratory deterioration. This allows control of the airway in a patient with a potentially unstable neck to be accomplished in as non-emergent an environment as possible.

IV. **Scoliosis**

A. **General**

1. Scoliosis is a structural disease of the vertebral column involving lateral curvature of the spine with rotation of the vertebra.

2. Scoliosis most frequently involves the thoracic and lumbar regions.

3. The severity of the disease is expressed in "degrees of lateral angulation." A larger degree of angulation represents more severe disease. The side of convexity of the curve designates it as a right or left curvature.

4. Idiopathic scoliosis, accounting for almost 75% of cases, occurs most frequently in adolescent girls. Other types are classified as nonstructural (caused by gait/posture), congenital, neuromuscular, and traumatic.

5. The degree of severity of scoliosis correlates directly with the degree of respiratory dysfunction. Curvatures of less than 60° are not usually associated with significant pulmonary involvement, whereas patients with curvatures of greater than 100° degrees are typically severely impaired.

6. Pulmonary function testing typically reveals a restrictive pattern due to the reduction in chest wall compliance, with reductions in all measures of lung capacity and volume. The greatest decrease is noted in the vital capacity. Blood gas analysis will reveal a lowered PaO_2, which is primarily due to the ventilation-perfusion mismatch that occurs. $PaCO_2$ is not usually altered unless an obstructive pulmonary component has also developed (more common in the elderly).

7. In patients with more severe thoracic disease, rib cage deformities lead to underdevelopment of the pulmonary vasculature. This is exacerbated by hypoxic pulmonary vasoconstriction and can lead to potentially significant elevations in pulmonary vascular resistance. Right ventricular hypertrophy and right atrial enlargement can occur as a result of these changes in pulmonary vascular resistance. Eventually patients develop irreversible pulmonary hypertension.

B. Preoperative management

1. The preoperative assessment should include information about the location and degree of scoliosis, as well as its etiology. Both location and degree of disease will play a role in determining the amount of pulmonary/cardiac involvement one can expect to find. Scoliosis due to concurrent neurologic motor deficits may alter the choice of muscle relaxants.

2. Physical exam will indicate necessary testing. Patients with limited exercise tolerance require further pulmonary function testing to ascertain the extent of pulmonary insufficiency. Patients who have vital capacities below 25 mL/kg are high operative risks.

3. Preoperative sedation is avoided in patients with significant pulmonary compromise.

C. Intraoperative management

1. Decisions regarding monitoring are guided by the extent of pulmonary and cardiac involvement. One should consider an arterial line for blood gas measurement in any patient with even moderately reduced pulmonary reserve. An arterial line is also necessary for closer monitoring of blood pressure when "deliberate hypotension" is employed to reduce intraoperative blood loss.

2. Pulmonary artery catheter monitoring should be reserved for those patients with pulmonary hypertension or significantly diminished right ventricular output.

3. No advantage can be demonstrated for any particular anesthetic induction or maintenance regi-

men. The underlying hemodynamic condition of the patient should be used to guide the choice and dose of agents.

4. Placement of spinal instrumentation involves traction to correct the curvature. Frequently SSEP monitors are utilized to monitor the sensory component of the spinal cord. However, SSEPs monitor only the posterior cord. It is possible that anterior cord elements might be damaged despite normal SSEPs. When SSEP monitoring is utilized one should limit inhalation anesthetics, which will interfere with signal interpretation (see above).

5. A wake-up test definitively confirms adequate blood flow to, and thus the function of the anterior, motor portion of, the spinal cord. This is accomplished by having the patient awaken and move the lower extremities in response to verbal command. With a multitude of short-acting muscle relaxants and maintenance anesthetics, it has become relatively simple to maintain a deep anesthetic until the time of the wake-up test and yet allow for a quick awakening at the appropriate time during the procedure.

D. **Postoperative management.** The spinal fusion and rodding procedure prevents further deterioration of pulmonary and cardiac parameters. These abnormalities are not typically corrected by the procedure. Careful consideration of the patient's baseline status helps to determine which patients are suitable candidates for early extubation.

SUGGESTED READING

Atkinson PP, Atkinson JLD. Spinal shock. *Mayo Clin Proc* 1996;71:384.

Chiles BW, Cooper PR. Acute spinal injury. *N Engl J Med* 1996;334:514.

Eltorai IM, Wong DH, Lacerna M, et al. Surgical aspects of autonomic dysreflexia. *J Spinal Cord Med* 1997;20(3):361–364.

Grande CM, Barton RB, Stene JK. Appropriate techniques for airway management of emergency patients with suspected spinal cord injury. *Anesth Analg* 1988;67:714–715.

Hastings RH, Marks JD. Airway management for trauma patients with potential cervical spine injuries. *Anesth Analg* 1991;73:471.

Marshall WK, Mostrom JL. Neurosurgical diseases of the spine and spinal cord: anesthetic considerations. In: Cottrell JE, Smith DS, eds. *Anesthesia and neurosurgery,* 3rd ed. St. Louis: Mosby, 1994:569–603.

Zelby AS, Mcallister WH. Complications of spinal cord trauma. In: Maull KI, Rodriguez A, Wiles CE, eds. *Complications in trauma and critical care.* Philadelphia: WB Saunders, 1996:214–231.

Pediatric Neuroanesthesia

Rukaiya K. A. Hamid and Philippa Newfield

I. **Intracranial physiology.** The development of the central nervous system (CNS) is incomplete at birth; maturation continues until the end of the first year of life. Cerebral blood flow (CBF) affects cerebral volume and in turn intracranial pressure (ICP). In children from 3 to 12 years of age the CBF is 100 mL/100 g/minute and is higher than in adults. The CBF in children from 6 to 40 months is 90 mL/100 g/minute and in newborns and premature infants it is about 40 to 42 mL/100 g/minute.

In the newborn autoregulation is easily impaired or abolished, which can lead to intraventricular hemorrhage (IVH) with grave consequences. Recent studies have demonstrated that hyperventilation restores autoregulation in the neonate and that CBF velocity changes logarithmically and directly with end-tidal carbon dioxide ($ETCO_2$) in infants and children. Under normal conditions ICP is much more dependent on CBF and cerebral blood volume (CBV) than CSF production, and all inhalational agents must be used with care, as they increase the CBF by producing vasodilatation.

II. **Anesthetic requirements.** The anesthetic requirements in pediatric patients vary with age and maturity. Neonates and premature infants have decreased anesthetic requirements relative to older children. The minimum alveolar concentration (MAC) for halothane for the premature infant is 0.6%, for the term neonate, 0.89%, and for the 2- to 4-month-old infant, 1.12%. The reasons for the lower requirements are the immaturity of the newborn's nervous system, the presence of maternal progesterone, and elevated levels of endorphins, along with the immaturity of the blood–brain barrier.

Under normal conditions the ICP is more dependent on CBF and CBV than on the production of CSF. Since all inhalational anesthetics produce vasodilatation and increase CBV, they must be used with great caution in children. The choice of anesthetic technique is based on the knowledge and the experience of the anesthesiologist, the condition of the patient, and the nature of the surgical procedure. Appreciation of the fact that neonates have a lower MAC and a more rapid uptake of the inhalational drugs is vital to the safe use of these drugs for induction of anesthesia in the pediatric neurosurgical patient.

The causes of rapid induction are:

A. The ratio of alveolar ventilation to functional residual capacity (FRC) is 5:1 in the infant and 1.5:1 in the adult.

B. The neonate has a greater cardiac output per kilogram of body weight compared to the adult.

C. More of the cardiac output of the neonate goes to the vessel-rich group of organs including the brain and the heart.

D. The infant has a lower blood-gas partition coefficient for volatile anesthetics and a lower anesthetic requirement.

The induction of anesthesia is very rapid with most inhalational agents and may cause hypotension. This may be hazardous in the premature, small for gestational age (SGA), or unstable patient, and the child who requires rapid control of the airway. Whatever the choice of drugs, sick neonates require resuscitation before the induction of anesthesia. Most neonates do well with an intravenous sedative-hypnotic, narcotic, and relaxant. The length of the operation and the need for postoperative ventilation must be taken into account when choosing the anesthetic technique in pediatric patients.

III. **Anatomy of the airway.** The newborn period is the first 24 hours of life. The neonatal period is the first 30 days of extrauterine life, and includes the newborn period. The most significant transition occurs within the first 24 to 72 hours after birth. All systems change, but the most important for the anesthesiologist are the circulatory, respiratory, and renal systems. The infant is an obligate nose breather. The immaturity in the coordination between respiratory efforts and the oropharyngeal motor and sensory input accounts in part for obligate nasal breathing. Conditions like congenital choanal atresia or simple nasal congestion can cause respiratory distress and asphyxia in the infant.

The oxygen demand in the infant is high: 7 to 9 mL/kg as compared to 3 mL/kg in the mature state. Infants have a high closing volume, high minute ventilation-to-FRC ratio, and soft pliable ribs. Therefore, even some degree of airway obstruction can have a major impact on the oxygen supply in the neonate. There are five major differences in the airway of the neonate as compared to the adult:

A. **Tongue.** In the infant the tongue is relatively large compared to the rest of the oral cavity and thus easily causes obstruction.

B. **Larynx.** The infant's larynx is anatomically higher in the neck, at C_{3-4}, as compared to an adult, at C_{4-5}. The larynx in the infant thus has a more rostral or superior location, making it more difficult to visualize.

C. **Epiglottis.** The epiglottis is narrow and angled away from the trachea, and it is more difficult to lift by the laryngoscope blade.

D. **Vocal cords.** The infant's vocal cords have a lower attachment anteriorly than posteriorly, sometimes making the larynx difficult to intubate as compared to an adult, in whom the axis of the vocal cords is perpendicular to the trachea.

E. **Subglottic area.** The narrowest portion of the infant's larynx is the nonexpandable cricoid cartilage. Hence, in an infant the endotracheal tube might pass through the trachea but still be tight at the subglottic region.

IV. Anesthetic considerations

A. **Preoperative assessment.** The preoperative assessment of a pediatric patient who has neurologic dysfunction involves establishing the degree of change in the cerebral compliance. The clinical presentation varies with the age of the patient as well as the rapidity and degree of change in the intracranial contents. Neonates might present with a history of irritability, lethargy, and failure to feed. They may have an enlarging head circumference, bulging fontanelle, or lower extremity motor deficits. Older children might have headache, nausea, vomiting, or change in the level of alertness. Fundoscopy might reveal papilledema. The evaluation also includes assessment of any fluid and electrolyte imbalance from lack of intake or active vomiting because of changes in the ICP.

B. **Premedication.** Sedative premedication should be avoided in all patients suspected of increases in ICP, as these drugs might further embarrass respiration, cause hypercarbia and cerebral vasodilatation, and lead to tonsillar herniation. Patients scheduled for the repair of vascular lesions whose ICP is normal may be sedated to control preoperative anxiety and avoid hypertension and rupture of the vascular abnormality.

C. **Monitoring.** Monitoring depends on the age and condition of the patient and the planned surgical procedure. Routine monitoring includes the use of the precordial stethoscope, electrocardiogram (ECG), oxygen saturation (SaO_2) by pulse oximeter, $ETCO_2$, indirect blood pressure (NIBP) measurement, esophageal stethoscope and temperature probe, and a peripheral nerve stimulator to monitor the degree of neuromuscular blockade. Direct blood pressure monitoring, at least two good peripheral intravenous catheters, and a urinary catheter are recommended for extensive and invasive surgical procedures.

V. Neuroanesthetic management

A. **Hydrocephalus**

1. **Definition.** Enlargement of the ventricles from increased production of CSF, decreased absorption by the arachnoid villi, or obstruction of the CSF pathways. Hydrocephalus is classified as communicating (nonobstructive) or noncommunicating (obstructive). The causes of the increased CSF collection can be congenital or acquired.

a. **Etiology**

(1) Congenital

(a) Stenosis of the aqueduct.

(b) Myelomeningocele, Arnold-Chiari malformation, spina bifida.

      (c) Dandy-Walker syndrome.
      (d) Mucopolysaccharidoses (obliteration of subarachnoid space).
      (e) Achondroplasia (occipital bone growth).
    (2) **Acquired**
      (a) Intraventricular hemorrhage.
      (b) Space-occupying intracerebral lesions.
      (c) Infections: abscess and meningitis.

Hydrocephalus causes an increase in the head circumference. Prevention of any further increase in intracranial contents is vital, as this may precipitate herniation. Drainage of CSF can also be a problem since ventricular arrhythmias may be associated with rapid removal of CSF. In some circumstances, epidural or subdural hemorrhage can result from a sudden reduction in the ICP. This can cause a change in the level of consciousness of the child, although the shunt is functioning.

2. **Surgical procedures**
   a. Ventriculoperitoneal (VP) shunt.
   b. Ventriculoatrial (VA) shunt.
   c. Ventriculopleural shunt.
   d. Ventriculojugular shunt.
   e. Ventriculostomy.
3. **Preoperative management**. Assess the patient for any effects of increased ICP such as nausea, vomiting, changes in the ventilatory pattern, irritability, decreased level of consciousness, bradycardia, or hypertension. A computed tomography (CT) scan might demonstrate increase in the size of the ventricles. Sudden neurologic deterioration in the pediatric patient is always a concern and must be treated quickly with emergency endotracheal intubation and hyperventilation, including monitoring with $ETCO_2$, until emergency surgical reduction in the ICP is achieved. This is sometimes accomplished by a direct needle puncture of the lateral ventricle and aspiration of CSF.
4. **Premedication.** Sedation is contraindicated as the resultant hypoventilation may increase ICP. EMLA cream may be used whenever possible to achieve intravenous access without causing distress to young patients.
5. **Anesthesia.** Inhalation induction is usually not attempted as all inhalation agents are cerebral vasodilators and might increase ICP. Modified rapid sequence induction is preferred to minimize the risk of aspiration due either to gastric hypotonia from effects of increased ICP or to a recent meal. Preoxygenation is followed by intra-

venous induction with barbiturate and a fast-acting nondepolarizing muscle relaxant such as rocuronium for intubation. Muscle relaxation is maintained throughout the procedure and an inhalation agent is introduced once adequate hyperventilation is achieved. Intravenous fluid is given at maintenance level and intravenous ceftriaxone or vancomycin is given (after checking sensitivity) slowly (over 60 minutes) and in a dilute solution to prevent any histamine release. At the end of the procedure, the stomach is suctioned and the trachea is extubated when the patient is fully awake. This is usually not a problem as long as the shunt is functioning well.

B. Craniosynostosis. Craniosynostosis is a congenital anomaly resulting from premature fusion of the cranial sutures. This can cause severe cranial deformity, depending on the involved sutures, and, rarely, intracranial hypertension and psychomotor retardation from abnormal brain growth. Males are more often affected than females. Sagittal synostosis accounts for nearly half of all cases of craniosynostosis. Surgery is usually performed in the first 6 months of life for best results.

1. Preoperative assessment. Patients are otherwise healthy but require assessment for any evidence of raised ICP. Hemoglobin is determined preoperatively and blood is made available for surgery. The surgeons are working in close proximity to major venous sinuses, so that sudden and massive blood loss is a possibility.

2. Monitoring. Includes ECG, SaO_2, $ETCO_2$, NIBP, and esophageal temperature as well as an arterial catheter for direct blood pressure and arterial blood gas (ABG) measurement and a precordial Doppler to monitor for venous air embolism. The patient must have adequate intravenous access (at least two good lines) and a urinary catheter to monitor urinary output.

3. Anesthesia. Induction of anesthesia is either inhalational or intravenous if a catheter is already in place. The endotracheal tube is well secured so that ventilation is undisturbed with head movements. Anesthesia is maintained with an inhalational agent, N_2O, oxygen, an intermediate-acting nondepolarizing relaxant, and a narcotic (fentanyl or morphine) for analgesia. A key point in the procedure is when the surgeons manipulate the sagittal sutures, due to the possibility of venous air embolism or massive bleeding. Body temperature is monitored closely and all intravenous fluids are warmed.

4. Postoperative Management. At the end of the procedure the patient is first awakened and then the trachea is extubated. The hematocrit is measured during recovery as blood loss continues from the surgical incision, and patients may need blood or blood products to control oozing. The maintenance of adequate urine output throughout the procedure serves as an indicator of the adequacy of regional organ perfusion.

C. **Intracranial Space-Occupying Lesions.** Intracranial tumors are the most common solid tumors of childhood and are the second most common pediatric cancer after the leukemias. Supratentorial tumors account for approximately half of all intracranial malignancies and arise from midline structures. Two-thirds of the infratentorial tumors are in the posterior fossa. The pathologic distribution includes gliomas (30%), medulloblastomas (30%), astrocytomas (30%), ependymomas (7%), and others (3%: acoustic neuromas, meningiomas, etc.). All intracranial tumors increase intracranial volume. Infratentorial lesions produce signs and symptoms of brain stem compression and intracranial hypertension from hydrocephalus.

1. **Preoperative Considerations.** Signs and symptoms of increased ICP including the need for the placement of a ventriculostomy or shunt before the definitive operation are noted. The most common presentation is with headache and vomiting for several days and sometimes weeks. Neonates and infants may have a history of poor feeding, irritability, or lethargy. The anterior fontanelle may bulge, eyes may exhibit "sunset sign" or cranium may be enlarged. There may be obvious engorgement of the scalp veins, and some patients may show changes in the level of consciousness or definite neurological deficits depending on the area of brain compression. Posterior fossa tumors may cause cranial nerve dysfunction along with signs and symptoms of increased ICP. Untreated space-occupying lesions of the brain lead to death because of brain stem herniation.

2. **Anesthetic Considerations.**
   a. The history is reviewed, including presence of seizures and measures to control them, and documented. A complete physical examination to identify any neurological deficits is also performed and noted.
   b. Patients require assessment for signs and symptoms of increased ICP and review of investigative procedures such as CT and magnetic resonance imaging (MRI) scans.
      Measures taken to control ICP including placement of ventriculostomy or shunt before the definitive operation are noted. Increased ICP can also be controlled by dexamethasone to reduce peritumoral edema,

fluid restriction, and the use of diuretics such as mannitol, furosemide, or hypertonic saline. Furosemide is particularly helpful as it also reduces CSF production.

c. Patients with increased ICP may have altered gastric emptying or dehydration and electrolyte imbalance from poor feeding, vomiting, and the syndrome of inappropriate antidiuretic hormone (SIADH) secretion.

d. Patient position is discussed with the surgeon and the head is positioned to avoid any obstruction to venous return. Blood is typed and crossmatched and available in the operating room.

e. Monitoring for operation for removal of intracranial tumors includes the use of all routine monitors and a urinary catheter. An arterial catheter for hemodynamic monitoring and blood chemistry determination is necessary for pediatric patients undergoing craniotomy. A central venous catheter is recommended when blood loss is expected or when there is a concern about SIADH. Head position and surgical approach also increase the risk of intraoperative air embolism.

3. **Anesthesia.** Induction is focused on measures to reduce the ICP. The recommended sequence is intravenous induction, hyperventilation, and gentle, brief laryngoscopy to secure the airway. Intraoperative concerns involve optimal positioning of the head, maintenance of body temperature, and adequate replacement of fluid and blood losses. The anesthetic technique (nitrous oxide; oxygen; low concentration of isoflurane; a non-histamine-releasing, nondepolarizing relaxant; and a short-acting narcotic) is designed to avoid oversedation and allow early assessment of neurologic function at the completion of surgery.

A smooth and prompt emergence from anesthesia is desirable. The decision to extubate the trachea of pediatric patients depends not only on the length of the procedure but on the intraoperative course of events, the extent of the tumor resection, the expected neurologic deficits, and the degree of postoperative control of ICP. Monitoring of ABG, blood chemistry, fluid balance, and neurologic function is continued in the postoperative period.

D. **Surgery for epilepsy.** Patients who require surgery for epilepsy have intractable seizures due to congenital disorders, birth trauma, tumors, or vascular malformations. Continual seizure activity has deleterious effects on the development of the brain and causes psychosocial dysfunction.

Perioperative risks arising from status epilepticus

include severe hypoxemia and sudden death. The use of large doses of anticonvulsants for the medical management of seizures may alter pharmacologic response because of enzyme induction, liver dysfunction, and jaundice.

1. **Preoperative assessment.** Determine the age of onset, type, and frequency of the seizures, and any deleterious effects on mental status and development. Recent changes in the level of consciousness and the appearance of new motor deficits must be recognized preoperatively. Liver function tests and a coagulation profile are performed preoperatively.

   When targeting important areas of the brain such as the motor cortex and the speech centers, surgery is performed under local anesthesia if the patient is a cooperative older child or adolescent. Small children will need general anesthesia. For awake procedures, it is essential to establish rapport with the patient and explain the state of dissociation, lack of pain (neuroleptanalgesia), and need for cooperation for the operation to be a success. No sedatives or anticonvulsants are administered for 48 hours if electrophysiologic studies are to be conducted intraoperatively. All patients receive dexamethasone for 48 hours to control brain swelling. Ultra-short-acting barbiturates are readily available to control seizure episodes in the perioperative period.

   Blood loss may be a concern from a large craniotomy, especially in the smaller patient, so blood must be available. The fluid warmer is used to maintain normothermia. The patient is well padded as these procedures may be lengthy.

2. **Monitoring.** Routine monitors, including a urinary catheter, are employed, and normocapnia is maintained during the procedure. Intravenous catheters, arterial catheters, and nerve stimulators are placed on the limbs not being used by the surgeons to observe motor function during the localization of the seizure focus. This is discussed with the surgeons in advance and explained to the patient.

3. **Anesthesia.** All inhalational anesthetics depress cerebral activity and are avoided during EEG studies. Enflurane additionally has seizure activation properties, especially in the presence of hypocarbia. The successful use of low concentrations of isoflurane in combination with narcotics has been reported in several centers. Nitrous oxide, oxygen, and a narcotic are also useful. Propofol induces dose-dependent changes in the EEG with an increase in beta activity at low infusion rates and an increase in delta activity, followed by burst suppression, at high infusion

rates. Etomidate is not recommended as it produces interictal spiking and might induce clinical seizures in these patients. A combination of droperidol and fentanyl can be used for neuroleptanalgesia during awake craniotomy in older, cooperative patients. Ketamine activates epileptogenic foci in epileptic patients and is not recommended.

Nondepolarizing relaxants have no effect on electrical activity. The dose requirements are higher due to the interaction with the anticonvulsant drugs. No muscle relaxant is used during the period of direct cortical stimulation so that motor activity may be observed by the surgeons.

4. **Postoperative management.** Careful monitoring of neurologic function is vital during the first 24 hours after the operation. There may be motor, memory, or speech dysfunction or increased seizure activity in the postoperative period. The hematocrit is monitored as blood loss from a large cranial incision can be considerable. Postoperative pain must be controlled to avoid episodes of hypertension. Short-acting barbiturates or propofol must be available to treat seizure activity.

E. **Head trauma.** Skull fractures occur at all ages as a result of birth injury, traffic accidents, playground accidents, domestic negligence, or abuse. They may be depressed, open, or basal skull fractures, and will increase morbidity and mortality if unrecognized.

1. Traumatic sequelae include epidural, subdural, and intracerebral hematomas, cerebral contusion, and edema with signs of intracranial hypertension.

   a. **Epidural hematomas.** Epidural hematomas account for 25% of all intracranial hematomas and are considered to be true medical emergencies. Most frequently caused by a tear in the middle meningeal artery, epidural hematomas can lead to decreasing level of consciousness, pupillary dilatation, hemiparesis, posturing, or coma. Patients require urgent surgical evacuation of the hematoma and achievement of intracranial hemostasis.

   b. **Subdural hematomas.** Subdural hematomas result from parenchymal contusion or blood vessel tears sustained during birth trauma or shaking, as with shaken baby syndrome. They can cause brain edema and progressive neurologic dysfunction.

   c. **Skull fractures.** Skull fractures are of concern if they involve major blood vessels. Depressed fractures require surgical elevation and might be associated with dural lacerations. Signs and symptoms depend on the extent of cortical injury. Basilar fracture might cause periorbital ecchymoses, hemotympanum, changes in the level of consciousness, and seizures.

2. **Preoperative considerations.** Assessment of neurologic injury and possible intracranial hypertension is by CT. The establishment of an airway, maintenance of adequate ventilation and circulation, and determination of the level of consciousness, associated injuries causing cardiovascular instability, and thermoregulatory problems are of paramount concern. The cervical spine is evaluated. Renal function must be investigated and the urine checked for hematuria. Blood for transfusion must be available. The need for preoperative evaluation of hematocrit, coagulation profile, and acid–base and electrolyte balance will depend on the type and extent of injury.

3. **Monitoring.** Routine monitors, urinary catheter, and arterial catheter for direct blood pressure monitoring are essential. Adequate intravenous access is necessary for volume resuscitation.

4. **Anesthesia.** The trachea is intubated with the head in "neutral position" to avoid any injury to the cervical spine, and ventilation is controlled to avoid increasing ICP. Rapid sequence induction of anesthesia follows volume resuscitation and is achieved by thiopental, narcotic, and a nondepolarizing muscle relaxant of rapid onset, the patient's volume status permitting. The dose of sedative-hypnotic is reduced in hypovolemic patients. Maintenance of anesthesia with nitrous oxide, oxygen, low-dose isoflurane, and narcotic allows prompt emergence for early neurologic assessment. Poor preoperative condition and adverse intraoperative events mitigate against early awakening and extubation.

5. **Postoperative care.** Control of ICP is vital. The patient may be sedated and mechanically ventilated in the intensive care unit postoperatively if there is concern about neurologic or other organ dysfunction.

F. **Meningomyelocele, encephalocele.** Embryologic neural tube fusion takes place during the first month of gestation. Failure of fusion causes herniation of the meninges (meningocele) or elements of the neural tube (myelomeningocele), and can occur at any level of the spinal cord. Abnormality occurring at the level of the head is referred to as encephalocele. Defects arising at higher levels in the spine can produce bowel, bladder, and lower extremity dysfunction. Most patients also have Arnold-Chiari malformation and hydrocephalus. Surgery is performed at the earliest opportunity (usually in the first week of life) to avoid infection of the CNS.

1. **Preoperative preparation.** Patients are evaluated for signs and symptoms of hydrocephalus and the presence of any airway problems due to a large encephalocele or thoracic myelomeningocele. There may be considerable evaporative losses with consequent problems in maintaining body temperature and fluid balance. Hematocrit must be checked preoperatively and blood made available for transfusion as blood loss may occur during repair of large defects. The defect should be well padded in the perioperative period to avoid further complications from compression, CSF leak, and bleeding.

2. **Monitoring.** Routine monitoring is used. Patients who are expected to incur blood loss should have adequate intravenous access for transfusion, an arterial line, and a urinary catheter.

3. **Anesthesia.** Intravenous access should be established before induction. Positioning and airway management may be particularly challenging with a large encephalocele. The patient is placed in the lateral or supine position with the encephalocele or myelomeningocele padded in a "donut" support. Intravenous atropine is given and the trachea intubated either awake or after intravenous barbiturate and a depolarizing or nondepolarizing relaxant. The eyes are taped, the patient turned to the prone position, and the limbs padded. No more relaxant is given if the surgeons plan to use nerve stimulation during surgery, and anesthesia is maintained with a low concentration of inhalation agent and a narcotic suited to the length of the procedure. Temperature, blood loss, and fluid balance are monitored closely during the procedure. The trachea is extubated after the patient awakens at the end of the procedure and neurologic integrity is confirmed. Infants who are at risk of postoperative apnea have oxygen saturation and apnea monitors in place for overnight observation.

G. **Craniofacial Surgery.** Cranial deformities are syndromes associated with premature closure of the cranial sutures. This may be one manifestation of a number of congenital syndromes and is often associated with anomalies involving the heart or other organs. Patients may be born prematurely and have respiratory dysfunction in addition to a difficult airway from the craniofacial deformity.

1. **Preoperative preparation**
   a. Detailed evaluation of the etiology of the craniofacial abnormality as well as the presence of associated anomalies is vital. Careful note

is made of any anticipated airway management problems. Previous anesthesia records are reviewed if the patient has had cardiac or other corrective surgeries in the past.

    b. The choice of laboratory investigations depends on the specific craniofacial defect and may include an echocardiogram or consultation.

    c. Consideration of tracheotomy for airway management in the perioperative period is an important aspect of patient evaluation.

    d. Massive blood loss is always a concern during these procedures. Therefore, adequate quantities of blood and blood products should be available.

    e. The operating room is prepared with the knowledge that these procedures are lengthy to facilitate maintenance of body temperature and airway humidity.

    f. Fluid warmers are used to warm infusions. Blood replacement is started early and continued in the postoperative period.

2. Monitoring involves the use of routine monitors; Doppler if the patient's head is positioned above the heart during surgery; direct arterial blood pressure measurement, which will also allow assessment of ABGs, hematocrit, and electrolytes; and urinary catheter.

3. Anesthesia

    a. Establishment of good intravenous access is important as these procedures tend to be prolonged and involve massive blood loss.

    b. Every attempt is made to keep the patient warm during surgery: increased ambient temperature, warming blanket, heated humidifier, fluid warmer.

    c. Fluid balance is maintained by monitoring hematocrit and urine output.

    d. Coagulation profile is checked after replacement of one blood volume, especially if continued loss and replacement are expected.

    e. Air embolism is a concern when there is extensive bone dissection.

    f. Resuscitation drugs should be available during the procedure.

        Anesthesia can be induced with any inhalational agent if airway problems are anticipated or with intravenous drugs if the patient has an intravenous catheter in place and there is no potential problem with the airway. The endotracheal tube must be well secured, especially if the patient will be operated in the prone position. Eyes should be lubricated and taped securely. All pressure points must be well padded. Intraoperative reduction of intracranial volume may be requested by surgeons to help with retraction of the frontal lobes during dissection of the orbital structures. Maintenance of anesthesia is usually with nitrous oxide, oxygen, a long-acting nondepolarizing relaxant, and a narcotic for analgesia.

4. **Postoperative care.** Postoperative intubation is continued mainly to ensure adequate ventilation. Problems might arise due to the length of procedure, expected fluid shifts from massive transfusion, and use of intraoperative narcotic. Postoperative transfusion might be required due to continued oozing from the surgical site.

VI.   Neuroradiology

A. **Anesthetic management of neurodiagnostic procedures.** Most pediatric patients require general anesthesia for neuroradiologic diagnosis such as CT scanning, MRI, angiography, and myelography, as well as radiation therapy procedures because of age (infants), anxiety, lack of understanding and cooperation, developmental delay, and inability to remain still for lengthy procedures. Sedation is employed in older, cooperative children undergoing short procedures that do not produce pain and discomfort.

1. **Magnetic resonance imaging** has an intense magnetic field from the large static magnet, so that no ferromagnetic objects can be brought into the room housing the magnet. The patient must be absolutely still and isolated within the tunneled scanning space (which may induce claustrophobia) during the examination. The procedure does not cause any pain to the patient and usually takes 45 minutes to 1 hour. All ferromagnetic objects must be removed from the patient as they may induce a motion artifact in the magnetic field. Patients are checked for metal objects such as aneurysm clips and cochlear implants. Intravenous propofol, either by bolus or by infusion, in combination with midazolam has proved successful and is commonly used to provide anesthesia for these procedures.

2. **Computed tomographic scanning** also requires understanding and cooperation on the part of the patient who will need to remain still throughout the procedure to secure high-quality diagnostic images. Sedation is used to enhance patient cooperation. Neonates may be scanned without any sedation because they will fall asleep but infants might need oral chloral hydrate for the procedure. Sedation is also required in older children who are mentally handicapped and/or uncooperative. Otherwise normal older children may undergo the procedure without sedation as long as they are assured it will be pain-

less. The CT scanning usually takes under an hour and may be performed without the help of the anesthesiologist in the case of an older patient.

   3. **Angiography** is mainly used as an adjunct to diagnostic CT and MRI scanning. Its main indication is for the detailed demonstration of arteriovenous malformations (AVMs) and Moya Moya disease, as well as the extent of tumor vascularity. Cerebral angiography is usually performed via the transfemoral route with injection of nonionic contrast agents and requires anesthesia in small children.

B. Periprocedural management

   1. Review the patient's history and any previous diagnostic or surgical procedures and their management.

   2. Check that the consent form has been signed and the patient has been fasting.

   3. Discuss the procedure with the parent and the older patient and develop rapport with the younger patient.

   4. Ensure adequate functioning of the anesthesia machine and suction apparatus, and the availability of equipment for difficulty in airway management and resuscitation.

   5. Apply all standard monitors routinely used in the operating room: ECG, BP, pulse oximeter, $ETCO_2$, temperature.

   6. Institute controlled ventilation and moderate hyperventilation for patients undergoing cerebral angiography to induce cerebral vasoconstriction in order to achieve good-quality images after the injection of the contrast.

   7. Since allergic or anaphylactic reactions are always a possibility with the contrast material used during CT, MRI, and angiographic procedures, document a history of any allergic reactions in the past and be prepared to treat a reaction if one occurs during the course of the procedure.

   8. Monitor patients in a recovery area until they are fully awake and stable before discharging them from the unit. Patients who exhibit an anaphylactic reaction might require intubation, ventilation, and overnight observation as laryngeal edema is a possible sequela of allergic reactions.

SUGGESTED READINGS

Berry FA. Neonatal anesthesia. In: Barash PG, Cullen BF, Stoelting RK, eds. *Clinical anesthesia.* Philadelphia: JB Lippincott, 1989:1253–1280.

Bissonnette B, Armstrong DC, Rutka TJ. Pediatric neuroanesthesia. In: Albin MS, ed. *Textbook of neuroanesthesia with neurosurgi-*

cal and neuroscience perspectives. New York: McGraw-Hill, 1997:1177–1246.

Coté CJ. Practical pharmacology of anesthetic agents, narcotics, and sedatives. In: Coté CJ, Ryan JF, Todres ID, Goudsouzian NG, eds. *A practice of anesthesia for infants and children*, 2nd ed. Philadelphia: WB Saunders, 1993:105–133.

Dierdorf SF, McNiece WL, Rao CC, Wolfe TM, Means LJ. Failure of succinylcholine to alter plasma potassium in children with myelomeningocele. *Anesthesiology* 1986;64:272.

Hamid RKA, Newfield GP. Anesthesia for pediatric spine procedures. In: Porter S, ed. *Anesthesia for surgery of the spine.* New York: McGraw-Hill, 1995:225–280.

Harris MM, Yemen TA, Davidson A, et al. Venous embolism during craniectomy in a supine infant. *Anesthesiology* 1987;67:816.

Todres ID, Gore R. Growth and development. In: Coté CJ, Ryan JF, Todres ID, Goudsouzian NG, eds. *A practice of anesthesia for infants and children*, 2nd ed. Philadelphia: WB Saunders, 1993: 7–29.

Trop D, Oliver A, et al. Seizure surgery. In: Albin MS, ed. *Textbook of neuroanesthesia with neurosurgical and neuroscience perspectives.* New York: McGraw-Hill, 1997:643–696.

Neurosurgery in the Pregnant Patient

David J. Wlody

Neurologic disorders requiring surgery during pregnancy are surprisingly common and most anesthesiologists eventually encounter a pregnant woman with such a disorder. The anesthetic management of these patients can be complicated by the significant maternal physiologic changes that occur during pregnancy. These changes may require alterations in anesthetic management that are in complete opposition to the techniques that would be appropriate for a nonpregnant patient with the same neurosurgical disorder.

Additionally, while maternal considerations must remain paramount, it is important to recognize that interventions that benefit the mother might have the potential to cause fetal harm. Thus, the major challenge of neuroanesthesia during pregnancy is to provide an appropriate balance between competing, or even contradictory, clinical goals.

In this chapter we will limit our discussion to the anesthetic management of women undergoing craniotomy for arteriovenous malformation (AVM) resection, aneurysm clipping, and resection of intracranial neoplasms. Because the anesthetic management of these procedures is discussed elsewhere in this book, this chapter will deal primarily with the ways in which anesthetic management is altered by pregnancy.

I. **Maternal physiologic alterations during pregnancy**
   A. **Neurologic changes**
      1. **Inhalation anesthetic requirements**. The minimum alveolar concentration (MAC) for inhalation anesthetics is decreased by approximately 30% to 40% during pregnancy, a change that occurs as early as the first trimester. This has been postulated to be a result of increased circulating endorphins. Alternatively, increased concentrations of progesterone, a hormone with known sedative effects, might account for decreased anesthetic requirements. As a result of the increased sensitivity to inhalation anesthetics, inspired anesthetic concentrations that would be appropriate in nonpregnant patients can lead to severe cardiopulmonary depression during pregnancy.
      2. **Local anesthetic requirements** for spinal and epidural anesthesia are decreased by 30% to 40% during pregnancy. This is in part due to the decreased volume of cerebrospinal fluid (CSF) in the lumbar subarachnoid space secondary to engorgement of epidural veins. Decreased local anesthetic requirements predate the onset of significant epi-

dural venous engorgement, however; a progesterone-induced increase in the sensitivity of neurons to the sodium blocking properties of local anesthetics is thought to be the cause.

B. Respiratory changes

1. **Upper airway mucosal edema**. Extracellular fluid accumulation produces soft tissue edema during pregnancy, particularly in the upper airway, where marked mucosal friability also develops. Nasotracheal intubation and the placement of nasogastric tubes should be avoided unless absolutely necessary, because of the risk of massive epistaxis. Laryngeal edema can reduce the size of the glottic aperture, leading to difficult intubation, particularly in pre-eclamptic individuals. A 6.0-mm endotracheal tube is appropriate for most pregnant patients.

2. **Functional residual capacity (FRC)** is decreased by as much as 40% at term. Closing capacity (CC) remains unchanged. In the supine position, when the FRC becomes further decreased, CC commonly exceeds the FRC leading to small airway closure, increased shunt fraction, and an increased potential for arterial desaturation. Additionally, because FRC represents the store of oxygen available during a period of apnea, decreases in FRC can be expected to lead to the more rapid development of hypoxemia when a patient becomes apneic, as occurs during the induction of anesthesia. Because oxygen consumption is increased by 20% during pregnancy, significant desaturation can occur even when intubation is performed expeditiously. This mandates at least four minutes of preoxygenation and denitrogenation with a tightly fitting face mask prior to induction of general anesthesia during pregnancy.

3. **Ventilation.** Significant increases in minute ventilation occur as early as the end of the first trimester. At term, minute ventilation increases by 50%, due to increases in both tidal volume (40%) and respiratory rate (15%). It is postulated that these increases are due to a progesterone-induced increase in the ventilatory response to carbon dioxide (CO_2). Because the increase in ventilation exceeds the increase in CO_2 production, the normal arterial partial pressure of CO_2 ($PaCO_2$) decreases to approximately 32 mm Hg. Increased renal bicarbonate excretion partially compensates for hypocarbia and pH increases only slightly, to approximately 7.42 to 7.44.

C. Cardiovascular changes

1. **Blood volume** increases by 35% during pregnancy. Because plasma volume increases to a greater extent than red cell mass (50% versus

20%), a dilutional anemia occurs. Normal hematocrit at term will range from 30% to 35%.

2. **Cardiac output**. Significant increases in cardiac output (CO) occur as early as the first trimester. Capeless and Clapp demonstrated a 22% increase in CO by 8 weeks gestation, which represents 57% of the total change seen at 24 weeks. Cardiac output rises steadily throughout the second trimester. After 24 weeks, it remains stable or increases slightly. Older studies demonstrating a decrease in CO in the third trimester reflect measurements made in the supine position and subsequent aortocaval compression (see below).

Cardiac output can increase by an additional 60% during labor. Part of this increase is due to pain and apprehension associated with contractions, an increase that can be blunted with the provision of adequate analgesia. There is a further increase in CO, unaffected by analgesia, that is due to autotransfusion of 300 to 500 mL of blood from the uterus into the central circulation with each contraction. Finally, CO will increase further in the immediate postpartum period, by as much as 80% above prelabor values, due to autotransfusion from the rapidly involuting uterus as well as by augmentation of preload secondary to alleviation of aortocaval compression.

3. **Aortocaval compression**. When pregnant women of 20 weeks gestation or greater assume the supine position, the enlarged uterus can compress the inferior vena cava against the vertebral column. When this occurs, venous return to the heart will decrease, sometimes to a marked extent, leading to decreases in CO and blood pressure. This has the potential to decrease uterine blood flow (UBF) to a level that can produce fetal asphyxia. Supine positioning may also produce aortic compression. If this occurs, upper extremity blood pressure might be normal but distal aortic pressure and thus uterine artery perfusion pressure will be significantly decreased. Because both regional and general anesthesia reduce venous return, the effects of aortocaval compression will be magnified in the anesthetized patient. Thus, the supine position must be avoided in pregnant patients undergoing anesthesia. Tilting the operating table 30° to the left will prevent significant aortocaval compression. This goal can also be achieved by placing a roll under the patient's right hip.

D. **Gastrointestinal changes**
1. **Gastric acid production.** Ectopic gastrin is produced by the placenta. This leads to increases in both the volume and the acidity of gastric secretions.

2. **Gastric emptying**. Progesterone decreases gastrointestinal tract motility through its smooth muscle relaxant effect. The pylorus can be obstructed by the rapidly enlarging uterus. These changes will slow gastric emptying and lead to increased gastric residual volume.

3. **Gastroesophageal sphincter**. The enlarging uterus causes elevation and rotation of the stomach, which interferes with the pinch-cock mechanism of the gastroesophageal sphincter. This increases the likelihood of gastric reflux.

4. **Pregnancy and aspiration pneumonia**. The changes described make it more likely that a pregnant patient will regurgitate and aspirate, and, if this occurs, that the pulmonary injury will be greater because of the increased volume and acidity of the gastric contents. These changes occur by the end of the first trimester, if not earlier. Thus, pregnant patients with an estimated gestational age of approximately 14 weeks or greater must be assumed to have a full stomach. They should therefore receive aspiration prophylaxis with either a nonparticulate antacid or a combination of an H_2 blocker and metoclopramide. Anesthetic induction will be influenced by the presence of a full stomach but, as described below, techniques designed to minimize the risk of aspiration might not be ideal for the patient with intracranial disease.

E. **Renal and hepatic changes**. Aldosterone levels are increased during pregnancy leading to an increase in total body sodium and water. This can cause increased edema in an intracranial neoplasm leading to worsening symptomatology or onset of symptoms from a previously unrecognized mass lesion. Renal blood flow and glomerular filtration rate increase by approximately 60% at term, paralleling the increase in CO. Thus, blood urea nitrogen (BUN) and creatinine are usually one half to two thirds the values seen in nonpregnant women. What would be considered a normal or only slightly elevated BUN and creatinine in nonpregnant women should be a cause for concern during pregnancy.

Slight increases in alanine aminotransferase (ALT), aspartic transaminase (AST), and lactate dehydrogenase (LDH) are not uncommon during normal pregnancy. Plasma cholinesterase levels are decreased but prolonged neuromuscular blockade does not occur in normal parturients receiving succinylcholine.

II. **Effects of anesthetic interventions on uterine blood flow**

A. **Determinants of uterine blood flow.** At term, normal UBF is approximately 700 mL/minute, which is approximately 10% of total maternal blood flow. The magnitude of UBF is determined by the equation:

UBF = (UAP − UVP)/UVR

where UAP is uterine arterial pressure, UVP the uterine venous pressure, and UVR the uterine vascular resistance. Alterations in any of these will influence UBF and therefore oxygen and nutrient delivery to the fetus.

B. Factors decreasing uterine arterial pressure
1. Hypovolemia
2. Sympathetic blockade
3. Aortocaval compression
4. Anesthetic overdose
5. Vasodilator overdose
6. Excessive positive pressure ventilation

C. Factors increasing uterine venous pressure
1. Vena caval compression
2. Uterine contractions
3. Uterine hypertonus
   a. Oxytocin overstimulation
   b. Alpha-adrenergic stimulation

D. Factors increasing uterine vascular resistance
1. Endogenous catecholamines
   a. Untreated pain
   b. Noxious stimulation (laryngoscopy, skin incision)
2. Preeclampsia
3. Chronic hypertension
4. Exogenous vasoconstrictors

Ephedrine is the drug of choice for treating maternal hypotension. Because of its mixed α and β effects, it increases maternal blood pressure (and therefore UAP) without increasing UVR. It therefore maintains UBF. The use of the pure α-agonist **phenylephrine** during pregnancy is controversial. In high doses, it increases maternal blood pressure but decreases UBF because it is a potent uterine artery vasoconstrictor. In low doses (50 to 100 μg) UBF is apparently well maintained.

III. Uteroplacental drug transfer and teratogenesis
  A. Drug transfer. A detailed consideration of the various mechanisms (active transport, facilitated diffusion, pinocytosis) by which substances are transported across the placenta is beyond the scope of this chapter. This discussion will concentrate on **passive diffusion**, the mechanism by which most anesthetic agents administered to the mother reach the fetus. This process does not require the expenditure of energy. Transfer can occur either directly through the lipid membrane or through protein channels that traverse the lipid bilayer.
    1. **Determinants of passive diffusion**
       a. **Concentration gradient** is the primary de-

terminant of the rate of transfer of drugs across the placenta. As an example, the initial rate of transfer of an inhalation agent is quite rapid. As the partial pressure of the agent increases in the fetus the rate of transfer will decrease.

b.   **Substances** with a low **molecular weight** cross the placenta more readily than those with a higher weight.

c.   **Drugs** with high **lipid solubility** readily traverse the placenta.

d.   **Ionization** limits placental transfer.

e.   **Membrane thickness** can be increased in certain pathologic states, including chronic hypertension and diabetes. The effects of these conditions on drug transfer are of less concern than the limitation of oxygen and nutrient transport that may result. This can lead to intrauterine growth restriction or, in severe cases, fetal demise.

2.   **Specific drugs**

a.   The **inhalation agents** freely cross the placenta due to their low molecular weight and high lipid solubility. The longer the period of fetal exposure to the agent (induction to delivery interval), the more likely the newborn is to be depressed.

b.   The **induction agents** including thiopental, etomidate, and propofol are highly lipophilic and un-ionized at physiologic pH. Placental transfer is quite rapid. Because most of the blood returning to the fetus from the umbilical vein passes through the fetal liver, extensive first-pass metabolism occurs and neonatal depression after an induction dose is uncommon.

c.   Both depolarizing and nondepolarizing **muscle relaxants** are highly ionized at physiologic pH. Placental transfer is minimal.

d.   The **opioids** freely traverse the placenta because of their high lipid solubility and low molecular weight.

e.   The **reversal agents** neostigmine and edrophonium are highly ionized and demonstrate minimal placental transfer.

f.   The **anticholinergic agents** atropine and scopolamine freely pass the placenta. **Glycopyrrolate** is highly ionized and thus crosses the placenta to a minimal degree.

g.   The commonly used **anticoagulants** heparin and warfarin have remarkably different placental transfer. Heparin, a highly ionized polysaccharide molecule, does not reach the fetus. Warfarin, which is uncharged and has a molecular weight of only 330, readily passes the placenta. Because warfarin can cause birth defects, its use is contraindicated during the period of organogenesis (see below).

h. **Antihypertensive agents.** The **beta blockers** that have been studied all cross the placenta. Labetalol appears to have the least placental transfer of this group of drugs. High-dose infusions of **esmolol** have been reported to cause persistent fetal bradycardia lasting up to 30 minutes after the termination of the infusion. The effect of a single bolus dose is not known but there are numerous case reports of its safe use as a bolus during anesthetic induction. **Sodium nitroprusside** (SNP) freely passes the placenta; this has implications for fetal toxicity (see below).

B. **Anesthesia during pregnancy and the risk of birth defects**
1. **Principles of teratology.** It is an established principle that any substance, if administered in large enough quantities for a prolonged period of time during critical periods of gestation, can produce fetal injury ranging from growth restriction to major structural anomalies to death. Thus, it should be a goal of anesthesiologists caring for pregnant women to minimize the exposure of their fetuses to potentially toxic substances. Nevertheless, our fears regarding the potential for injury should be tempered by the following realizations:

●Most anesthetics are administered for such a brief period of time that the potential for toxicity is minimal.

●There is no convincing **human** evidence that any of the commonly used anesthetics are dangerous to the fetus.

●Maternal hypotension and hypoxemia pose a much greater risk to the fetus than any anesthetic drugs.

●Maternal well-being must be our paramount concern. If avoiding a potentially teratogenic drug leads to a poor maternal outcome or maternal death, fetal outcome will be equally compromised.

2. **Evaluation of teratogenic potential.** Because of the ethical and logistical difficulties inherent in large-scale prospective studies of the teratogenic effects of anesthetics in humans, we must rely on more indirect evidence to evaluate the teratogenic potential of these drugs. The principal investigative tools used are small animal studies, retrospective studies of the offspring of women who underwent anesthesia during pregnancy, and, in the case of inhalation anesthetics, studies of operating room personnel who were exposed to low-level waste anesthetic gases during pregnancy. In

the discussion of specific drugs that follows, reference will be made to the studies supporting or opposing their teratogenic potential.

3. **Specific drugs**

   a. Animal studies of the potent **inhalation anesthetics** have given conflicting results. Reproductive effects appear to be dose-related. These effects are more likely to be due to the physiologic disturbances (hypothermia, hypoventilation, poor feeding) produced by the anesthetic state rather than the anesthetic agent itself. When animals are exposed to inspired concentrations that do not impair feeding behavior or level of consciousness, reproductive effects are minimal. Neither studies of operating room personnel exposed to trace anesthetics nor studies of women undergoing surgery during pregnancy support any teratogenic potential for the potent inhaled anesthetics. Pregnancy loss is increased in women undergoing surgery but this is primarily due to the underlying condition requiring surgery and the increased incidence of preterm delivery in women undergoing surgery in close proximity to the uterus.

   b. **Nitrous oxide** has clearly been shown to increase structural abnormalities and fetal loss in rats. This was initially thought to be a result of inhibition of the enzyme **methionine synthetase** and subsequent decreases in levels of methionine and tetrahydrofolate. This mechanism has been called into question because maximal inhibition of methionine synthetase activity occurs at levels of anesthetic exposure that do not produce teratogenic effects. More recent evidence suggests that the fetal effects of nitrous oxide are due to α-adrenergic stimulation and subsequent decreases in UBF. This is reversed by the simultaneous administration of a potent inhalation agent. Studies of operating room personnel exposed to trace nitrous oxide levels and of women undergoing nitrous oxide anesthesia fail to show any teratogenic potential.

   c. **Muscle relaxants** do not have any teratogenic potential at clinically appropriate doses.

   d. **Opioids** have not been shown to be teratogenic in either human or animal studies.

   e. Several human studies have suggested that chronic **benzodiazepine** therapy during pregnancy increases the incidence of cleft lip and cleft palate. These studies have been faulted for failure to control for concomitant exposure to other potentially teratogenic substances. There is little evidence to suggest that a single dose of a benzodiazepine during pregnancy poses any risk to the fetus.

    f. There is no human evidence suggesting that clinically useful **local anesthetics** are teratogenic. Chronic **cocaine** abuse has been linked to birth defects.

    g. Coumadin therapy during pregnancy has been linked to ophthalmologic, skeletal, and central nervous system abnormalities, presumably due to microhemorrhages during organogenesis. Because **heparin** does not cross the placenta, it is the drug of choice in women requiring anticoagulation during pregnancy.

IV. Epidemiology of intracranial disease in pregnancy and the effect of pregnancy on intracranial disease

    A. Subarachnoid hemorrhage: aneurysm and arteriovenous malformation. There are numerous causes for subarachnoid hemorrhage (SAH) during pregnancy including hypertensive intracerebral hemorrhage, vasculitis, and bacterial endocarditis, but by far the most common are aneurysm rupture and bleeding from an AVM. The overall incidence of SAH during pregnancy appears to be approximately 1 in 10,000, which is similar to the incidence in the general population. Approximately 4% to 5% of maternal deaths are due to SAH and it has been reported to be the fourth most common nonobstetric cause of death after trauma, malignancy, and cardiac disease.

    In 1990, Dias and Sekhar published a review of 154 published cases of SAH during pregnancy. The ratio of aneurysms to AVMs was approximately 3:1. There was no link between increasing parity and the incidence of hemorrhage. In both AVMs and aneurysms, there was an increasing incidence of hemorrhage with advancing gestational age. This may be due to increases in cardiac output or possibly hormonal influences on vascular integrity. Interestingly, few women bled during labor and delivery, which is consistent with the observation that more than 90% of all hemorrhages in nonpregnant patients occur at rest. Thirty-four percent of these patients had hypertension, proteinuria, or both, suggesting that the differentiation of SAH and preeclampsia may be difficult on clinical grounds alone

    B. Neoplastic lesions. The incidence of intracranial neoplasms does not appear to be appreciably different in pregnant compared with nonpregnant women. However, as mentioned previously, some tumors appear to grow more rapidly or become symptomatic during pregnancy. This may be due to increased edema secondary to increased sodium and water retention, as well as increased blood volume in vascular tumors such as meningiomas.

    There is considerable evidence that there are hormonal influences on the growth of brain tumors, particularly meningiomas. The incidence of meningioma is higher in women than in men but decreases significantly after menopause. Progesterone receptors have been identified in both meningiomas and gliomas. Accelerated tumor growth during pregnancy is likely due in part to the high levels of circulating progesterone seen during pregnancy.

V. Management of anesthesia for craniotomy during pregnancy

  A. Timing of surgery in relation to delivery

   1. General concerns. Whenever craniotomy during pregnancy is contemplated, the physicians caring for the pregnant woman must decide whether the pregnancy will be allowed to proceed to term or whether simultaneous operative delivery will occur. This will be determined by the gestational age of the fetus, with 32 weeks commonly used as the cutoff. Prior to this time, pregnancy is allowed to continue; after 32 weeks, cesarean delivery is performed and followed by immediate craniotomy. This is not because viability begins at 32 weeks but rather because at this time the risks of preterm delivery are felt to become less than the risks to the fetus of such maternal therapies as controlled hypotension, osmotic diuresis, and mechanical hyperventilation.

   2. Aneurysm clipping. Dias and Sekhar demonstrated a significant improvement in survival for both mother and fetus when aneurysm clipping was performed after SAH, when compared with nonsurgical management. Therefore, in patients with good SAH grades, aneurysm clipping should be performed as soon as possible to prevent rebleeding. Clipping of unruptured contralateral aneurysms can be delayed until the postpartum period.

   3. Arteriovenous malformation resection. Resection of unruptured AVMs can be delayed until after delivery with no apparent increase in maternal mortality. Conversely, resection of symptomatic AVMs is usually performed regardless of gestation. The management of women with ruptured AVM who are neurologically stable is controversial. Dias and Sekhar showed improved maternal outcome with early surgery but this difference did not reach statistical significance. Thus, the question of early surgery for ruptured AVM during pregnancy remains unanswered at this time.

   4. Neoplasm resection. Resection of a histologically benign neoplasm such as a meningioma can be delayed until after delivery but only if frequent follow-up and careful monitoring for neurologic deterioration can be assured. Surgery for presumed malignant tumors and for those masses producing worsening neurologic deficits should occur regardless of pregnancy.

B. Anesthetic management

1. Sedative **premedication** may be appropriate in extremely anxious patients, but the risk of hypoventilation, hypercarbia, and subsequent increases in intracranial pressure (ICP) should be considered and guarded against. It might be more appropriate to defer the administration of sedative medications until the patient arrives in the preoperative holding area, where careful observation can be maintained. Because pregnant patients must be considered to be at increased risk of regurgitation and aspiration of gastric contents, medications to decrease the acidity and/or the volume of the gastric contents should be administered. This can include 30 mL of a nonparticulate antacid, metoclopramide 10 mg, and an H_2 blocker such as ranitidine 150 mg.

2. Anesthetic **induction** in the pregnant patient with intracranial pathology provides the clearest example of the need to reconcile competing clinical goals. A rapid sequence induction that is designed to prevent aspiration does little to prevent the hemodynamic response to intubation that can be catastrophic for the patient with an intracranial aneurysm or increased ICP. At the same time, a slow neuroinduction with thiopental, narcotic, a nondepolarizing muscle relaxant, and mask ventilation does little to decrease the risk of aspiration. This technique can also be expected to lead to neonatal depression should cesarean section be performed as part of a combined procedure.

   One acceptable technique for anesthetic induction is described below (Table 18-1); there are obviously other approaches that are equally acceptable. As described previously, aspiration prophylaxis is mandatory. Cricoid pressure should be maintained from loss of consciousness until intubation is confirmed. If cesarean delivery is performed as part of a combined procedure, the phy-

Table 18-1. Anesthetic induction for craniotomy

Thiopental 5–7 mg/kg

Fentanyl 3–5 μg/kg

Lidocaine 75 mg

Rocuronium 0.9–1.2 mg/kg

Mask ventilation with cricoid pressure, 100% O_2

sician caring for the newborn should be made aware of the likelihood of neonatal depression and the need to provide respiratory support.

3. In addition to the standard maternal monitors, **fetal heart rate (FHR) monitoring** can be extremely useful during craniotomy, not because an ominous FHR indicates when cesarean delivery should be performed but rather because it should lead to a rapid search for potentially reversible causes of decreased uteroplacental perfusion, such as hypotension or hypoxemia. Fetal heart rate monitoring usually becomes technically feasible by approximately 20 weeks gestation. Note that decreases in short- and long-term variability, as well as a decreased baseline FHR, are commonly seen even in the healthy, uncompromised fetus whose mother is receiving general anesthesia.

4. **Anesthetic maintenance** is not appreciably different between the pregnant and nonpregnant patient undergoing craniotomy (Table 18-2). As is the case during induction of anesthesia, every effort should be made to maintain hemodynamic stability, as well as to avoid increases in cerebral blood volume that could interfere with surgical exposure. As stated previously, potentially teratogenic agents should be avoided but the commonly used anesthetics do not appear to fall into this category.

5. **Adjuvants to surgery**
   a. Osmotic diuresis with **mannitol** is commonly used for decreasing brain bulk and facilitating exposure during craniotomy. Because mannitol has been demonstrated in both animal and human studies to produce fetal dehydration, some have advised against the use of this agent during pregnancy. However, the doses utilized in these early studies were considerably higher than those currently in clinical use. There is no evidence that mannitol 0.5 to 1.0 g/kg has any significant adverse effect on fetal fluid balance.
   b. In addition, **maternal hyperventilation** can facilitate surgical exposure by decreasing ce-

Table 18-2.   Anesthetic maintenance for craniotomy

Fentanyl 1–2 μg/kg/h

Isoflurane 0.5–1.0% ± nitrous oxide

Nondepolarizing muscle relaxant

Thiopental 5–6 mg/kg/h for "tight brain"

rebral blood volume. Severe hypocarbia may impair fetal oxygen delivery, however, by shifting the maternal oxygen–hemoglobin dissociation curve to the left. Hyperventilation can also decrease maternal cardiac output by increasing intrathoracic pressure. Modest hyperventilation to a $PaCO_2$ of 28 to 30 mm Hg should provide adequate surgical conditions without significantly compromising the fetus.

c. **Controlled hypotension** is becoming less common during aneurysm surgery because of the growing use of temporary clip occlusion of proximal vessels. There will be situations, however, when this technique becomes necessary. Because UBF varies directly with perfusion pressure, severe hypotension can lead to fetal asphyxia. Blood pressure should therefore be lowered only to that level deemed necessary for maternal well-being, and for as brief a duration as possible. Fetal heart rate monitoring might alert the anesthesiologist to the development of fetal hypoxia and lead to the restoration of blood pressure if the need for hypotension is not critical at that time.

An additional concern is present when **SNP** is chosen as the hypotensive agent. Because of the limited ability of the fetal liver to metabolize cyanide, it is possible for fetal intoxication to occur in the absence of any signs of maternal toxicity. There are several case reports of the safe use of SNP during pregnancy. Nevertheless, the duration of administration should be limited to that period deemed essential to maternal well-being and the total dose of SNP should be limited through the administration of additional agents such as a beta blockers and inhalation anesthetics..

d. It has been suggested that mild **hypothermia** (33°C to 35°C) has cerebral protective effects. This level of hypothermia has no significant fetal effects. More profound levels of hypothermia, however, can cause fetal arrhythmias and should be avoided.

6. **Emergence.** Prior to the removal of the endotracheal tube, the pregnant patient should be fully awake and her airway reflexes should be intact to minimize the risk of aspiration. An awake patient will also facilitate early neurologic evaluation and eliminate the need for emergent radiologic evaluation of persistently obtunded patients. At the same time, however, every effort should be made to prevent coughing and straining on the tube because

this may lead to catastrophic intracranial hemor-rhage. This may be accomplished through the ad-ministration of lidocaine 75 to 100 mg and/or fen-tanyl 25 to 50 μg at the end of surgery. Because placement of the head dressing is associated with movement that produces airway stimulation, it is appropriate to maintain neuromuscular blockade until the dressing has been secured. These guide-lines do not apply to the patient who was obtunded preoperatively or who had a significantly compli-cated intraoperative course (bleeding, brain swell-ing). Such patients should retain their endotra-cheal tubes until their neurologic status can be evaluated.

SUGGESTED READINGS

Capeless EL, Clapp JF. Cardiovascular changes in early phase of pregnancy. *Am J Obstet Gynecol* 1989;161:1449.

Cohen SE. Physiologic alterations of pregnancy: anesthetic implica-tions. *American Society of Anesthesiologists Refresher Courses in Anesthesiology* 1993;21:51.

Cohen SE. Nonobstetric surgery during pregnancy. In: Chestnut DH, ed. *Obstetric anesthesia*. St. Louis: Mosby-Year Book, 1994: 273–293.

Dias MS, Sekhar LN. Intracranial hemorrhage from aneurysms and arteriovenous malformations during pregnancy and the puerpe-rium. *Neurosurgery* 1990;27:855.

Donaldson JO. *Neurology of pregnancy,* 2nd ed. London: WB Saun-ders, 1989.

Herman NL. The placenta: anatomy, physiology, and transfer of drugs. In: Chestnut DH, ed. *Obstetric anesthesia*. St. Louis: Mosby-Year Book, 1994:57–75.

Induced Hypotension

Wiebke Gogarten and Hugo Van Aken

I. **Definition and indications.** Induced or deliberate hypotension is defined as lowering mean arterial blood pressure (MAP) to 50 to 65 mm Hg in normotensive, anesthetized patients. It is established to decrease blood loss during surgery, improve surgical conditions, and decrease the need for blood transfusions. In aneurysm surgery, induced hypotension is used to lower the risk of aneurysm rupture due to wall tension. Alternative techniques of lowering aneurysm wall tension include local hypotension with positioning of a temporary clip on the proximal feeding artery.

   Lowering MAP to 50 to 65 mm Hg can decrease blood loss by 50% in a number of different operations. However, there is high interpatient variability, making the effect of induced hypotension on blood loss less predictable in individual patients. In reducing blood loss, the position of the surgical field might even have a greater impact than absolute MAP. If possible, the surgical field should be elevated, thereby decreasing arterial pressure, improving venous drainage, and decreasing blood loss. The most important criterion for inducing hypotension is patient benefit. However, outcome improvement has not consistently been shown and the margin of safety is reduced during periods of induced hypotension.

II. **General considerations.** Potential hazards of induced hypotension include myocardial and cerebral ischemia. Mortality due to induced hypotension is mainly evoked by inadequate organ blood flow and is in the range of 0.02% to 0.06%. A safe lower limit of blood pressure (BP) has not yet been conclusively established. Hypovolemia and anemia should be corrected before inducing hypotension as hypovolemic hypotension is more frequently associated with organ dysfunction than normovolemic hypotension. Blood pressure control is also facilitated in normovolemic patients.

III. **Cerebral effects of induced hypotension**

   A. **Cerebral autoregulation.** Cerebral autoregulation ensures a stable cerebral blood flow (CBF) over a wide range of systemic MAP (50 to 150 mm Hg) in normotensive patients. Below this threshold, CBF becomes dependent on MAP, which should not be lowered any further. Even within the range of cerebral autoregulation, abrupt changes in MAP lead to transitory changes in CBF of 3 to 4 minutes in duration. In patients with intracranial pathology, subarachnoid hemorrhage (SAH), or cerebral trauma, cerebral autoregulation may be impaired, putting these patients at increased risk of cerebral ischemia during induced hypotension. Patients with cerebral vasospasm have impaired autoregulation and are more prone to cerebral ischemia during induced hypotension. The incidence of vasospasm may be increased, borderline ischemic brain tissue compromised, and autoregulation further impaired. On the other hand, intraoperative hypertension in patients with SAH may increase the risk of bleeding and rupture. Vasodilator therapy and volatile anesthetics can also adversely affect cerebral autoregulation.

B. Carbon dioxide reactivity. During normotension, changes in the partial pressure of carbon dioxide ($PaCO_2$) are followed by changes in CBF in a linear way, with each mm Hg increase in $PaCO_2$ leading to a 3% increase in CBF. However, this increase in CBF can provoke a cerebral steal with blood diverted away from already ischemic, maximally dilated cerebral regions to normal areas of the brain. The $PaCO_2$ reactivity of cerebral vessels is diminished during hypotension, SAH, cerebral trauma, and cerebrovascular disease. Hypocarbia should be avoided in order not to decrease CBF further during induced hypotension.

Patients with increased intracranial pressure (ICP) should not undergo induced hypotension until the dura has been opened because decreases in blood pressure in this setting expose the brain to an increased risk of ischemia.

IV. Implications for organ perfusion. A reduction in MAP during induced hypotension is achieved through a reduction in systemic vascular resistance (SVR), cardiac output (CO), or both. Lowering the CO, however, can have a major impact on organ blood flow and oxygen delivery. Therefore, it is preferable to induce hypotension by predominantly reducing SVR through the use of vasodilators. To maintain organ blood flow, it is crucial to assess volume status frequently and avoid hypovolemia.

A. Heart. Reflex tachycardia and low MAP with exhausted coronary vasodilatory reserve can provoke myocardial ischemia. Vasodilatation with adenosine and sodium nitroprusside can result in coronary steal. More appropriate for patients with coronary artery disease are drugs that do not induce reflex tachycardia (esmolol, labetalol, urapidil); reduce metabolic requirements (esmolol, anesthetics); or improve blood flow to ischemic myocardium (nitroglycerin).

B. Lungs. Reduced CO during hypotension can lead to an increase in dead space and, concomitantly, in $PaCO_2$. Vasodilator therapy can increase pulmonary shunt through inhibition of hypoxic pulmonary vasoconstriction with a decrease in oxygen saturation. Pulmonary gas exchange should be controlled by periodic blood gas analysis.

C. **Kidneys.** Resting arteriolar tone is low and there is diminished capacity to vasodilate in response to hypotension. Below a MAP of 75 mm Hg, renal blood flow and glomerular filtration decline, resulting in oliguria. In normovolemic patients, normal urine production rapidly recovers after discontinuation of induced hypotension. A combination of labetalol and isoflurane better preserves renal function than isoflurane alone.

D. **Liver.** During induced hypotension, hepatic blood flow is diminished because it is directly dependent on systemic arterial pressure and autoregulation does not exist. Baroreflex activation, surgical stress response, and exogenous vasopressors can also reduce hepatic blood flow. Hypotensive drugs that maintain CO should be preferred. Therefore, it is prudent to maintain MAP at 50 to 60 mm Hg. Within this range, changes in hepatic function are unlikely to occur.

V. **Monitoring**
   A. Besides electrocardiography (ECG), pulse oximetry, and end-tidal CO_2, monitoring should include invasive arterial BP measurement. Measurement of urine output is mandatory in longer procedures. In order to calculate cerebral perfusion pressure (CPP) accurately (MAP-ICP), pressure transducers should be zeroed to the level of the external auditory meatus.
   B. The electroencephalogram (EEG) is profoundly influenced by anesthetics and therefore not very useful for monitoring cerebral integrity intraoperatively. Moreover, electrode placement in close vicinity to the operative field is usually not possible. Sensory and brain stem evoked potentials are more resistant to anesthetic influences and therefore more suitable during neurosurgical procedures.

VI. **Contraindications.** Absolute or relative contraindications to induced hypotension include:

Cerebrovascular disease
Coronary artery disease (angina, myocardial infarction)
Peripheral vascular disease
Uncontrolled arterial hypertension
Renal dysfunction
Liver dysfunction
Hypovolemia
Severe anemia
Low intracranial compliance, increased ICP

Patients with stenotic vessels or existing organ dysfunction are at increased risk of inadequate organ perfusion during induced hypotension. Uncontrolled hypertension shifts the CBF autoregulation curve to the right and puts these patients at increased risk for major morbidity and mortality when lowering blood pressure beneath the threshold for critical CBF. However, if hypertension is

controlled, cerebral autoregulation returns to normal
values. Therefore, deliberate hypotension is considered
safe in patients with controlled hypertension.

VII.   Drugs commonly used for induced hypotension
(Table 19-1)

  A.   Volatile anesthetics. Volatile anesthetics have
been widely used for induced hypotension. A major
advantage is their rapid onset of action and their
easy controllability. Volatile anesthetics decrease cerebral metabolic rate with a favorable influence on
global cerebral oxygen supply/demand ratio. Nevertheless, they should not be used as the sole agent
to induce hypotension in patients with intracranial
pathology, as their use can increase CBF, cerebral
blood volume, and ICP.

   1.   Halothane. Halothane is predominantly a myocardial depressant with less effect on SVR. Increases in CBF and ICP are more pronounced
and reduction in cerebral oxygen metabolic demand is less than that of isoflurane. It is therefore best avoided in neurosurgical procedures.

   2.   Isoflurane. Isoflurane causes a decrease in SVR
with little effect on CO. However, isoflurane administration in concentrations of greater than 1
MAC (mean alveolar concentration) results in
direct dilatation of cerebral vessels, an impairment of cerebral autoregulation, and an increase
in CBF and concomitantly in ICP. The use of low
concentrations of isoflurane combined with intravenous agents is more appropriate to induce
hypotension. Animal studies show a greater increase in cerebral edema during induced hypotension with isoflurane compared with labetalol.

   3.   Sevoflurane. Sevoflurane has a similar hemodynamic profile compared with isoflurane. Cerebral CO_2 reactivity is maintained with 1 MAC
sevoflurane. There is a similar increase in ICP
and reduction in CPP compared with isoflurane.
Due to its lower blood gas solubility, titration
and onset of hypotension are facilitated.

   4.   Desflurane. Desflurane induces the same
changes in CBF, autoregulation, and ICP as
isoflurane. There are few studies on desflurane
and induced hypotension; therefore, general
statements on its suitability cannot be made. In
animal models, desflurane decreases CPP and
CBF. Care should be taken not to raise the concentration too quickly to avoid increases in sympathetic tone with resultant hypertension and
tachycardia.

  B.   Intravenous agents. Drugs suitable for induced
hypotension possess a predictable, dose-dependent
effect with fast onset and recovery and minimal effects on blood flow to vital organs, and can be titrated as needed. They should not impair cerebral

Table 19-1. Drugs and dosages commonly used for induced hypotension

Drug	Dosage	Hemodynamic Changes	Adverse Reactions
Nitroprusside	1–8 µg/kg/min max. 1.5 mg/kg w.o. thiosulfate	SVR↓↓, MAP↓↓, HR↑↑, CO(↑↑), ICP↑↑, CBF↑↑	Cyanide toxicity, renin↑, angiotensin↑↓, tachyphylaxis, rebound hypertension
Nitroglycerin	0.1–7 µg/kg/min	SVR↓↓, PVR↓↓, MAP↓↓, CO(↓↓), HR↑↑, ICP↑↑ CBF↑↑	Headache, nausea, vomiting
Hydralazine	2.5–20 mg i.v., 1–2 µg/kg/min	SVR↓↓, MAP↓↓, HR↑↑, CO↑↑, ICP↑↑, CBF↑↑	Renin, angiotensin↑↑, slow onset 5–15 min, coronary steal
Trimethaphan	1–20 mg i.v., 0.5–10 mg/min	SVR↓↓, MAP↓↓, HR(↑↑), CO⇔, ICP⇔, CBF⇔	Tachyphylaxis, pupillary dilatation, histamine release, urinary and gastrointestinal atony, inhibition of pseudocholinesterase
Esmolol	0.25–0.5 mg/kg load, 50–200 µg/kg/min	SVR↑↑, MAP↓↓, HR↓↓, CO↓↓	Heart block, congestive heart failure, bronchospasm
Nicardipine	1–4 µg/kg/min	SVR↓↓, MAP↓↓, HR(↑↑), ICP⇔	Headache, flushing, nausea, vomiting, phlebitis
Phentolamine	1–5 mg i.v., 1–20 µg/kg/min	SVR↓↓, MAP↓↓, HR↑↑, CO↑↑, ICP(⇔)	Histamine release, epinephrine reversal, dysrhythmias, renin↑↑
Urapidil	20–50 mg i.v., 2–10 µg/kg/min	SVR↓↓, MAP↓↓, CO↑↑, HR⇔, ICP⇔, CBF⇔	Headache, dizziness, nausea, fatigue
Labetalol	20–50 mg i.v., 2 mg/kg/min	SVR↓↓, MAP↓↓, HR↑↑, CO↓↓	Heart block, bronchospasm
Prostaglandin E_1	0.05–0.4 µg/kg/min	SVR↓↓, PVR↓↓, MAP↓↓, ICP⇔	Inhibition of platelet aggregation
Adenosine	6 mg i.v./12 mg i.v., 100–140 µg/kg/min	CO↑↑, HR↑↑, SVR↓↓, ICP⇔	Renin↓↓, renal blood flow↓↓, atrioventricular block, cardiac arrest

SVR, systemic vascular resistance; MAP, mean arterial pressure; HR, heart rate; CO, cardiac output; ICP, intracranial pressure; CBF, cerebral blood flow; PVR, pulmonary vascular resistance; ⇑, parameter increases; ⇓, parameter decreases; ⇔, parameter remains unchanged; (⇑) or (⇓) or (⇔), parameter changes slightly or remains the same.

autoregulation or increase brain bulk. Most vasodilators also dilate cerebral vessels with an increase in CBF or a restoration of CBF at prehypotension levels, with the exception of the ganglionic blocker trimethaphan. The influence of vasodilator therapy on ICP is less critical, if hypotension is induced slowly.

1. **Sodium nitroprusside (Nipride, Nipruss).** Sodium nitroprusside (SNP) is commonly used for induced hypotension. It possesses a fast onset and short duration (1 to 3 minutes) with easy titration. The main action is on arteriolar tone; only 65% to 70% of the dose is recovered in venous plasma. Cardiac output is decreased in hypovolemia but increased in normo- or hypervolemia. Intracranial pressure can be increased. Side effects include cyanide toxicity, reflex tachycardia, tachyphylaxis, and rebound hypertension. If SNP is used, it is prudent to determine the rate of administration and absolute dose given accurately.

   Tachyphylaxis is influenced by stimulation of renin-angiotensin and activation of the sympathoadrenal system and can be prevented by pretreatment with beta blockers or angiotensin-converting enzyme (ACE) inhibitors, e.g., enalapril, 2.5 mg i.v., 60 minutes before initiation of hypotension. This regimen can also diminish rebound hypertension on discontinuation of SNP, which should be tapered rather than stopped abruptly.

   a. **Cyanide toxicity.** In plasma, free cyanide ions (CN^-) are released from nitroprusside and cyanide toxicity is directly dependent on the amount of SNP used. Signs of cyanide toxicity are metabolic acidosis during induced hypotension, decreased arteriovenous oxygen difference (e.g., increased venous oxygen saturation), tachycardia, shock.

   The presence of free cyanide ions inhibits cytochrome oxidase and oxidative phosphorylation, resulting in tissue hypoxia. Cyanide production also occurs in vitro due to photodegradation. Therefore it is essential to protect SNP from light. In doses exceeding 2 μg/kg/minute or 1.5 mg/kg totally, sodium thiosulfate should be administered concomitantly to reduce cyanide toxicity. If cyanide toxicity is suspected, SNP must be discontinued.

   b. **Therapy of cyanide toxicity**
      (1) **Sodium thiosulfate** 150 mg/kg i.v. The enzyme rhodanese converts CN^- and thiosulfate to thiocyanate, which is significantly less toxic and is excreted by the kidneys.

(2) **Hydroxycobalamin** 0.1 mg/kg i.v. Hydroxycobalamin and CN^- form cyanocobalamin (vitamin B_{12}).

2. **Nitroglycerin (Nitrolingual, Nitrostat, Perlinganit).** Nitroglycerin is a direct vasodilator of venous capacitance vessels. Arteriolar vasodilatation is less pronounced. Half-life is short and toxic metabolites are not produced. Response depends on the patient's volume status. Cardiac output may decrease if preload is reduced. Administration induces reflex tachycardia. Induced hypotension with nitroglycerin is less rapid and predictable than with SNP, and only moderate levels of hypotension (e.g., 60 mm Hg) are achieved. In patients with diminished intracranial compliance, use of nitroglycerin is contraindicated until the dura is opened. Patients are at risk of developing increased cerebral blood volume and significant brain edema. Intracranial pressure is increased and CPP decreased during nitroglycerin infusion, while CO_2 reactivity is maintained. Half-life is 1 to 3 minutes. Compared to SNP, nitroglycerin is less toxic, less effective, and less controllable.

3. **Hydralazine (Apresoline, Nepresol).** Hydralazine is a direct arteriolar vasodilator and acts via smooth muscle relaxation, thereby significantly reducing SVR without causing any change or only a mild increase in cardiac output and heart rate (HR). The advantages include selective vasodilatation with more dilatation of coronary, cerebral, renal, and splanchnic beds as opposed to vessels in skin and muscles. Blood pressure will only be lowered by 20 to 30 mm Hg due to an activation of baroreceptor reflexes. Coronary vasodilatation and reflex tachycardia can lead to coronary steal with myocardial ischemia. Hydralazine can also cause a significant rise in ICP. On discontinuation, rebound hypertension does not occur. Onset of action is rather slow with a peak effect 5 to 15 minutes after intravenous administration; elimination half-life is 4 hours. Long-term usage is associated with a lupus erythematosus–like syndrome, skin rash, drug fever, pancytopenia, and peripheral neuropathy.

4. **Trimethaphan (Arfonad).** Trimethaphan is a sympathetic and parasympathetic ganglionic blocker that acts via direct vasodilatation and histamine release. It has been widely used for induced hypotension. Onset of action is fast (1 to 2 minutes) and half-life short (5 to 10 minutes) due to rapid inactivation by plasma cholinesterases and renal excretion. Mean arterial pressure is decreased without decrease in CO. Heart rate

remains unchanged or increases (reflex). Tri-methaphan does not dilate cerebral vessels. Therefore ICP increases are less than with SNP. Trimethaphan is suitable for inducing hypotension as an adjunct to other vasodilators (e.g., SNP) in order to reduce side effects and achieve better control of BP. Nonspecific ganglionic blockade results in tachycardia, mydriasis, cycloplegia, reduced gastrointestinal motility, and urinary retention. Inhibition of pseudocholinesterase by trimethaphan may prolong the action of succinylcholine. The resulting gastrointestinal and bladder atony as well as a rapid development of tachyphylaxis are major drawbacks. Due to the induced mydriasis, pupil size cannot be evaluated in neurologic patients during the action of trimethaphan.

5. **Esmolol (Brevibloc).** Esmolol is a short-acting β_1 blocker with a very rapid onset of action and a beta half-life of 9 minutes. Elimination occurs by red blood cell esterases, which are not influenced by cholinesterase inhibitors. It possesses no intrinsic sympathetic activity. Plasma renin activity decreases slightly during administration, improving the induced hypotension. Because of myocardial depression, decreased HR, and increased SVR, cardiac output is decreased markedly. Therefore, it should only be used to induce mild reductions in BP or in combination therapy.

6. **Nicardipine (Cardene).** Nicardipine is a dihydropyridine calcium channel blocker that dilates peripheral, coronary, and cerebral arterial vessels. Cardiac output and myocardial contractility are maintained or even increased and tachycardia is not induced. Intracranial pressure and CO_2 reactivity remain unchanged. Nicardipine has been shown to reduce neurologic deficit from cerebral vasospasm after SAH and improve cognitive function after coronary artery bypass graft. Careful titration is mandatory because induced hypotension resists conventional antihypotensive treatment. The potency of nicardipine is comparable to that of SNP, but rebound hypertension is lacking. Alpha and beta half-life are 3 and 14 minutes, respectively. With longer infusions, phlebitis can be induced in peripheral veins.

7. **Phentolamine (Regitine).** Phentolamine is a competitive antagonist at α_1-, α_2-, and 5-hydroxytryptamine (5-HT) receptors and induces primarily arterial vasodilatation with little effect on venous tone. The resulting hemodynamic changes are decreased SVR and MAP with an increase in HR and contractility. Reflex tachy-

cardia can be blunted by beta blockade. Half-life is 19 minutes with an unknown elimination. In patients treated with alpha blockers, coadministration of epinephrine can lead to a significant fall in BP, known as epinephrine reversal. Although CPP is reduced temporarily, ICP does not change significantly. Hypotension starts 2 minutes after intravenous administration and lasts for 10 to 15 minutes.

8. **Urapidil (Ebrantil).** Urapidil (not available in the United States) is a peripheral (α_1-adrenergic receptor antagonist as well as a weak β_1-antagonist, resulting in peripheral vasodilatation with a decrease in SVR and BP. Significant sympathetic activation and reflex tachycardia are inhibited by stimulation of central serotonergic 5-HT1A receptors. Intracranial pressure, CBF, and cerebral compliance remain unchanged. The maximum decrease of BP is 20 to 30 mm Hg. Therefore, urapidil is suitable if moderate degrees of hypotension are desired or in combination with volatile anesthetics or other hypotensive drugs. This technique is commonly practiced in European countries. Potentially adverse reactions include dizziness, nausea, and fatigue. Rebound hypertension and tachyphylaxis do not occur. Onset begins within 5 minutes of intravenous administration and half-life is 3 hours.

9. **Labetalol (Normodyne, Trandate).** Labetalol is an α_1-, β_1-, and β_2-blocking agent (α/β ratio 1:7). Hypotension results due to a decrease in myocardial contractility and SVR. Heart rate remains unchanged and ICP is not increased. Onset of action occurs 5 minutes after intravenous administration and the effect lasts for approximately 4 hours, making it less suitable for intraoperative titration. Combined with volatile anesthetics or other vasodilators, a remarkable synergism results and organ blood flow is better preserved than during induced hypotension with volatile anesthetics alone. Caution should be exercised in cases involving hypovolemia and severe blood loss, as adrenergic responses will be masked during administration of labetalol.

10. **Prostaglandin E_1 (PGE$_1$, Prostin VR, Alprostadil).** Prostaglandin E_1 induces direct vasodilatation via specific prostaglandin receptors on vascular smooth muscle cells. Onset of action begins immediately and inactivation occurs enzymatically in most tissues, especially the lung, with a high first-pass effect. During anesthesia, the hypotensive effect of PGE$_1$ can be prolonged after discontinuation of the drug. In neurosurgical patients, local CBF and CO_2 reactivity re-

main unchanged. The PGE_1 only exhibits inhibition of platelet aggregation in dosages higher than currently used.

11. **Adenosine (Adenocard, Adrecar).** Adenosine, an endogenous nucleoside, acts as an agonist at cardiac A_1 purinoreceptors as well as A_2 receptors in arteriolar vessels. This leads to a decrease in sinoatrial and atrioventricular node conduction and a reduction in SVR and BP. The CO and HR are increased reflexly. Rebound hypertension does not occur. An indirect mechanism includes the release of nitric oxide. Inactivation is rapid through deamination in plasma and erythrocytes with an ultrashort half-life of 10 seconds. Due to this ultrashort half-life, hemodynamic changes occur only transiently.

Adenosine dilates cerebral and coronary vessels, and impairs autoregulation. Side effects include flushing, chest discomfort, bronchospasm, transient complete heart block, and asystole. These side effects usually last for seconds and do not require therapeutic intervention. Nevertheless, a pacemaker and a defibrillator should be available if adenosine is used. The effects of adenosine are antagonized by theophylline. Due to renal arteriolar constriction with reduced renal blood flow and filtration, adenosine should not be used over a long period of time or in patients with impaired renal function.

VIII. **Management of induced hypotension**

Elevate surgical field

Ensure adequate anesthesia

Maintain normovolemia

Regard contraindications

Add small doses of a vasodilator (e.g., SNP, urapidil)

Avoid rapid changes in BP

Avoid reflex tachycardia with small doses of a beta blocker

If ICP is raised, avoid hypotension until the dura has been opened

SUGGESTED READINGS

Abe K. Vasodilators during cerebral aneurysm surgery. *Can J Anaesth* 1993;40:775.

Drummond JC, Shapiro HM. Cerebral physiology. In: Miller RD, ed. *Anesthesia.* New York: Churchill Livingstone, 1994:689–729.

Inglis A, Fitch W. Physiology and metabolism of the central nervous system: anaesthetic implications. In: Van Aken H, ed. *Neuro-anaesthetic practice.* London: BMJ, 1995:1–22.

Kitaguchi K, Ohsumi H, Kuro M, Nakajima T, Hayashi Y. Effects of sevoflurane on cerebral circulation and metabolism in patients with ischemic cerebrovascular disease. *Anesthesiology* 1993;79:704.

Larach DR, Solina AR. Cardiovascular drugs. In: Hensley FA, Martin DE, eds. *A practical approach to cardiac anesthesia.* Boston: Little, Brown, and Co, 1995:32–95.

Law JA, Gelb AW. Anaesthetic management of aneurysms and arteriovenous malformations. In: Van Aken H, ed. *Neuro-anaesthetic practice.* London: BMJ, 1995:193–213.

Van Aken H, Miller ED Jr. Deliberate hypotension. In: Miller RD, ed. *Anesthesia.* New York: Churchill Livingstone, 1999 (in press).

20A

Anesthetic Management of Diagnostic and Therapeutic Interventional Neuroradiologic Procedures

Shailendra Joshi and William L. Young

The endovascular approach has opened new options in the treatment of vascular and nonvascular intracranial and spinal diseases. Although such procedures seem to be technically simple they carry a low but significant morbidity. Approximately 1% to 3% of the patients may develop neurologic symptoms after conventional cerebral angiography.

I. **Neurovascular access and methods**
   A. **Vascular access.** Interventional neuroradiologic (INR) procedures typically involve placement of catheters in the arterial circulation of the head or the neck, usually through the transfemoral route. As illustrated in Fig. 20A-1, transfemoral access is accomplished by the placement of a large introducer sheath into the femoral artery, usually 7.5-Fr in size. Through the introducer sheath a 7.0-Fr coaxial catheter is positioned by fluoroscopic control into the the carotid or vertebral artery. Finally, a 1.5- to 2.8-Fr superselective microcatheter is introduced into the cerebral circulation. The superselective catheter can be used to deliver drugs, embolic agents, or balloons to the desired location. The transfemoral placement site is usually infiltrated with local anesthetic agent, which can result in femoral nerve block. Transfemoral venous access can be used to reach the dural sinuses and in some cases the arterial side of the arteriovenous malformations (AVMs) as well. Direct percutaneous puncture is used to access superficial venous malformations.
   B. **Imaging technology.** Necessary radiologic imaging methods include high-resolution fluoroscopy and high-speed digital subtraction angiography (DSA) with road mapping functions. Digital subtraction angiography enables visualization of only those vessels that are opacified by contrast injection. The road mapping function enables the radiologist to observe the advance of the catheter against the background map of the patient's cerebral vessels. Digital subtraction angiography involves subtraction of images obtained before and after injection of radiocontrast. Any displacement of the cerebral vessels due to movement of the head profoundly degrades DSA images. Hence,

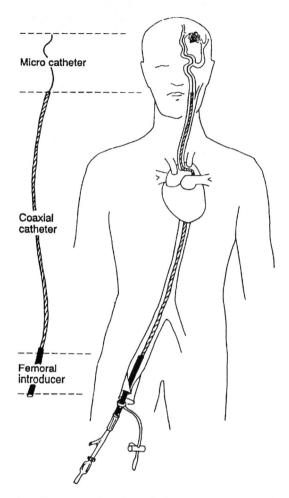

Fig. 20A-1.   Representation of a typical arrangement of transfemoral coaxial catheter system showing the femoral introducer sheath, the coaxial catheter, and the microcatheter. [From Young WL. *Clinical neuroscience lectures.* Munster, IL: Cathenart Publishing, 1999 (in press), with permission.]

it is critical that the patient remains immobile during the procedure.
C. **Materials for embolization or infusion.** The nature of the disease, the purpose of embolization, the size and penetration of emboli and vessels, and the permanency of occlusion are among the factors taken into consideration for agent selection. The ideal

choice and the combination of agents is controversial. Embolic agents include balloons, coils, silastic pellets, and glue.

N-Butyl cyanoacrylate (NBCA) glue used for embolization is available as a liquid monomer that rapidly polymerizes in contact with ionic solutions such as blood and saline.

II.   **Anesthetic considerations.** In general, most INR procedures can be undertaken with intravenous sedation, which ensures patient comfort yet enables repeated neurologic assessments. The primary goals of anesthesia are not only to render the patient immobile but also to control the level of sedation and manipulate hemodynamics. Children, uncooperative patients, and prolonged procedures such as those on the spinal cord might require general anesthesia.

Briefly, the three primary functions of the anesthesiologist in the interventional suite are (a) provision of a physiologically stable and immobile patient, (b) manipulation of systemic blood pressure as dictated by the needs of the procedure, and (c) emergent care of catastrophic complications.

III.   **Conduct of anesthesia for interventional neuroradiologic procedures**

   A.   **Preoperative assessment.** A careful assessment of the airway has to be made. A history of snoring may suggest that partial airway obstruction might occur with sedation. Snoring results in movement artifacts that may degrade the quality of images during cerebral angiography. Patients with a history of adverse reaction to radiocontrast drugs require pretreatment with steroids and antihistaminic drugs. In the population with occlusive cerebrovascular disease, patients might require adequate treatment of hypertension, heart failure, or angina. Preoperative communication should exist with the INR team to develop a clear strategy for sedation and hemodynamic interventions that might be needed during the procedure.

   B.   **Preoperative investigations.** Routine guidelines for laboratory investigations are applicable to INR procedures. Of particular interest is the baseline coagulation screen since anticoagulation will be required for the procedure.

   C.   **Premedication.** Anxiolytics may be administered depending on the condition of the patient. Minimal premedication is required for INR procedures. Calcium channel blockers, such as nimodipine, are routinely used by neuroradiologists to decrease intraoperative vasospasm.

   D.   **Room preparation.** The INR suite should be equipped exactly like a standard anesthesia operating room. Suction, gas evacuation, oxygen, and nitrous oxide should be available from the wall outlets. Ideally, the anesthesia machine should have the capacity to provide carbon dioxide for deliberate hypercapnia. Long or extension tubing from the anesthesia circuit is desirable. Rapid access to all critical equipment should be possible at all times during the procedure. Induction and emergency drugs must be prepared for immediate use.

E. **Patient positioning.** Because INR procedures may last for several hours, it is essential that the patient be made as comfortable as possible prior to the start of sedation. After the femoral introducer sheath has been inserted, a pillow can be placed under the patient's knees to obtain modest amounts of flexion so as to improve patient comfort during prolonged periods of lying in the supine position.

F. **Intravenous access.** During INR procedures the patients are often moved cephalad toward the image intensifier and away from the anesthesiologist so that the position of the catheters can be checked. This limits access to venipuncture sites and injection ports during the procedure. Therefore, adequate vascular access and sufficient length of tubing should be in place before the start of the procedure. In adults, two intravenous cannulae are usually placed for this purpose; one cannula is at least 18 gauge in size. The anesthetic and vasoactive agents should be in line before the patient is draped.

G. **Monitoring**
  1. **Arterial pressure.** Because of the need for manipulating systemic hemodynamics and at times the emergent need for hemodynamic interventions, it is mandatory to obtain direct systemic arterial pressure measurements during INR procedures. This is most conveniently achieved by transducing the side arm of the femoral introducer sheath. It must be realized that if a relatively large coaxial catheter passes through the introducer, the arterial pressure trace will be "damped." Despite damping, the mean pressure will still be reliable in such a situation. To avoid excessive damping of the femoral arterial trace, the introducer sheath should be at least 1/2 Fr larger than the coaxial catheter. An alternative strategy for arterial blood pressure monitoring is to insert a radial arterial line. Rarely, radial artery cannulation may be desirable when systemic pressures are to be monitored before the femoral introducer sheath is placed, such as during induction of general anesthesia for coiling of intracranial aneurysms.

     For a typical intracranial procedure, in addition to the systemic arterial pressure, two other pressures may be measured in real time: the internal carotid or vertebral artery pressure through the coaxial catheter and the distal cerebral arterial pressure through the microcatheter or a balloon-tipped catheter. The coaxial catheter pressure is monitored so as to detect any thrombus formation or vasospasm at the catheter tip as evidenced by a damped arterial trace. A high volume of heparinized flush is passed continuously through the coaxial tip to discourage thrombus formation; hence, the pressure reading characteristically increases by 10 to 20 mm Hg when recorded through the coaxial catheter.

The distal cerebral arterial pressure measurements made through the microcatheter are useful during embolization of AVMs (see therapeutic embolization of AVMs below). When a balloon catheter is used for internal carotid artery (ICA) occlusion, pressure measurements at the tip of the catheter provide the stump pressure (see test occlusion below).

The setup for measuring arterial pressures is shown in Fig. 20A-2. The pressure transducers and access stopcocks for blood withdrawal and zeroing are mounted, depending on the institutional preferences, either on the sterile field or toward the anesthesiologist.

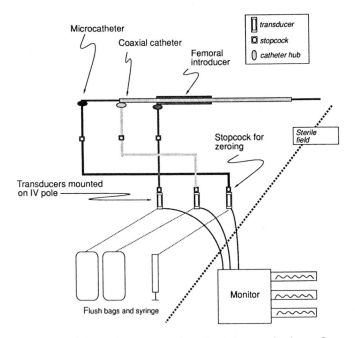

Fig. 20A-2.   Schematic representation of pressure monitoring and the continuous flush systems. [From Young WL. *Clinical neuroscience lectures.* **Munster, IL: Cathenart Publishing, 1999 (in press), with permission.]**

2. **Other systemic monitoring.** Other monitors include five-lead electrocardiogram, preferably with ST segment trending and respiratory trace, automated blood pressure cuff, end-tidal carbon dioxide, and peripheral temperature monitors. Two pulse oximeter probes are placed on each of the great toes and are useful for qualitatively comparing distal pulses in the lower limbs. Loss of oximeter pulse trace on the side of the femoral introducer sheath might give an early warning of thromboembolism, vasospasm, or mechanical obstruction.

3. **Central nervous system monitoring.** During many procedures, neurologic examination provides adequate monitoring of central nervous system integrity. Adjuncts that are especially useful during general anesthesia or planned proximal occlusions include electroencephalogram, somatosensory and motor evoked potentials, transcranial Doppler (TCD) ultrasound, and ^{133}Xe cerebral blood flow (CBF) monitoring.

4. **Urinary output.** Most patients undergoing INR procedures will require bladder catheterization to assist in fluid management and to increase patient comfort. Increased diuresis might occur during the procedure due to an increase in intravascular volume as a result of continuous flushing of the intravascular lines and osmotic load due to radiocontrast or mannitol injection. The timing and volume of contrast injected should be noted by the anesthesia team.

5. **Laboratory tests.** A baseline arterial blood gas (ABG) at the time of arterial puncture is useful to assess the gradient between PaO_2 and SaO_2 as well as the $PaCO_2$–$PETCO_2$ gradient. Activated clotting time (ACT) is used to monitor coagulation. The patients are given large quantities of fluids and dye, and can diurese considerably, so that a baseline hematocrit determination is helpful.

H. **Dynamic sedation.** Primary goals of anesthetic choice for conscious sedation are alleviating pain and discomfort, anxiolysis, and patient immobility. At the same time, one must allow a rapid decrease in the level of sedation when neurologic testing is required. The procedures are not generally painful, with the exceptions being sclerotherapy and chemotherapy. There is an element of pain associated with distention or traction on the vessels; contrast injection into the carotid artery is frequently described as "burning." Discomfort might be due to prolonged periods of lying still, bladder catheterization, and, to a lesser extent, the femoral puncture site. The procedure might be psychologically stressful due to the potential risk of stroke during the procedure. Patient immobility, whether by conscious effort or by deep sedation, is essential. Movement not only can degrade the quality of images but can also result in vascular injury.

Anesthetic agents are selected to meet the above goals. Our primary approach to conscious sedation is to establish a base of neurolept anesthesia by titration of 2 to 4 μg/kg of fentanyl, 2.5 to 5 mg of droperidol, and 3 to 5 mg of midazolam after intravenous access and monitoring have been established and oxygen administration has begun. A small bolus of propofol can be useful just as the bladder catheter is passed in males. The bolus dose of propofol also helps the anesthesiologist assess the airway under deep sedation and determine when nasopharyngeal airway is required. Placement of the nasopharyngeal airway after anticoagulation can result in troublesome bleeding and is best avoided.

When the patient is in final position, draping is begun and a propofol infusion is started at very low doses (10 to 20 μg/kg/minute) and then increased slowly to render the patient immobile yet breathing spontaneously. A variety of other sedation regimens and variations are certainly possible. However, the choice must be based on the experience of the practitioner and the requirements of the procedure.

I. **General anesthesia with tracheal intubation.** There is no evidence or suggestion that general anesthesia with endotracheal intubation should differ in the INR suite from its usual intraoperative application, be it for adult or pediatric cases. A theoretical argument can be made for eschewing the use of nitrous oxide because of the possibility of introducing air emboli into the cerebral circulation. The primary reason for employing general anesthesia is to reduce motion artifacts and to improve the quality of images. This is especially pertinent to INR treatment of spinal pathology in which extensive multilevel angiography must sometimes be performed. Because chest excursion during positive pressure ventilation can interfere with road mapping, radiologists frequently request apnea for DSA for spinal procedures.

J. **Anticoagulation.** Careful management of coagulation is required to prevent thromboembolic complications due to the presence of foreign bodies (catheters) and endothelial injury due to the passage of microcatheters. After placement of the femoral introducer sheath, a baseline ACT is obtained. Heparin (5,000 U/70 kg) is given and another ACT obtained. The target ACT is 2 to 3 times the baseline value. Sometimes, when the INR procedure is aborted, the anticoagulant effect of heparin is reversed with protamine and the femoral artery catheter is removed in the angiography suite.

K. **Deliberate hypotension.** Two primary indications for deliberate hypotension are to decrease flow through an arteriovenous fistula during injection of glue and to test the cerebrovascular reserve of the patient undergoing carotid occlusion. In most instances, the level of sedation is decreased to permit neurologic examination during deliberate hypotension. Induction of hypotension in awake or minimally sedated patients can be fairly challenging. Large doses of hypotensive drugs might be required to reduce the blood pressure in minimally sedated patients. Adrenergic blocking drugs that do not directly affect CBF might be preferable to drugs that are potential cerebral vasodilators. Typically, high doses of esmolol (1 mg/kg bolus followed by an infusion ≈0.5 mg/kg/minute) are required in these patients. Supplemental labetalol might be required during esmolol infusion. Agents such as sodium nitroprusside and nitroglycerin may also be used. Hypotension may lead to nausea and vomiting. Supplemental doses of antiemetic drugs, e.g., droperidol 1.25 mg or ondansetron 4 mg, may be given before decreasing the blood pressure.

L. **Deliberate hypertension.** During cerebral arterial occlusion, planned or inadvertent, systemic blood pressure might need to be increased to augment collateral blood flow. The extent to which the blood pressure has to be raised depends on the condition of the patient and the nature of the disease. Typically, during deliberate hypertension the systemic blood pressure is raised by 30% to 40% above the baseline or until ischemic symptoms resolve. Electrocardiogram and ST segments should be inspected for myocardial ischemia. Phenylephrine is the first-line agent for deliberate hypertension. Dopamine might be useful in patients who have a low heart rate (3).

M. **Deliberate hypercapnia.** Deliberate hypercapnia ($PaCO_2$ 50 to 60 mm Hg) may be employed during the treatment of venous malformations of the head and neck. The rationale for employing hypercapnia is to increase cerebral venous outflow relative to extracranial venous drainage and to create a pressure gradient that would divert sclerosing agents away from the intracranial veins. This is usually achieved by decreasing minute ventilation. Alternatively, carbon dioxide may be added to inspired gases.

N. **Radiation safety.** There are three sources of radiation in the INR suite: direct radiation from the x-ray tube, leakage (through the collimator's protective shielding), and scattered (reflected from the patient and the area surrounding the body part to be imaged). It must be realized that the amount of exposure drops off proportionally to the square of the distance from the source of radiation (inverse square law). It should also be realized that DSA delivers considerably more radiation than fluoroscopy. While working in the INR suite all persons should wear lead aprons and thyroid shields and have exposure badges.

Table 20A-1.   Management of neurologic catastrophes[a]

Initial resuscitation: Communicate with radiologists. Call for assistance. Secure the airway and hyperventilate with 100% O_2. Determine if problem is hemorrhagic or occlusive.

> *Hemorrhagic:* Immediate heparin reversal (1 mg protamine for each 100 U heparin given) and low-normal pressure.

> *Occlusive:* Deliberate hypertension, titrated to neurologic examination, angiography, or physiologic imaging studies (e.g., TCD, CBF).

Further resuscitation: Head-up 15° in neutral position. Titrate ventilation to a $PaCO_2$ of 26 to 28 mm Hg. Give 0.5 g/kg mannitol, rapid intravenous infusion. Anticonvulsants: phenytoin (give slowly, 50 mg/min) and phenobarbital. Titrate thiopental infusion to electroencephalogram burst suppression. Allow body temperature to fall as quickly as possible to 33 to 34°C. Consider dexamethasone 10 mg.[b]

---

[a]These are only general recommendations, and drug doses must be adapted to specific clinical situations and in accordance with a patient's preexisting medical condition. In some cases of asymptomatic or minor vessel puncture or occlusion, less aggressive management might be appropriate.

[b]Steroids are of dubious value in the treatment of focal cerebral ischemia but might have a place in reducing mass effect from a hemorrhage, if clinically appropriate.

TCD, transcranial Doppler; CBF, cerebral blood flow.

IV.   Management of neurologic catastrophes. Complications arising from cerebrovascular instrumentation can be rapid and dramatic and require a multi-disciplinary approach. A catastrophe plan such as that shown in Table 20A-1 should be clearly defined by the anesthesia team for every INR procedure. Drugs and equipment required to secure the airway should be available without any delay. Protamine should be available for immediate injection if the decision is made to reverse heparin. There should be effective communication between the INR team and the anesthesiologist. Appropriate neurology and neurosurgical consultants should be contacted as soon as possible. It is the primary responsibility of the anesthesia team to secure the airway and ensure adequate ventilation. Simultaneously with airway maintenance it is essential to communicate with the INR team to determine if the problem is occlusive or hemorrhagic.

   A.   Occlusive catastrophes. In case of vascular occlusion, a method to increase distal perfusion either by blood pressure augmentation or by thrombolysis is the primary strategy. Both therapies may be combined. Thiopental, if used for induction of anesthesia, may provide some degree of cerebral protection despite vascular occlusion.

   B.   Bleeding catastrophes might be heralded by headache, nausea, vomiting, and vascular pain related to the area of vascular perforation. The radiologist might see the contrast extravasate seconds before the patient becomes symptomatic. In the case of vessel puncture, heparin reversal before withdrawing the offending wire or the catheter back into the lumen of the vessel will keep the perforation partially blocked until the hemostatic function is restored. As soon as an intracranial hemorrhage is diagnosed, immediate reversal of heparin is indicated. Protamine (1 mg for every 100 U of heparin) is given without undue regard to systemic blood pressure. Later an ACT may be done to adjust the final dose. With active bleeding the blood pressure should be kept as low as possible. Once bleeding is controlled, the target blood pressure should be discussed with the radiology team. If vascular occlusion has been used to control hemorrhage, the INR team may ask for deliberate hypertension.

V. Transport and postprocedural considerations. After intracranial and spinal procedures patients are usually observed in the intensive care unit for the first 24 hours. Groin should be monitored for bleeding from the puncture site. After AVM embolization there might be minimal tissue edema that could lead to some deterioration in the neurologic status during the course of the first evening after the procedure.

VI. Specific procedures
   A. Superselective anesthesia and functional examination (SAFE) is routinely performed before therapeutic embolizations to minimize the risk of occluding a nutritive vessel to eloquent regions, either in the brain or the spinal cord, which may happen if the microcatheter tip is proximal to the origin of nutritive vessels. However, not all authors recognize the need for SAFE before embolization. The level of sedation should be decreased before testing by stopping the propofol infusion. In rare instances it might be necessary to use naloxone or flumazenil to antagonize other intravenous agents. A baseline focused neurologic examination under residual light sedation is performed by the INR team.

   Sodium amobarbital (30 mg) or lidocaine (30 mg) mixed with contrast is injected through the superselective catheter and an angiogram of the drug/contrast mixture is obtained. Sodium amobarbital is used for investigating the gray matter. Lidocaine can be used to evaluate the integrity of the white matter tracts, especially in the spinal cord. Injection of lidocaine into cortical areas particularly close to the motor strip can cause seizures. Seizure activity can result in transient neurologic deficit. Postictal paralysis may confuse interpretation of the test. For this reason the barbiturate is usually given first, followed by lidocaine. If the amobarbital test is negative, it can protect against seizure but will not interfere with the assessment of lidocaine's effect on white matter tracts.

B. **Superselective angiography and therapeutic embolization of arteriovenous malformations.** Typically, patients who present for embolization have large, complex, parenchymatous AVMs, which are composed of several discrete fistulae with multiple feeding arteries. The goal of the therapeutic embolization is to obliterate as many of the fistulae as possible.

Although in rare cases INR treatment is aimed at total obliteration, embolization is usually employed as an adjunct in preparation for surgery or radiotherapy and can be beneficial in several ways. First, embolization may facilitate surgery by obliterating deep feeding arteries that are difficult to approach surgically and thereby reduce the surgical risk. Second, staging obliteration of arteriovenous shunts also theoretically allows the surrounding brain to accommodate to the alterations in hemodynamics and may prevent normal perfusion–pressure breakthrough. Third, obliteration of high-flow feeders can be of benefit in patients with progressive neurologic deficits or intractable seizures, ostensibly by diminishing steal but more likely by decreasing mass effect. Finally, approximately 10% of AVM patients harbor intracranial aneurysms. Such aneurysms appear to increase the risk of spontaneous hemorrhage from AVMs. Obliteration of intranidal aneurysms during the initial embolization may decrease the rate of recurrent hemorrhage during the course of treatment.

The procedure can last 4 to 5 hours depending on the complexity of the lesions. A variety of embolic materials have been used to obliterate AVM fistulae, such as polyvinyl alcohol particles, coils, or silk threads. The best and probably the most lasting results are achieved with NBCA glue.

When the catheter is placed in position for potential glue injection, SAFE is performed. If SAFE is positive, i.e., focal neurologic deficits develop, then the catheter is repositioned or embolization of that pedicle is aborted. If the test is negative, glue or another embolic material can be injected. Controlled deposition of glue is necessary to decrease complications from obstruction of AVM venous drainage or pulmonary embolism. Flow arrest through the fistula is desired during glue injection to permit polymerization and solidification of NBCA glue. Techniques for flow arrest include deliberate hypotension, balloon occlusion of the proximal vessel, or circulatory pause with adenosine or controlled ventricular fibrillation. In most instances deliberate hypotension suffices for achieving flow arrest. Typically the mean systemic blood pressure is reduced to ≈50 mm Hg to achieve such a flow arrest.

Measurement of immediate postembolization pressure has been suggested as a means of following the course of hemodynamic changes and predicting post-procedure complications. A large increase in feeding artery pressure after embolization may be associated with intracranial hemorrhage. Because AVM feeding arteries supply normal vascular territories to a variable degree, abrupt restoration of normal perfusion pressure to a chronically hypotensive vascular bed might overwhelm the autoregulatory capacity and result in hemorrhage or swelling (normal perfusion pressure breakthrough). It is for this reason that the target range for posttreatment blood pressure is at or slightly below the patient's normal blood pressure.

C. **Embolization of spinal cord lesions.** Embolization can be used for intramedullary spinal AVMs, dural fistulae, or tumors invading the spinal canal. For cases performed under general anesthesia with endotracheal intubation, an intraoperative "wake-up test" may be requested. The wake-up test must be explained to the patient the night before and on the day of surgery. A nitrous oxide/narcotic anesthetic technique with concurrent propofol may be employed for the procedure. Neuromuscular block, if required, should be readily reversible for the wake-up test. For selected lesions, somatosensory and motor evoked potentials can be helpful in both anesthetized and sedated patients. When motor evoked potentials are monitored the neuromuscular block should be titrated to the monitoring needs.

D. **Carotid test occlusion and therapeutic carotid occlusion.** Test occlusion of the carotid artery is undertaken prior to anticipated sacrifice of the vessel or when temporary carotid ligation might be required during surgery. During test occlusion, a catheter with a distal balloon and a lumen is placed in the ICA. A baseline neurologic examination is done. Flow velocity can be measured over the middle cerebral artery by TCD ultrasound, if available, and the CBF can be measured by intracarotid ^{133}Xe injection technique. Baseline femoral and carotid artery pressures are noted. The balloon is then inflated and the pressure in the carotid artery distal to the balloon recorded. Inflation of the balloon might cause headache and at times an increase in the systemic blood pressure. Aggressive treatment of hypertension is probably not warranted as it may decrease collateral perfusion pressure. The anesthesiologist should be prepared to treat bradycardia with atropine. The neurologic examination is repeated a few minutes after occlusion, and TCD and ^{133}Xe CBF measurements are also repeated. After ^{133}Xe washout data have been obtained, radioactive tracer for single-photon emission computerized tomography (SPECT) studies may be injected. This provides a snapshot measurement of regional CBF during ICA occlusion. Since SPECT tracers usually have a long half-life and bind avidly to cerebral tissues, the imaging part of a SPECT study may be undertaken in the nuclear medicine department after the patient leaves the INR suite.

To assess the cerebrovascular reserve, if the patient does not demonstrate any neurologic impairment during the initial ICA occlusion, the systemic blood pressure is decreased. During the reduction of the systemic blood pressure, neurologic examination is repeated at frequent intervals. The distal ICA (stump) pressure at which neurologic deterioration occurs or whether the patient starts yawning—often a sign of impending cerebral ischemia—is noted along with the corresponding TCD flow velocity. Depending on the clinical condition of the patient, another ^{133}Xe measurement is obtained. If overt neurologic symptoms develop the balloon is immediately deflated, hypotensive agents are discontinued, and, depending on the clinical situation, vasopressors might be required to increase the blood pressure to normal levels.

Although a uniform guideline for interpreting the results of test occlusion has yet to be formulated, occurrence of a new neurologic deficit, a significant asymmetry on SPECT imaging, or a 25% to 30% reduction in ^{133}Xe CBF or TCD after occlusion may be considered as relative indications for an extracranial to intracranial bypass procedure prior to sacrifice of the carotid artery.

E. **Aneurysm ablation.** Sometimes aneurysms of the cerebral vessels, such as giant or fusiform aneurysms, cannot be safely treated by conventional neurosurgical methods. Additionally, some patients with medical diseases or poor neurologic grade might not be surgical candidates. Endovascular ablation of these lesions might still be possible in such patients. There are two basic approaches for endovascular obliteration of intracranial aneurysms: (a) the occlusion of the proximal parent artery, such as the carotid artery which has been discussed above, and (b) obliteration of the aneurysmal sac. Endovascular obliteration of the aneurysmal sac is usually done using the Guglielmi detachable coil. Several coils may be required to obliterate a large aneurysm. These procedures may be prolonged and frequently require general anesthesia with endotracheal intubation. The anesthesiologist should be prepared for aneurysmal subarachnoid hemorrhage (SAH) spontaneously or as a result of intravascular manipulations. It must be remembered that even after coil placement there may be areas of the dome that are still in contact with arterial blood. Therefore, careful attention to postprocedure blood pressure control is warranted.

F. **Angioplasty.** Balloon dilatation of cerebral vessels may be indicated for vasospasm after SAH and for atherosclerotic cerebrovascular disease.

1. **Angioplasty for *cerebral vasospasm*** is usually undertaken in patients who despite maximum medical management continue to have ischemic neurologic symptoms. These patients are often in extremis and are therefore frequently intubated, receiving vasopressor agents, and have either an external ventricular drain or other intracranial pressure monitoring device in place. Angiography is first undertaken to demonstrate that there is a significant degree of spasm in large proximal vessels (anterior, middle, and posterior cerebral arteries). A balloon catheter is guided under fluoroscopy into the spastic segment and inflated to distend the constricted area mechanically. If deliberate hypertension is being used to ameliorate a focal neurologic deficit before angioplasty, after angiographic demonstration of a significantly widened spastic segment, blood pressure should be reduced to the normal range.

2. **Angioplasty for *atherosclerosis*.** At present, patients with advanced age or poor medical condition are considered as candidates for cervical and intracranial angioplasty. These patients might require balloon dilatation or placement of a vascular stent. Angioplasty carries the risk of distal thromboembolism and vascular dissection. The procedure can be undertaken either under general anesthesia or under minimal sedation depending on the patient's medical condition, his or her ability to cooperate during the procedure, and the anticipated technical difficulty in negotiating the stenosed segment. Deliberate hypertension might be required for augmenting collateral blood flow. Considerations for general anesthesia are similar to those for carotid endarterectomy.

G. **Thrombolysis for acute stroke.** It is possible to recanalize the occluded vessel in acute thromboembolic stroke by superselective intraarterial delivery of thrombolytic agents close to the embolus. Neurologic deficits can be reversed if the treatment is completed within 6 hours of the onset of ischemic symptoms in the carotid territory and within 24 hours of onset of symptoms in the vertebrobasilar territories. Anesthetic consideration in these patients include those for the elderly and for patients with widespread arterial disease. Patients with acute thromboembolic stroke are spontaneously hypertensive and in the face of nonhemorrhagic focal neurologic deficits should not have their blood pressure aggressively treated. After clot lysis the blood pressure should be maintained in the normal range and ideally titrated to some index of CBF to prevent hyperperfusion injury.

H. **Treatment of other central nervous system vascular malformations**
   1. **Dural arteriovenous malformations.** Dural

AVMs may be fed by multiple intracranial and extracranial arteries and multistage embolization is usually performed. Superselective anesthesia and functional examination is usually performed, as in the case of intracranial AVMs. *N*-Butyl cyanoacrylate is the usual embolic agent. Both transarterial and transvenous approaches are used to provide access to the dural sinuses.

2. **Carotid cavernous fistulae.** Skull base trauma is the most common etiology of carotid cavernous fistula. Treatment usually consists of balloon occlusion of the lesion. Traumatic fistulae can also occur between the vertebral artery and the paravertebral veins. Such arteriovenous fistulae can lead to chronic hypotension of the surrounding normal vascular territories. Their obliteration might result in normal perfusion-pressure breakthrough. Therefore, after obliteration of these lesions the blood pressure should be maintained 10% to 20% below the patient's normal pressure.

3. **Vein of Galen malformation.** These are relatively uncommon but complicated lesions that usually present in infancy and childhood. These patients may have congestive heart failure, intractable seizures, hydrocephalus, and mental retardation. Several approaches have been attempted including transarterial and transvenous methods. Concerns during general anesthesia for INR therapy are the same as for surgical treatment. In the setting of congestive heart failure, preexisting right-to-left shunts, and pulmonary hypertension, a relatively small glue embolus can be fatal.

I. **Intraarterial chemotherapy and embolization of tumors.** Preoperative embolization as a means of decreasing blood loss during surgery can be performed for many hypervascular intracranial or spinal tumors. Superselective administration of chemotherapeutic agents can be used for treating neoplasms refractory to conventional treatment. Paragangliomas can cause catecholamine release from the tumor during embolization, and means of treating hypertensive crisis should be at hand.

VII. **Conclusions.** Interventional neuroradiologic procedures offer a new approach to several intracranial and spinal diseases. To some extent the risk/benefit ratio of INR procedures remains to be elucidated against traditional surgical approaches. Anesthetic management of these lesions, though similar to traditional operative approaches, is beset with hazards and requires certain accommodations.

SUGGESTED READINGS

1. Pile-Spellman J, Young WL, Hacein-Bey L. Perspectives on interventional neuroradiology. In: Maciunas RJ, ed. *Endovascular neurological intervention.* Park Ridge, IL: AANS, 1995:279–284.

2. Young WL, Pile-Spellman J, Hacein-Bey L, Joshi S. Invasive neuroradiologic procedures for cerebrovascular abnormalities: anesthetic considerations. *Anesth Clin North Am* 1997;15(3): 631–653.
3. Duong H, Hacein-Bey L, Vang MC, Pile-Spellman J, Joshi S, Young WL. Management of cerebral arterial occlusion during endovascular treatment of cerebrovascular disease. *Probl Anesth: Controv Neuroanesth* 1997;9:99–111.
4. Schell RM, Cole DJ. Cerebral protection and neuroanesthesia. *Anesth Clin North Am* 1992;10:453–469.
5. Young WL, Pile-Spellman J. Anesthetic considerations for interventional neuroradiology (review). *Anesthesiology* 1994;80:427–456.

20B

Diagnostic Neuroradiology

Patricia H. Petrozza

The introduction of the first computed tomography (CT) scanners in 1975 revolutionized the imaging of potential neurosurgical lesions. Since that time, the diagnostic armamentarium of the neuroimaging radiologist has consistently expanded. While diagnostic procedures involve limited pain, an anesthesiologist will be involved in cases where sedation is anticipated to be difficult for a myriad of reasons, such as the presence of extremes of age, claustrophobia, serious neurologic or systemic illness, and the inability of a particular patient to cooperate with the necessity of remaining motionless to achieve high-quality images.

Many radiology departments have recently adopted guidelines for the sedation of children formulated by the American Academy of Pediatrics Committee on Drugs (Table 20B-1). Patient selection, dietary precautions, equipment, monitoring, and discharge criteria are incorporated in these guidelines and strict selection criteria minimize sedation-related side effects. Still, 10% to 15% of sedation attempts fail and screening prior to the procedure often reveals those patients with anticipated airway difficulties or serious medical conditions for whom the presence of an anesthesiologist becomes advisable.

I. **General considerations.** Once involved in the neuroradiologic procedure the anesthesiologist faces the usual problems of providing anesthesia in an environment foreign from the operating room. Nonferromagnetic equipment and monitoring modalities will be required in the magnetic resonance imaging (MRI) suite, and most neuroradiographic procedures require that the anesthesiologist be positioned at a distance from the patient. Additionally, the issue of contrast media with their attendant osmolar effects and potential for toxic reactions must be considered. Finally, the design of modern medical facilities often requires that patients be either recovered by qualified personnel in an area adjacent to the radiologic suite or transported over relatively large distances through the medical center to the regular postanesthesia care unit (PACU).

   A. **Evaluation.** A proper preoperative evaluation should be performed on each patient scheduled for a diagnostic procedure. In addition to past medical history, experience with sedatives and anesthetics, the existence of allergies, and determination of the patient's medications, particular attention must be directed to the neurologic examination. Patients should be carefully evaluated for signs of increased intracranial pressure (ICP), preexisting neurologic

Table 20B-1. Sedation techniques for small children

Agent	Dose	Route	Onset (min)	Peak effect (min)
Chloral hydrate	20–75 mg/kg (2 g max)	p.o., p.r.	20–30	30–90
Pentobarbital sodium	2–4 mg/kg 5–7 mg/kg (120 mg max)	i.v. i.m.	5–10	60–90
Midazolam	0.02–0.15 mg/kg 0.3–0.75 mg/kg	i.v. p.o., p.r.	1–5 (i.v.)	20–30
Methohexital[a]	1–2 mg/kg 20–30 mg/kg	i.v. p.r.	5 10–15	45

[a] Might exacerbate temporal lobe seizures.

deficits, and, in the case of the emergency patient, concomitant spine or other major organ system injury.

B. **Equipment.** Equipment available in the radiology suite should include adequate supplies of medical gases, suction apparatus, age-appropriate drugs and airway equipment, and monitoring equipment for oxygen saturation, electrocardiogram (ECG), and blood pressure compatible with the imaging modality.

II. **Computed tomography**

A. **Basic considerations.** Ionizing radiation is delivered to the patient during performance of computed tomography (CT). Radiation detectors are permanently fixed 360° around the CT gantry. For each image, an x-ray tube rotates in a circle within the detector ring emitting a beam of ionizing radiation that passes through the body. The quantity of the x-ray beam that is attenuated or absorbed as it passes through the patient's tissues is recorded by the multiple detectors. This information from various angles is electronically integrated and the average attenuation value of each point in space is expressed in Hounsfield units.

Attenuation by a substance is directly related to its electronic density. Thus, structures are hypodense (of lower attenuation), isodense (of similar attenuation), or hyperdense (of higher attenuation) relative to brain parenchyma. Attenuation of vascular structures is increased by the use of iodinated contrast agents. While CT axial images are initially displayed, high-resolution thin images can be transformed into coronal or sagittal sections through computer reformatting. Currently, many CT examinations can be completed within 5 minutes.

Computed tomographic scanning is relatively insensitive for viewing structures within the posterior fossa due to image degradation by artifact produced by the interface of bone and brain parenchyma. This modality remains, however, the choice for the detection of skull fractures and acute subarachnoid hemorrhage in the emergent setting. Spiral acquisition CT is becoming more popular because larger anatomic regions can be imaged and this is particularly useful in the trauma situation. Unlike conventional CT scanning, in spiral acquisition the patient is moved at a continuous, constant speed through the scanning field while the x-ray tube rotates continuously. Computed tomographic angiography also takes advantage of spiral acquisition during the intravenous bolus administration of iodinated contrast medium.

Single-photon emission computed tomography (SPECT) provides information on cerebral metabolism and blood flow. Various radiopharmaceuticals are injected and a rotating gamma camera SPECT system produces tomographic brain imaging. Initial studies utilizing newly developed stable radiopharmaceutical compounds show promise in the localization of epileptogenic foci.

B. Management

  1. **Sedation.** With the current rapid CT scanners, very few adults or school-age children require sedation for CT scanning. Occasionally, intravenous midazolam in titrated doses of 0.5 mg may be effective or an infusion of propofol at a dose of 25 to 100 μg/kg/minute will sedate an anxious adult patient for the brief procedure. If an adult or older child manifests symptoms of increased ICP or serious airway compromise, it might be best to proceed with general anesthesia rather than attempt sedation. Several suggested techniques for the sedation of small children are listed in Table 20B-1. In addition to concerns with equipment, monitoring, and airway management, it must be remembered that the temperature of children within the cold radiology suite environment must be carefully guarded.

  2. **General anesthesia.** In the clinical situation where increased ICP is a critical factor, intravenous induction of general anesthesia in children can be accomplished through an indwelling catheter, the insertion of which has been facilitated by the prior application of EMLA (lidocaine 2.5% and prilocaine 2.5%) cream to one of the patient's hands. In adults, an induction utilizing thiopental (3 to 4 mg/kg) or propofol (1 to 2 mg/kg) followed by succinylcholine (1 mg/kg) with the addition of a small amount of narcotic such as fentanyl (50 to 100 μg) and lidocaine (1 mg/kg) to deepen the anesthetic is appropriate for endotracheal intubation. In small children, the issue

of an undiagnosed muscular dystrophy discourages the use of succinylcholine. An induction utilizing either rocuronium (0.6 to 1.0 mg/kg) or mivacurium (0.2 to 0.25 mg/kg) is often indicated. Anesthesia in children is maintained with an intravenous infusion of propofol (25 to 100 μg/kg/minute) or low concentrations of inhaled anesthetics. Rapid arousal at the end of the procedure is desirable. An infusion of remifentanil (0.05 to 0.1 μg/kg/minute) is an alternative in adults.

III. **Magnetic resonance imaging.** Magnetic resonance imaging (MRI) occurs when protons on water molecules within the patient's body are excited through a combination of a strong magnetic field and intermittent radiofrequency (RF) pulses. Additional magnetic fields are applied that create gradients and excite the protons to different orientations within the basic magnetic field. In the excited state, these protons gain energy and shift from a low energy state to a high energy state. This process is termed resonance. When the RF pulse is turned off, the protons lose energy in two ways: T1, the longitudinal relaxation time, and T2, the transverse relaxation time. Fortunately, no ionizing radiation is employed with MRI, but a large, powerful, external magnetic field is necessary.

Standard MRI sequences include T1-weighted images, proton density, and T2-weighted images, as well as T1 images with the intravenous administration of gadolinium contrast material. Additional imaging sequences include gradient echo, magnetic resonance angiography (MRA), magnetization transfer, perfusion imaging, and diffusion weighting. Through constant technological improvement, MRI is becoming more accurate in difficult clinical scenarios. Currently, areas optimally imaged by MRI include the pineal gland region, sella and parasellar structures, the limbic system, cranial nerves, internal auditory canal, the cerebellopontine angle, leptomeninges, and the posterior fossa.

While MRA provides images of arterial and dural sinus blood flow, magnetic resonance spectroscopy (MRS) is utilized with more frequency for the functional evaluation of patients. Magnetic resonance spectroscopy can provide noninvasive biochemical measurements of specific brain metabolites. Water and fat suppression techniques are employed to allow visualization of the small metabolic peaks in the MRS spectrum. Peak areas are proportional to the amount of chemical activity in the sample. MRS is helpful in the early detection of stroke.

The frequency of adverse reactions to gadolinium-based MRI contrast agents of all types is much lower than the frequency of adverse reactions to iodinated contrast material. However, gadolinium reactions can range from mild skin erythema to severe life-threatening reactions including periorbital edema as well as respiratory distress. In patients who report a previous gadolinium-based contrast reaction, pretreatment with corticosteroids and possible use of a different gadolinium-based contrast agent might be useful.

A. **Monitoring.** The MRI suite presents a hostile environment to the anesthesiologist. Several of the safety considerations are summarized below.

1. Metallic objects within the patient might be affected depending on their metallic properties. Implants are subject to magnetic flux which can induce electrical currents and cause local heating and movement. Most commonly, the hazards of metallic implants must be assessed by the radiologist. External metal wires, such as ECG leads and temperature probes, can burn the skin, and monitoring modalities especially designed for use in the MR scanner are available.

2. Small, loose metal objects can be pulled toward the magnet and are obviously dangerous. Large objects such as oxygen cylinders can be pulled into the magnet with considerable force and can be a serious threat to both patient and health care personnel. In general, no metallic objects are allowed in the scanning room unless they are securely fixed well away from the magnet.

3. Noise is a problem in the MR scanner due to torque on loops of wire that have gradient currents induced in them during the RF pulses. This causes vibration and audible noise, thus hampering communication. Noise during scans can average 95 decibels in a 1.5- tesla scanner.

4. Radiofrequency heating from induced currents is a potential problem, particularly in small infants. Periodic assessment of body temperature must be conducted. Infants might also become cold within the magnet due to the cool ambient temperature.

5. The anesthesiologist must find a point of least distortion by orienting monitors in various positions relative to the magnetic field. Most ECG artifacts cannot be eliminated and monitors should have good artifact suppression characteristics. In addition to having an MR-compatible ECG monitor, it is important to twist the ECG cables, keeping the electrodes close together, and position the electrodes near the center of the imager to get the best images and reduce the possibility of burns.

   Currently, specialized equipment compatible with MRI is available for blood pressure, end-tidal carbon dioxide ($ETCO_2$), Doppler, and oximeter monitors. There are compatible anesthesia machines and ventilators as well. Plastic laryngoscopes are available; however, the batteries in the handle might still be pulled into the magnetic field. Problems remain in terms of patient accessibility, hypothermia, and concern that obesity might limit the physical placement of a patient within the magnet's bore.

B. Anesthetic management. Many sedative techniques have proven quite reasonable for MR scanning including scanning of infants shortly after a meal to take advantage of postprandial drowsiness. However, it is often the case when an anesthesiologist is called to assist with MRI that the patient might be complicated neurologically, manifest serious illness, or have significant airway difficulties. In general, securing the airway with an endotracheal tube and then supplying ventilatory assistance through a long circuit assures an optimum combination of monitoring and anesthetic delivery. Certain centers have utilized laryngeal masks with propofol infusions to achieve the same goals. However, the concern for patient accessibility weighs in favor of assuring adequate control of the airway as an initial step.

IV. Positron emission tomography. Positron emission tomography (PET) images can demonstrate biochemical or physiologic processes involved in cerebral metabolism. The patient receives an intravenous injection of short-lived radionuclide, such as fluorodeoxyglucose (FDG), and is then imaged in a specialized detector system. The radionuclide emits positrons and energy is detected by sensitive detectors around the head. Computerized reconstruction procedures produce tomographic images, and information from PET can be overlaid on CT or MR images to improve anatomic localization of the activity detected. Positron emission tomography might provide localizing information when the MRI is normal in a patient with seizures who is under consideration for focal resective treatment.

A. Anesthetic considerations. Positron emission tomography scans are still considered investigational in many circumstances. Anesthetic considerations include the necessity to provide all appropriate monitoring equipment, medical gases, drugs, suction, and airway equipment in a remote location. Unlike MRI, PET scanners do not require nonferromagnetic monitors and patient visualization is easier. The injection of FDG, however, renders the patient "radioactive" for 24 hours. A common protocol includes two 15- to 20-minute initial scans, with follow-up scans in 2 to 3 hours.

V. Cerebral angiography. Cerebral angiography continues to be important in the evaluation of subarachnoid hemorrhage and carotid artery disease. The safest and most widely used arterial access is the common femoral artery, and the use of a transfemoral catheter has replaced direct carotid arterial puncture. Digital subtraction angiography reduces the required volume of intraarterial contrast and the overall duration of the procedure. Unfortunately, an incidence of neurologic problems related to angiography itself still remains. In a prospective study of 1,002 angiograms, the overall ischemic event rate within 0 to 24 hours of the procedure was 1.3%, and it was 2.5% in patients studied for cerebrovascular disease. Other catheter complications include transient global amnesia, cortical blindness, and multiple cholesterol emboli syndrome.

A. **Anesthetic management.** On the uncommon occasion that anesthesiologists are asked to participate in diagnostic angiography, it must be remembered that contrast medium causes vasodilatation and a burning discomfort. Often the degree of sedation for patients must be increased in anticipation of contrast injection. As always, the possibility of a reaction to the contrast material must not be overlooked.

VI. **Myelography.** Myelography is utilized to define the contents of the thecal sac and any intrinsic or extrinsic impressions. Contrast agents are introduced directly into the subarachnoid space, bypassing the blood–brain barrier. The newest myelographic contrast agents are low-osmolar, nonionic, and mix well with cerebrospinal fluid. Main complications related to myelography include headache, contrast-related complications, subdural or epidural contrast injection, spinal canal hematoma, meningitis, seizures, and various forms of neurologic deficits. Among the anesthetic considerations is careful positioning of infants and children while the myelogram table is rotated to achieve good flow of the contrast agent.

VII. **Contrast agents.** In addition to CT, iodinated agents are used for catheter angiography and myelography. High-osmolar contrast agents (HOCAs) are ionic monomers at concentrations ranging from 60% to 76% by weight. This material possesses 5 to 8 times the osmolality of human serum. Nonionic monomers and dimers as well as ionic dimers are considered low-osmolar contrast agents (LOCAs) when they have between 2 and 3 times the osmolality of human serum. The LOCAs have greater hydrophilia and less tendency for tissue binding, thus making them more biologically inert. Despite the higher cost, LOCAs are used for most neurodiagnostic procedures.

Iodinated contrast agents are nephrotoxic. After an initial mild vasodilatation, the renal vascular tree undergoes prolonged vasoconstriction. Patients with preexisting renal insufficiency, diabetes mellitus, and low cardiac output syndromes are at risk for developing contrast agent–induced nephrotoxicity.

Responses to iodinated contrast material might range from a warm flushing with a metallic taste during contrast injection to an anaphylactoid reaction. Large multiinstitutional studies have demonstrated that patients given nonionic contrast material have a 1 in 10,000 chance of having a very severe reaction. Patients likely to have a problem with contrast include those with previous idiosyncratic contrast reactions, patients with asthma or multiple food and medication allergies, and patients with a number of other diseases including preexisting azotemia and cardiac disease. The use of corticosteroids such as methylprednisolone in two 32-mg oral doses, one 6 to 24 hours before and the other 2 hours before the injection of contrast material, markedly reduces the chance of a severe reaction to contrast. Additionally, some centers add antihistamines to the steroid regimen.

Not infrequently, a few hives about the face, neck, and chest might be the only reaction a patient manifests to contrast. Often the only therapy necessary in such cases is reassurance with perhaps a dose of 50 mg of intravenous diphenhydramine. A severe reaction to contrast, manifested by respiratory difficulties, hypotension, and generalized skin irritation, requires therapy with an intravenous dose of epinephrine (100 μg). Equipment must be available in a radiology suite for immediate airway control and additional adjuncts such as β_2-agonists including albuterol and others might be useful for treating bronchospasm. Occasionally, large volumes of fluid as well as vasoactive drugs may be necessary to support blood pressure. A prolonged stay in the intensive care setting might be necessary to stabilize the patient.

SUGGESTED READINGS

Cohan RH, Leder RA, Ellis JH. Treatment of adverse reactions to radiographic contrast media in adults. *Radiol Clin North Am* 1996;34:1055–1076.

Frush DP, Bisset GS III, Hall SC. Pediatric sedation in radiology: the practice of safe sleep. *AJR* 1996;167:1381–1387.

Kuzniecky RI. Neuroimaging in pediatric epilepsy. *Epilepsia* 1996; 37(Suppl 1):S10–S21.

Murphy KJ, Brunberg JA, Cohan RH. Adverse reactions to gadolinium contrast media: a review of 36 cases. *AJR* 1996;167:847–849.

Patterson SK, Chesney JT. Anesthetic management for magnetic resonance imaging: problems and solutions. *Anesth Analg* 1992; 74:121–128.

Zalduondo FM, Heinz ER. Neuroradiology: neuroradiologic procedures. In: Albin MS, ed. *Textbook of neuroanesthesia*. New York: McGraw-Hill, 1997:735–805.

III

Intensive Care

Respiratory Care of the Neurosurgical Patient

Karen B. Domino

Arterial hypoxemia commonly occurs in patients with central nervous system (CNS) injury. Hypoxemia is especially associated with a poor neurologic outcome after head injury. Prompt recognition and treatment of pulmonary disorders is therefore important in the management of neurosurgical patients.

I. **Respiratory disorders**
   A. **Clinical physiology of oxygen transfer.** Arterial hypoxemia might be secondary to a decreased alveolar oxygen tension (PaO_2) or an increased alveolar–arterial oxygen tension difference [$P(A-a)O_2$] (Fig. 21-1). Inspired gas is mixed with gas in the functional residual capacity (FRC) to make up alveolar gas. Mixed venous blood equilibrates with alveolar gas and is distributed to the systemic circulation as mixed arterial blood. The $P(A-a)O_2$ is due to (a) diffusion, (b) ventilation–perfusion ($\dot{V}A/\dot{Q}$) imbalance, and (c) pulmonary shunt.
   B. **Causes of decreased PaO_2.** PaO_2 might be reduced because of either diminished inspired PO_2 (PiO_2) or diminished alveolar ventilation from respiratory depression, increased respiratory deadspace, or mechanical impairment.
      1. **Respiratory depression.** Respiratory depression might be central (due to CNS disease, narcotics, or sedatives) or peripheral (due to neuromuscular disease or muscle relaxants).
         a. **Head injury.** Variations in depth and rate of spontaneous respirations occur in 60% of patients with brain injury. Five respiratory patterns are observed after head injuries (Fig. 21-2).
            (1) **Normal breathing.** Breathing might be normal, such as in an awake patient with a small, unilateral lesion.
            (2) **Cheyne-Stokes ventilation.** Cheyne-Stokes ventilation is a periodic breathing pattern in which hyperpnea alternates with apnea. It is associated with severe, bilateral injuries in the cerebral hemispheres or basal ganglia. The breathing waxes from breath to breath in a smooth crescendo and, once the peak is reached, wanes in a smooth decrescendo. The hyperpneic phase lasts longer than the apneic phase. The

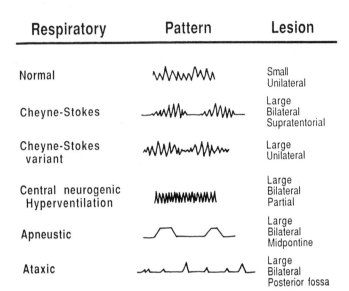

Respiratory	Pattern	Lesion
Normal		Small Unilateral
Cheyne-Stokes		Large Bilateral Supratentorial
Cheyne-Stokes variant		Large Unilateral
Central neurogenic Hyperventilation		Large Bilateral Partial
Apneustic		Large Bilateral Midpontine
Ataxic		Large Bilateral Posterior fossa

Fig. 21-1.   Respiratory patterns associated with closed head injury. (Reprinted with permission from Plum F, Posner JB. *The diagnosis of stupor and coma*, 2nd ed. Philadelphia: FA Davis Co, 1972.)

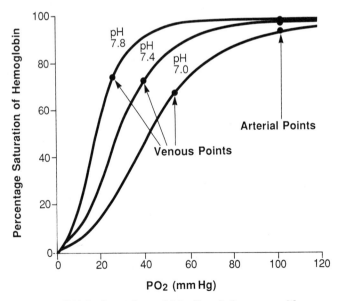

Fig. 21-2.   Shift in the oxyhemoglobin dissociation curve with change in blood pH.

Cheyne-Stokes variant is similar, but it has less of an apneic phase and is associated with large unilateral injuries.

(3) **Central neurogenic hyperventilation.** Central neurogenic hyperventilation is a sustained, regular, rapid, fairly deep hyperpnea. It occurs with a large pontine lesion, systemic hypoxia, or metabolic acidosis.

(4) **Apneustic breathing.** Apneustic breathing occurs with large bilateral midpontine lesions. There is a brief 2- to 3-second pause at the end of inspiration, alternating irregularly with expiratory pauses. It has a very poor prognosis.

(5) **Ataxic respiration.** Ataxic respiration is an irregular breathing in which shallow and deep breaths alternate randomly with irregular pauses. It is associated with medullary compression and has a very poor prognosis. The irregularity distinguishes it from Cheyne-Stokes ventilation.

b. **Spinal cord injury.** High cervical spinal cord lesions might impair ventilation because of partial or complete loss of innervation of the diaphragm (C_3–C_5). Patients with lesions below C_6–C_7 have an intact diaphragm, but loss of intercostal and abdominal muscle function reduces FRC and creates paradoxical ventilation (chest retraction on inspiration and expansion during expiration), loss of cough, and reduced ability to handle secretions. Expiratory reserve volume is markedly decreased. With a C_5–C_6 lesion, ventilation might be inadequate and forced vital capacity (FVC) decreases to 30% of predicted. Improvement of FVC occurs with time because of strengthening of the accessory muscles (clavicular portion of pectoralis major and sternocleidomastoid), development of spasticity (which stops the paradoxical chest wall motion), improvement of diaphragmatic function, and decreased usage of narcotics and sedatives. At 5 months after injury, FVC reaches 60% of predicted values.

2. **Increased airway deadspace.** Deadspace is increased with drug administration (such as atropine and nitroprusside for deliberate hypotension), mechanical ventilation with positive endexpiratory pressure (PEEP), hypovolemia, hypotension, hypocapnia, and cardiopulmonary disease.

3. **Mechanical impairment.** Airway obstruction from oropharyngeal soft tissue, uncleared secretions, hemoptysis, foreign bodies, or bronchospasm might cause a mechanical impairment to effective alveolar ventilation. Restriction of free chest movement in surgical positioning, surgical retraction on chest and abdomen, and restrictive lung disease might also reduce alveolar ventilation.

C. **Causes of increased P(A-a)O$_2$.** The P(A-a)O$_2$ might be increased by both intrapulmonary and extrapulmonary factors. Pulmonary disorders can increase P(A-a)O$_2$ due to increases in (a) diffusion limitation, (b) shunt, or (c) $\dot{V}A/\dot{Q}$ inequality. Most pulmonary disorders increase $\dot{V}A/\dot{Q}$ mismatch and shunt and seldom affect diffusion capacity. Decreases in cardiac output and a respiratory or a metabolic alkalosis are important extrapulmonary factors that increase P(A-a)O$_2$ in the presence of lung disease.

1. **Pulmonary etiologies of increased P(A-a)O$_2$.** Increased P(A-a)O$_2$ might result from primary lung injuries (e.g., pulmonary contusion, flail chest, pneumothorax, hemothorax, tracheobronchial disruptions, diaphragmatic disruption), secondary lung injuries (e.g., aspiration, atelectasis, pneumonia, pulmonary edema from heart failure, adult respiratory distress syndrome, or fat/air embolism), or neurologic disease. Pulmonary etiologies for hypoxemia should be ruled out prior to assuming neurologic etiologies.

   a. **Primary lung injuries**

      (1) **Pulmonary contusion.** A pulmonary contusion might occur after penetrating lung injury or after severe blunt injury due to the deceleration of the lung against the rib cage. Rib fractures are present in 50% of cases of pulmonary contusion. The presentation of pulmonary contusion is progressive respiratory failure. The chest radiograph findings lag behind the patient's clinical condition.

      (2) **Flail chest.** Flail chest occurs when there is abnormal movement of the chest wall due to fractures of three or more ribs in two places on the same side. The free-floating rib segment reduces the stability of the chest wall, resulting in increased work of breathing. The chest wall develops paradoxical motion such that the flail segment moves inward with negative inspiratory pressure and outward during exhalation. Pulmonary dysfunction with a flail chest is caused initially by the underlying lung injury. Delayed pul-

monary dysfunction occurs because splinting and hypoventilation due to pain might lead to atelectasis and pneumonia.

(3) Pneumothorax. An open pneumothorax results in the "sucking" of air through the defect during inspiration. A tension pneumothorax may occur when air that enters the pleural cavity during inspiration cannot leave during expiration. A tension pneumothorax causes a mediastinal shift, decreased venous return, and severe hypotension. A tension pneumothorax is associated with marked decrease in pulmonary compliance, increased peak airway pressures, hypoxemia, hypotension, or cardiovascular collapse. Tracheal deviation away from the side of the pneumothorax might be present. Chest wall movement and breath sounds might be diminished or absent on the side of the pneumothorax.

Cardiovascular collapse is unlikely in the absence of a tension pneumothorax; however, gas exchange abnormalities (especially hypoxemia) and increased peak airway pressures are common with a pneumothorax of greater than 20%. In the presence of cardiovascular collapse, emergency decompression is required. Insertion of a 14-gauge catheter into the second intercostal space, midclavicular line, will release the tension pneumothorax while a chest tube is being prepared for more definitive treatment.

(4) Hemothorax. A hemothorax can cause cardiopulmonary dysfunction by compression of lung tissue, reduction in venous return, and severe hypovolemia. As the hemothorax can accommodate 30% to 40% of the blood volume, the most common clinical presentation is hypovolemia. The signs of a massive hemothorax are similar to a tension pneumothorax except that neck veins are collapsed and the hemothorax is dull to percussion. About 500 mL of blood must be present to detect a hemothorax on chest radiograph. Treatment involves fluid resuscitation and insertion of a chest tube. A thoracotomy is indicated only for severe bleeding.

(5) **Tracheobronchial disruption.** The clinical signs of tracheobronchial disruption vary depending on the location of the injury. Rupture of the proximal trachea results in hemoptysis and airway obstruction. Rupture of the distal trachea and main bronchi causes subcutaneous or mediastinal emphysema. Rupture of distal bronchi might cause a pneumothorax, bronchopleural fistula, and massive air leak. The diagnosis of a tracheobronchial injury is dependent on bronchoscopy, although chest radiographs may be suggestive. Treatment is often surgical.

(6) **Traumatic disruption of the diaphragm.** Most diaphragmatic ruptures occur on the left side because of the protection of the right side by the liver. Left-sided diaphragmatic hernias might be associated with an increased risk of aspiration of gastric contents. Because of the severity of concurrent injury, including the presence of a pulmonary contusion, gas exchange might not improve dramatically after decompression and reinflation of the lung with surgical repair of the diaphragmatic hernia.

b. **Secondary lung injuries**

(1) **Gastric aspiration.** Aspiration of gastric contents occurs frequently in the head trauma patient due to loss of consciousness, intoxication from alcohol and street drugs, and abdominal injury. Aspiration of large volumes of fluid with low pH or particulate matter results in a more severe injury. Aspiration of large foreign bodies, such as gravel, gum, or teeth, might also cause bronchial obstruction, atelectasis, and hypoxemia. Treatment of aspiration is primarily supportive and may involve mechanical ventilation depending on the severity of the lung injury. Antibiotics are indicated with aspiration of food particles.

(2) **Atelectasis.** Atelectasis is also common in the neurosurgical patient. Hypoventilation due to pain, altered level of consciousness, obstruction due to mucous plugs or aspiration of particulate matter, or compression of adjacent lung by pneumothorax, hemothorax, or pleural effusion can contribute to the

formation of atelectasis in the immediate or late posttrauma period.

(3) **Pneumonia.** Pneumonia is a common late pulmonary complication following head and spinal cord injury. Sedation and coma depress the gag reflex and impair the cough reflex. Impairment in mucociliary clearance, abnormalities in surfactant metabolism, impairment in alveolar macrophage function, and iatrogenic insults such as endotracheal intubation, mechanical ventilation, administration of cimetidine and antacids, and suctioning in an intensive care unit (ICU) contribute to the development of pneumonia. The etiology of pneumonia is the aspiration of oropharyngeal secretions that are colonized by pathogenic bacteria. Antibiotic treatment should be guided by antibiotic sensitivities from sputum obtained by bronchoscopy or bronchoalveolar lavage.

(4) **Pulmonary edema.** The development of pulmonary edema is a serious cause of pulmonary dysfunction in the neurosurgical patient. Pulmonary edema can be either cardiogenic or noncardiogenic in etiology. The chest radiograph reveals diffuse alveolar infiltrates regardless of the etiology.

   (a) **Cardiogenic pulmonary edema.** Pulmonary edema can occur in the neurosurgical patient as a result of a cardiogenic etiology. Left ventricular dysfunction due to myocardial ischemia or infarction, adverse drug reaction, tachyarrhythmias, severe hypertension, or fluid overload such as associated with hypervolemic therapy for treatment of cerebral vasospasm might result in pulmonary edema. Older patients are at greater risk; however, myocardial ischemia due to severe anemia and hypotension, fluid overload, and excessive mannitol dosage can precipitate pulmonary edema in the younger patient. Treatment involves diuresis, fluid restriction, and supportive care.

   (b) **Noncardiogenic pulmonary edema.** A noncardiogenic etiology of pulmonary edema is more common in the younger traumatized patient population. The differential diagnosis of noncardiac pulmonary edema in this population includes anaphylactic or anaphylactoid reactions, aspiration of gastric contents, pulmonary contusion, air or fat embolism, near-drowning, sepsis, disseminated intravascular coagulation, acute lung reexpansion, postobstructive or negative pressure pulmonary edema, acute opioid reversal, or CNS pathology. Neurogenic pulmonary edema is an important cause of noncardiogenic pulmonary edema in the neurosurgical patient. Treatment is predominantly supportive.

(5) **Fat embolism syndrome.** Fat embolism is a multisystem disorder characterized by respiratory failure, neurologic deficits, and petechial rash. The clinical presentation of the syndrome is variable in the severity and distribution of organ involvement. Pulmonary dysfunction is always involved but ranges from mild pulmonary shunting to full-blown adult respiratory distress syndrome (ARDS).

The clinical presentation of fat embolism syndrome is often delayed by 24 to 72 hours after trauma or surgical repair of the fracture. Fat globules are released from the bone marrow with traumatic fractures and during surgical repair of fractures. Inflammation is caused by the breakdown of fat emboli into free fatty acids by lipase. As treatment is supportive and consists of mechanical ventilation for respiratory failure, the primary aim is prevention of fat embolism by early surgical fixation.

(6) **Adult respiratory distress syndrome.** Adult respiratory distress syndrome is a clinical syndrome of diffuse lung injury that results in noncardiogenic, high-permeability pulmonary edema. It is a severe complication of trauma with a mortality rate in excess of 50%. However, only about 10% of patients dying from ARDS die from respiratory failure and hypoxemia per se. Most of the mortality of ARDS is due to multiple organ failure or sepsis.

Adult respiratory distress syndrome usually develops within the first 72 hours of the initiating event, with 60% to 70% of cases occurring within the first 24 hours. **Risk factors** for the development of ARDS in traumatized patients include sepsis syndrome, documented aspiration of gastric contents, multiple emergency transfusions, pulmonary contusion, and multiple major fractures. The incidence of ARDS is dramatically increased by the presence of multiple risk factors.

The **pathophysiology** of ARDS involves the development of noncardiogenic pulmonary edema due to increased pulmonary capillary permeability. Significant abnormalities of pulmonary vascular permeability may persist for 1 to 2 weeks after the onset of ARDS. Pulmonary capillary wedge pressures are usually normal or minimally elevated. Pulmonary hypertension develops due to elevated pulmonary vascular resistance, primarily from arteriocapillary obstruction, rather than pulmonary vasoconstriction. Pulmonary compliance is decreased. The common pathologic findings of ARDS are the end result of a complex sequence of cellular and biochemical changes that lead to damage of endothelial cell membranes. Treatment is predominantly supportive using mechanical ventilation and PEEP.

(7) **Pulmonary embolism.** Pulmonary emboli are common in critically ill neurosurgical patients. Pulmonary emboli usually originate from venous thrombosis in lower extremities, although they might originate from pelvic or prostatic venous plexuses or the right ventricle. Pulmonary embolism causes acute pulmonary hypertension, right ventricular failure, and a reduction in cardiac output. Smaller pulmonary emboli should be considered in patients with unexplained tachypnea and chest pain. Usually PaO_2 is normal and $PaCO_2$ is decreased in the tachypneic patient with small pulmonary emboli. Massive pulmonary embolism causes acute cardiorespiratory failure. Definitive treatment is predominantly sup-

portive and involves anticoagulation. Diagnosis requires a pulmonary arteriogram. If anticoagulation is contraindicated after intracranial or spinal cord operation or injury, a Greenfield filter may be placed in the inferior vena cava.

c. **Neurogenic etiologies of increased P(A-a)O$_2$**

(1) **Reduced functional residual capacity.** The FRC is often reduced after head and spinal cord injury. Head trauma patients might exhibit a reduction in FRC and pulmonary compliance and an increase in pulmonary shunting without evidence of pulmonary disease on the chest radiograph. The FRC is also reduced in patients with spinal cord injury at the cervical and thoracic levels.

(2) **Neurogenic pulmonary edema.** Classic neurogenic pulmonary edema has immediate onset and becomes clinically recognizable 2 to 12 hours after brain or spinal cord injury. Neurogenic pulmonary edema is generally of short duration. It resolves within hours to days if the patient survives the associated injuries. The pathogenesis of neurogenic pulmonary edema is complex and is not completely understood (2).

(3) **Neurogenic alterations in $\dot{V}$A/$\dot{Q}$ matching.** Hypoxemia and increased pulmonary shunting have been observed in animals and patients with CNS disorders in the absence of pulmonary disease. The etiology of these changes in $\dot{V}$A/$\dot{Q}$ regulatory mechanisms is multifactorial. Brain thromboplastin is released into the blood with head trauma causing deposition of fibrin microemboli and platelet aggregates in the pulmonary capillaries. Neutrophil accumulation and release of vasoactive substances might also cause abnormalities of local perfusion and ventilation. Patients with increased fibrin spit products are more likely to develop respiratory failure after head trauma.

2. **Extrapulmonary factors.** Two extrapulmonary factors commonly contribute to hypoxemia in neurosurgical patients with lung disease. These include (a) hyperventilation to reduce intracranial pressure (ICP) and (b) excessive intravascular

volume depletion due to diuretics and fluid restriction.

a. **Respiratory alkalosis.** Hyperventilation to induce hypocapnia results in a decrease in venous return and decrease in cardiac output. Hypocapnia increases pulmonary shunt, especially in the presence of lung disease. The mechanism is unclear but might be related to hypocapnic bronchoconstriction and inhibition of hypoxic pulmonary vasoconstriction (HPV). In addition, the oxyhemoglobin dissociation curve shifts to the left, resulting in a lower PO_2 for any given oxygen saturation (see Fig. 21-2). This is especially noticeable at PO_2 equal to or less than 70 mm Hg.

b. **Hypovolemia and decrease in PO_2.** PaO_2 will be lower when the mixed venous oxygen tension (PO_2) is decreased, as may occur with decreased cardiac output, increased oxygen consumption, or severe anemia with increased oxygen extraction. The effect of PO_2 can be quite significant, especially when there are areas of low $\dot{V}A/\dot{Q}$ and shunt (Fig. 21-3). For instance, in the presence of $\dot{V}A/\dot{Q}$

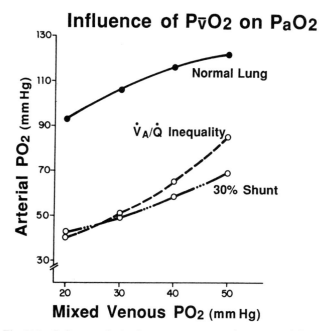

Influence of $P\bar{v}O_2$ on P_aO_2

Fig. 21-3. Influence of mixed venous oxygen tension on arterial oxygen tension. From Dantzker DR. Ventilation-perfusion inequality in lung disease. *Chest* 1987;91:749–754.

mismatch, PaO_2 = 80 mm Hg when PO_2 is 50 mm Hg. If PO_2 is decreased to 20 mm Hg due to decreased cardiac output, then PaO_2 will decrease to 40 mm Hg, without any change in degree of $\dot{V}a/\dot{Q}$ inequality or shunt. Therefore, low cardiac output due to hypovolemia or myocardial depression will increase $P(a\text{-}a)O_2$ and might result in hypoxemia, especially in the presence of pulmonary disease.

II. **Respiratory care**
   A. **Administration of oxygen.** All head trauma patients should be considered hypoxic until proven otherwise. A PaO_2 value of greater than 60 mm Hg might be necessary to maintain adequate cerebral oxygenation in head-injured patients. Supplemental O_2 should be administered.
   1. **Mask/nasal O_2**
      a. **Nasal prongs.** Nasal prongs used at flows of 6 L/minute or less can deliver a fraction of inspired oxygen (FiO_2) of 24% to 44%. The FiO_2 varies depending on the patient's inspiratory flow rate, with lower FiO_2 occurring during high inspiratory flow rates.
      b. **Venturi mask.** The Venturi mask can provide an FiO_2 of 24% to 40%. Although the FiO_2 is specified when ordering the use of a Venturi mask, the exact FiO_2 might be significantly less when the patient has high minute ventilation.
      c. **Nonrebreather mask.** The nonrebreather mask can provide a higher FiO_2, although the amount of O_2 delivered is also dependent on the patient's minute ventilation. Therefore, elective endotracheal intubation is necessary when a high FiO_2 is required.
   2. **Endotracheal intubation**
      a. **Endotracheal intubation is indicated in the neurosurgical patient for the following conditions:**
         (1) Inability to protect the airway or clear secretions.
         (2) Need to reduce ICP by control of ventilation.
         (3) PaO_2 less than 60 mm Hg in spite of supplemental O_2.
         (4) $PaCO_2$ greater than 50 mm Hg.
         (5) pH less than 7.2.
         (6) Respiratory rate greater than 40/minute or less than 10/minute.
         (7) Tidal volume less than 3.5 mL/kg.
         (8) Vital capacity less than 10 to 15 mL/kg.
         (9) Muscle fatigue.
         (10) Airway compromise.
         (11) Hemodynamic instability.

       b. Nasotracheal intubation. Nasotracheal intubation is absolutely contraindicated in the presence of a basilar skull fracture. Prolonged nasotracheal intubation might increase the risk of sinusitis and subsequent sepsis due to obstruction of sinus drainage. Awake nasotracheal intubation might increase ICP in the head trauma patient.

       c. Orotracheal intubation. Orotracheal intubation is preferable for urgent intubation in the presence of increased ICP, hypoxemia, and/or hemodynamic instability. In the hemodynamically stable patient, sodium thiopental (3 to 5 mg/kg) and succinylcholine (1.5 mg/kg) can be used to prevent coughing and increases in ICP. Alternatively, rocuronium (1 to 1.5 mg/kg) can be used for muscle paralysis. Etomidate (0.1 to 0.3 mg/kg) or lidocaine (1 to 1.5 mg/kg) should be used in the less stable patient. In patients with a full stomach, a modified rapid sequence induction with cricoid pressure and ventilation by mask should be used to avoid marked increases in ICP due to hypoxemia and hypercarbia. The head and neck should be stabilized by an assistant (manual in-line stabilization) to prevent head movement in the presence of potential cervical spine injury.

   3. Tracheotomy. Endotracheal intubation is well tolerated for prolonged periods. However, tracheotomy might be indicated in the presence of high spinal cord injury (C_{3-4} and above), multiple facial fractures, persistent vegetative state, or for patient comfort during prolonged ventilatory failure.

 B. Mechanical ventilation. Mechanical ventilation is used to improve gas exchange following endotracheal intubation. The ventilation parameters that are set include (a) mode of ventilation [assist-controlled, intermittent mandatory ventilation (IMV), and pressure support ventilation (PSV)]; (b) FiO_2; (c) respiratory rate; (d) tidal volume; (e) inspiratory pressure limit; and (f) PEEP. Vital signs should be monitored and arterial blood gases should be measured 30 minutes after changing ventilator settings. Due to the potential for the development of oxygen toxicity, the lowest FiO_2 with satisfactory oxygenation ($PaO_2 = 70$ mm Hg or oxygen saturation of above 90%) should be used. Positive end-expiratory pressure should be titrated to allow decreases in FiO_2 to 0.6 or less because of concern for oxygen toxicity. Deliberate hypercapnia ventilation techniques usually should not be used in patients with significant head trauma and high ICP.

   1. Assist-controlled ventilation. With assist-controlled ventilation, the ventilator delivers a positive pressure breath at a preset rate and tidal volume in the absence of respiratory efforts. Controlled ventilation is used in the operating room and occasionally in the ICU in selected patients without ventilatory efforts due to neuromuscular blockade, high cervical spinal cord injury, absent ventilatory drive, drug overdose, or brain death. The ventilator also delivers a breath when triggered by the patient's inspiratory effort. Unfortunately, this may cause hyperventilation and a respiratory alkalosis. Therefore, the IMV mode should be used in the ICU in the presence of spontaneous respiratory efforts.

2. **Intermittent mandatory ventilation.** With IMV, the patient receives positive pressure ventilation at a preset tidal volume and rate, while allowing spontaneous ventilations. It is the primary method for primary ventilatory support in the ICU because it maintains spontaneous respiratory activity and results in fewer hemodynamic and pH complications. The work of the spontaneous breathing is increased in the IMV mode because of the presence of a demand valve.

3. **Pressure support ventilation.** In contrast to assist-controlled ventilation and IMV, a level of pressure (rather than volume) is set at which every spontaneous breath is augmented. Airway pressure is maintained at a preset level until the patient's inspiratory flow decreases below a certain level. Tidal volume is determined secondarily by the level of set pressure, the patient's effort, and pulmonary compliance.

4. **Positive end-expiratory pressure.** Positive end-expiratory pressure is used to increase arterial oxygenation by increasing FRC and alveolar ventilation, which decreases intrapulmonary shunting and ventilation–perfusion abnormalities. Application of PEEP might decrease the need to give high, potentially toxic concentrations of oxygen. Positive end-expiratory pressure also increases $PaCO_2$ due to increased deadspace ventilation. It decreases venous return, cardiac output, and systemic arterial blood pressure, especially with levels of greater than 5 cm H_2O. Intravenous hydration might require augmentation with the application of PEEP.

Positive end-expiratory pressure can increase ICP in patients with reduced intracranial compliance by decreasing cerebral venous outflow. Positive end-expiratory pressure at 10 cm H_2O improves oxygenation and usually causes clinically inconsequential increases in ICP in patients with severe head trauma. Up to 30 cm H_2O of PEEP has been used to treat hypoxemia with minimal adverse effect on ICP. However, because larger, potentially serious increases in ICP and clinical deterioration have been observed in some head-injured patients with PEEP, ICP should be monitored.

The variable clinical responses to PEEP in head-injured patients might be secondary to PEEP's effect on other hemodynamic and respiratory variables. Positive end-expiratory pressure may affect ICP less in patients with the stiffest lungs, who presumably are the ones who need PEEP the most. Increases in ICP due to PEEP can be reduced by elevating the head 30° and by concurrent mannitol administration. Abrupt removal of PEEP might also increase ICP.

5. **Monitoring of patients receiving mechanical ventilation.** The efficacy and safety of mechanical ventilation in patients is evaluated by the monitoring of gas exchange, airway pressures, breathing patterns, hemodynamic function, and chest x-rays.

   a. **Gas exchange.** Evaluated by measuring the arterial oxygen tension or saturation, the arterial carbon dioxide tension, and arterial blood pH.

   b. **Airway pressure.** Monitored by observing the peak inspiratory pressure, the plateau (end-expiratory occlusion) pressure, PEEP (external and auto-PEEP), and the waveform of pressure.

   c. **Breathing pattern.** Monitored by the minute ventilation, tidal volume, and respiratory frequency.

   d. **Hemodynamic function.** Monitored by the blood pressure, cardiac output, pulmonary artery occlusion pressure, and urine output.

   e. **Chest x-ray.** Used to assess the endotracheal tube position, signs of barotrauma, and signs of pneumonia.

C. **Weaning.** Weaning can be attempted when the patient is clinically stable.

1. **Clinical parameters to be met before attempting weaning.**

   a. Cause for instituting mechanical ventilation is sufficiently resolved. Pneumonia, bronchospasm, and other lung disease should be adequately treated before instituting weaning.

   b. PaO_2 of 60 to 70 mm Hg or SaO_2 of more than 90% on FiO_2 of 0.4 with PEEP less than or equal to 5 cm H_2O.

   c. Respiratory parameters:

     (1) Tidal volume of more than or equal to 5 mL/kg.

     (2) Respiratory rate less than or equal to 35 breaths/minute.

(3) Vital capacity more than or equal to 10 to 15 mL/kg.

(4) Inspiratory force of -25 cm H_2O.

d. $PaCO_2$ of less than or equal to 50 mm Hg.

e. Absence of sepsis or fever.

f. Appropriate neurologic and muscular status.

g. Correction of metabolic and/or electrolyte disorders.

h. Hemodynamic stability.

2. **Weaning techniques.** Weaning may be accomplished by use of the IMV mode, pressure support mode, or intermittent spontaneous breathing with a T piece. Weaning is usually faster for patients with neurologic disease than for those with chronic obstructive pulmonary disease.

   a. **Intermittent mandatory ventilation mode.** Weaning is accomplished by reducing the rate of the mandatory breaths, generally by 2 to 4 breaths per minute at least 2 times per day. Intermittent mandatory ventilation has the theoretical advantage of a smooth transition from full ventilatory assistance to spontaneous ventilation. However, IMV can increase the duration of weaning compared to the pressure support mode and the T-piece trial. This may be due to an increased work of breathing imposed by the demand valve systems and the resistance of external ventilator circuits and humidifiers. The trachea can be extubated once patients tolerate mechanical rates of 4 to 5 breaths per minute without signs of clinical deterioration for periods of 2 to 24 hour. Continuous positive airway pressure may be continued once the patient is breathing spontaneously.

   b. **Pressure support ventilation.** Weaning is accomplished by progressively reducing the level of pressure support, generally by steps of 2 to 4 cm H_2O twice a day. Pressure support ventilation improves the efficacy of spontaneous ventilation and reduces external respiratory work during weaning. The combination of pressure support and PEEP may be especially useful in the weaning of chronic obstructive pulmonary disease patients. Evidence of tolerance to a level of pressure support that is less than or equal to 8 cm H_2O is required before extubation.

   c. **Spontaneous breathing with T piece.** Intermittent use of the T piece allows periods of respiratory effort to be alternated with periods of rest. The T piece has very little resistance to gas flow and does not increase the work of breathing. This may be especially useful in patients who do not tolerate weaning using the IMV mode. Weaning can be accomplished by a once-daily trial of spontaneous ventilation, followed by extubation if the patient tolerates at least 2 hours of spontaneous breathing.

REFERENCES

1. Domino KB. Pulmonary function and dysfunction in the traumatized patient. *Anesth Clin North Am* 1996;14:59.
2. Malik AB. Mechanisms of neurogenic pulmonary edema. *Circ Res* 1985;57:1.
3. Kolley MH, Schuster DP. Ventilator-associated pneumonia: clinical considerations. *AJR* 1994;163:1031.
4. Tobin MJ. Mechanical ventilation. *N Engl J Med* 1994;330:1056.
5. Mancebo J. Weaning from mechanical ventilation. *Eur Respir J* 1996;9:1923.

Cardiovascular Therapy

Steven J. Allen and C. Lee Parmley

I. **Basic considerations.** The crucial goal of cardiovascular therapy in perioperative neurosurgical patients is to provide sufficient metabolic substrate to the threatened central nervous system (CNS). As glucose is usually not a problem our attention is directed to oxygen delivery. Cardiovascular therapy can affect CNS swelling and result in irreversible injury. Therefore, while maintaining oxygen delivery out of the left ventricle is important, care must be exercised not to compromise intracerebral hemodynamics.

   A. **Autoregulation** refers to the interdependence of cerebral blood flow (CBF) and mean arterial blood pressure (MAP). The range of MAP over which nonhypertensive patients exhibit autoregulation is 50 to 150 mm Hg. Chronically hypertensive patients have altered autoregulation and will not maintain CBF at MAPs in the low end of the normal range. A similar alteration of autoregulation is seen with sympathetic activation induced by shock or surgery.

      1. When autoregulation is impaired, CBF will become more dependent on the blood pressure; minor swings in MAP might have significant impact on intracerebral hemodynamics.

      2. Many conditions such as head injury and tumors might result in generalized or regional disruption of autoregulation.

   B. **Intracranial pressure.** As the intracranial compartment is essentially a closed space, intracranial pressure (ICP) is determined by the intracranial volume, composed of cerebrospinal fluid (CSF), cerebral parenchyma, and cerebral blood volume (CBV). Increases in any of these components can contribute to intracranial hypertension (ICH) and result in decreased cerebral perfusion pressure (CPP).

   C. **Cerebral perfusion pressure** = MAP − ICP. In most organs, venous pressure generates the back pressure that determines the pressure drop across an organ. As venous pressure tends to be negative in the brain, parenchymal pressure (ICP) generates the back pressure for determining CPP. It is CPP that determines CBF both globally and regionally in the CNS. Normal CBF is 50 mL/100 g brain tissue/minute and will decrease only if CPP falls from a normal value of approximately 80 mm Hg to below 50 mm Hg, unless autoregulation is altered.

II. **Cerebral oxygen delivery** is a function of the quantity of oxygen carried in arterial blood (CaO_2) and CBF. Cerebral blood flow is related to CPP, and since blood pressure is a function of cardiac output (CO) and systemic vascular resistance (SVR), clearly cardiac output is an important parameter to manipulate in order to preserve CBF and cerebral oxygen delivery. The normal awake brain consumes 3.3 mL O_2/100 g/minute, a value reduced by about one third during anesthesia.

A. **Cardiac Output**

1. **Determinants of cardiac output.** The CO is a result of four basic factors: contractility, preload, heart rate (HR), and afterload.

   a. **Preload** is impractically monitored, but best determined by measuring left ventricular end-diastolic volume (LVEDV) by either angiography or echocardiography. Pulmonary artery occlusion pressure (PAOP) is more frequently used as a reliable estimate of left atrial pressure.

   b. **Contractility.** Ejection fraction measured by either angiography or echocardiography is frequently used to assess contractility, which can also be assessed by evaluating the magnitude of the CO for a given preload condition.

   c. **Heart rate.** CO = HR × stroke volume. When preload and/or contractility limits stroke volume, increase in HR often acts to maintain CO.

   d. **Afterload.** Mean aortic pressure is the afterload against which the left ventricle ejects a stroke volume. We use MAP in neuroanesthesia as a close approximation.

B. **Cardiac failure** occurs when cardiac output is insufficient for adequate oxygen delivery. Traditional causes include cardiomyopathies from infarction, ischemia, and chronic hypertension; dysrhythmias; increased afterload from arterial hypertension; and outflow obstruction from pulmonary embolus. Neurologic critical care patients have additional considerations.

1. **Hypovolemia** causing insufficient preload.

   a. **Blood loss.** Surgical and traumatic causes should be considered including scalp lacerations.

   b. **Osmotic diuretic** administration might result in excessive intravascular volume contraction.

   c. **Fluid restriction** instituted to minimize cerebral swelling can lead to hypovolemia and end-organ compromise.

   d. **Diabetes insipidus** associated with severe traumatic brain injury and pituitary surgery might result in significant urine output leading to hypovolemia.

2. **Central nervous system causes**

   a. Spinal cord injury and injury to the brain stem vasomotor center can result in hypotension due to decreased sympathetic tone.

        b. Neurogenic cardiomyopathy has been described in patients following subarachnoid hemorrhage and acute traumatic brain injury. Electrocardiographic changes might be consistent with ischemia and myocardial dysfunction.

    3. Drug-induced. Occasionally aggressive therapy with calcium entry blockers or beta blockers might result in suboptimal myocardial performance.

C. Blood pressure

    1. Mean arterial blood pressure = CO × SVR (systemic vascular resistance). Cardiac output is discussed above.

    2. Hypotension in the presence of normal intravascular volume and cardiac function occurs because of decreases in SVR.

        a. Hypotension secondary to high cervical cord injury.

        b. Brain stem damage involving the vasomotor center results in hypotension. Such an insult is usually lethal.

        c. Fever/sepsis

III. Drugs used in cardiovascular therapy

A. Guidelines for administration of vasoactive drugs

    1. Use a calibrated pump for all infusions.

    2. Inject into the intravenous line as close to vein insertion as possible.

    3. Avoid using systolic blood pressure as the goal of therapy, as this value is prone to fluctuation from a number of causes, not all of which are related to the patient's cardiovascular condition. Mean arterial pressure is a more reliable variable.

    4. Potent vasoactive drugs should be administered in a graded fashion starting with a dose below that thought to be therapeutic.

B. Adrenergic drugs. See Table 22-1 for action of adrenergic receptors, and see Tables 22-2 and 22-3 for relative adrenergic action and dosing recommendations. Sympathomimetic drugs appear to have little influence on the vascular tone of cerebral vessels. However, if MAP is raised above the upper threshold of autoregulation, CBF will increase. There is some evidence that β-agonists might increase the cerebral metabolic rate for oxygen and secondarily raise CBF.

    1. Epinephrine (adrenalin) possesses α and β properties that are dose-related. Its primary uses are in cardiopulmonary resuscitation, anaphylaxis, and refractory hypotension. Toxicity from epinephrine is due to arrhythmias and sequelae of vasoconstriction.

    2. Dobutamine is a synthetic drug with predominantly β_1 activity. Compared to other agents it

Table 22-1. Action of adrenergic receptors

Receptor	Site	Action
α_1	Postsynaptic Vasculature Heart	Vasoconstriction
α_2	Presynaptic Peripheral and central nervous system, liver, pancreas, kidney, eye	Vasodilatation
β_1	Heart	Contractility Chronotropy
β_2	Heart Vascular and bronchial smooth muscle	Contractility Chronotropy Smooth muscle relaxation
Dopaminergic	Presynaptic Renal and splanchnic circulation, brain stem	Smooth muscle relaxation Nausea and vomiting

tends to produce less tachycardia and elevation of pulmonary vascular pressures for the same degree of inotropic enhancement. It does not have any dopaminergic agonist action.

3. **Dopamine** has α, β, and dopaminergic properties in a dose-related fashion. Its primary uses are hypotension, inotropic support, and renal protec-

Table 22-2. Adrenergic agonist and phosphodiesterase inhibitor drugs

Name	Receptors	Dosage
Epinephrine	β_2 $\beta_1 + \beta_2$ α	1–2 μg/min 2–10 μg/min >10 μg/min
Norepinephrine	α, β_1	4–12 μg/min
Dopamine	Dopaminergic β α	0–3 μg/kg/min 3–10 μg/kg/min >10 μg/kg/min
Dobutamine	β_1	2.5–10 μg/kg/min
Phenylephrine	α, β_1 (slight)	0.1–0.5 μg/kg/min
Ephedrine	α, β_1	5- to 10-mg bolus
Isoproterenol	β_1, β_2	0.5–10 μg/min
Amrinone	Inhibition of phosphodiesterase	0.75 mg/kg load, then 5–10 μg/kg/min
Milrinone	Inhibition of phosphodiesterase	50–75 mg/kg load, then 0.5–0.75 μg/kg/min

Table 22-3. Adrenergic antagonists

Name	Receptor Blocked	Dosage
Phentolamine	α	5–10 mg i.v.
Esmolol	β	0.15–1 mg/kg i.v. bolus, then 50–300 µg/kg/min
Labetalol	$\beta > \alpha$	5–20 mg i.v., then 2 mg/min
Metoprolol	β	2.5–15 mg i.v.
Propranolol	β	0.25–5 mg i.v. bolus

tion. Low doses inhibit renal sodium reabsorption, resulting in a natriuresis. In high doses, dopamine's α properties predominate. There is evidence that it can produce mild cerebral vasodilatation.

4. **Phenylephrine** is a synthetic drug whose chief characteristic is its relative selectivity for α receptors. When used to increase MAP, there is often a baroreceptor-mediated reflex decrease in HR. It is preferable to use when cardiac index (CI) is sufficient but MAP is below the goal.

5. **Isoproterenol** is a synthetic drug that has remarkable β selectivity. Administration is associated with tachycardia, decreased MAP, and improvement of bronchospasm.

6. **Norepinephrine** (Levophed) has some β activity but mostly used as an α-adrenergic agonist. Its primary use is treatment of refractory hypotension.

C. **Adrenergic antagonists (Table 22-3)**

1. **Esmolol** is an ultra-short-acting (9 to 10 minutes duration) β-specific competitive antagonist. Its quick onset and short duration render it suitable for rapid intervention in the treatment of tachyarrhythmias in the perioperative period.

2. **Metoprolol** is a cardioselective β antagonist that has a longer duration of action than esmolol. It is most commonly used to treat angina and acute myocardial infarction but may be used intravenously in the perioperative period to control tachycardia. All beta blockers possess the risk of inducing bronchospasm and/or heart failure.

3. **Labetalol** blocks both α and β receptors with greater β effects than α. However, a reduction in MAP usually occurs when the dosage is sufficient to decrease HR. It also has a longer duration of action than either esmolol or propranolol.

4. **Propranolol** was the original clinically available beta-blocking agent. It is nonselective and has a relatively short onset, but because liver metabolism of the drug differs widely from patient to patient, dosing is variable. Curiously, it shifts the hemoglobin–oxygen dissociation curve to the right.

5. **Phentolamine** specifically competes for both α_1 and α_2 receptors. Because of its duration of action, it is not frequently used as an antihypertensive in acute perioperative situations.

D. **Phosphodiesterase inhibitors (Table 22-2)**

1. **Amrinone** is a nonadrenergic, nonglycosidic compound that enhances contractility and promotes pulmonary and arterial vasodilatation. Its action is thought to be inhibition of phosphodiesterase, which leads to increased intracellular concentrations of cyclic AMP. It has little potential for cardiac arrhythmias but has a long half-life (hours) and might induce thrombocytopenia as well as hypotension.

2. **Milrinone** is similar to amrinone but might have less thrombocytopenia and, in our experience, less hypotension.

E. **Vasodilators (Table 22-4)**

1. **Sodium nitroprusside** (SNP) is a potent, rapid-onset, short-acting agent that results in greater arteriolar than venular vasodilatation via release of nitric oxide. Sodium nitroprusside administration is associated with activation of the renin-angiotensin system and reflex tachycardia may interfere with blood pressure reduction. There are occasional patients who demonstrate relative resistance to SNP. These patients are at particular risk for developing cyanide toxicity.

2. **Nitroglycerin** (NTG) is a rapid-onset, short-acting agent that induces vasodilatation via nitric oxide. Nitroglycerin results in greater venular than arteriolar vasodilatation and is less potent than SNP but has little toxicity.

Table 22-4. Vasodilators

Name	Dosage
Sodium nitroprusside	0.5–10 μg/kg/min
Nitroglycerin	5–50 μg/min
Trimethaphan	1–15 mg/min
Hydralazine	0.1–0.2 mg/kg
Nicardipine	5–15 mg/kg

3. **Trimethaphan** decreases MAP by ganglionic blockade. Unlike SNP or NTG, it does not result in cerebral vasodilatation and does not increase ICP. The drawbacks include dilated pupils and tachyphylaxis.

4. **Hydralazine** is a vascular smooth muscle relaxant with no effects on contractility or chronotropy. Its use is frequently accompanied by reflex tachycardia.

5. **Nicardipine** is a calcium entry blocker that reliably decreases MAP when given as an intravenous infusion. Due to its low toxicity, it may be an acceptable alternative to SNP when MAP is not critically high.

6. **Adenosine** is an ultrafast-acting vasodilator agent that produces decreased MAP and increased CI due to decreased SVR. Heart block is a potential side effect of its use.

IV. **Goal-directed pharmacologic intervention for cardiovascular dysfunction.** The two goals of cardiovascular therapy in neurosurgical patients—adequate CPP and sufficient CO to maintain oxygen delivery—might require different drug regimens. Optimal fluid therapy should be instituted either prior to or in conjunction with drug therapy.

A. **Raising MAP** might be indicated in a number of clinical settings.

1. **Decreased SVR** due to impaired sympathetic tone, sepsis/fever, or anesthetic drugs might be associated with inadequate MAP. Cardiac output might be normal or even high while CPP is too low to optimize cerebral perfusion. Phenylephrine is a vasoconstrictor agent that should be considered in this setting.

2. **Increasing CPP** by raising MAP might be needed to protect cerebral perfusion following carotid endarterectomy and cerebral vasospasm. With ICH (intracerebral hemorrhage) following head injury, it may be desirable to increase MAP to maintain CPP and prevent cerebral hypoperfusion if ICP cannot be controlled.

3. **Anaphylactic reactions.** Hypotension accompanying an allergic reaction should be treated with epinephrine.

4. **Cardiopulmonary resuscitation.** Drugs should be administered according to advanced cardiac life support guidelines.

5. **Therapy.** Mean arterial pressure may be increased by administering an agent with vasoconstrictive properties that work by direct and/or indirect adrenergic stimulation (see Table 22-2) with varying effect on HR. Pulmonary artery pressure and PAOP will also tend to rise, even if there has been no change in intravascular volume status.

6. **Precautions**
   a. **Myocardial risks.** In a patient with coronary artery disease, increasing MAP (afterload) might increase myocardial oxygen demand sufficiently to outstrip delivery, causing myocardial ischemia and failure.
   b. **Left ventricular dysfunction.** Increasing MAP might decrease CO if left ventricular (LV) dysfunction exists. Thus, CO monitoring might be indicated when hypertension is being induced in patients suspected of having LV dysfunction.
   c. **Hypovolemia** should be treated with augmentation of intravascular volume rather than further masked with the use of adrenergic drugs that will increase the risk of end-organ ischemia.
   d. **Impaired renal function.** Pharmacologically increasing MAP might cause vasoconstriction of renal vessels and could result in deterioration of renal function if perfusion is marginal.

B. **Increasing CO** might be indicated in a number of clinical settings.
   1. **Low CO due to cardiomyopathy.** This may arise from ischemia, viral disease, or drug overdose. Goals that have been recommended for inotropic therapy are:
      a. MAP of more than 80 mm Hg.
      b. Mixed venous saturation (SvO_2) of more than 65%.
      c. Cardiac index (CO/body surface area) of more than 3.5 L/m^2/minute.
      d. Evidence of adequate end-organ perfusion. Monitoring urine output might be unreliable once diuretics are administered.
   2. **Cerebral vasospasm.** Supernormal CO might reduce the risk of permanent neurologic deficit.
   3. **Therapy.** If CO is insufficient after intravascular volume has been optimized, inotropic drugs should be administered.
      a. **Beta agonists** are the first-line drugs as their onset and duration allow rapid titration of effect. Empiric therapy should be replaced by goal-directed dosing as soon as appropriate monitoring is available.
      b. **Phosphodiesterase inhibitors.** Amrinone and milrinone may be used as adjunct agents to further enhance CO.
      c. **Digoxin** possesses mild to moderate inotropic activity, can be given orally or intravenously, and can increase CO by 10% to 20% in otherwise stable chronic heart failure patients.

4. **Precautions**
   a. In high enough doses all adrenergic drugs will cause tachycardia, and in patients with coronary artery disease, ischemia may develop. Heart rates above 120 should be avoided.
   b. When doses of the adrenergic agents reach the range where α activity predominates, renal perfusion may be compromised, risking renal failure.
   c. While digoxin is useful in the management of chronic cardiac failure, its onset is not immediate nor is it easily titratable. Undocumented previous digoxin administration, hypokalemia due to diuretics, and onset of renal failure increase the risk of digoxin toxicity.

C. **Lowering MAP** may be indicated in a number of clinical settings
   1. **Hypertension**
      a. **Unclipped aneurysm.** Hypertension in the presence of an unclipped cerebral aneurysm is believed to be a significant risk factor for rebleeding.
      b. **Disrupted cerebral microvascular membrane.** In the presence of disruption of the blood–brain barrier, hypertension can exacerbate the formation of vasogenic edema and blood pressure control should be considered.
   2. **Surgical exposure.** Iatrogenic hypotension may be requested by surgeons to enhance exposure, reduce risk of aneurysm rupture, or assist with the control of bleeding.
   3. **Therapy**
      a. **Analgesics.** Clearly, the control of pain might be sufficient to return the MAP to a more acceptable level.
      b. **Vasodilators.** Although many vasodilator agents are available, the patient's comorbid problems and the urgency of the situation often guide the choice. Regardless, a target MAP should be chosen concomitantly with starting therapy. In the absence of pre-existing hypertension, MAP, measured at the level of the external auditory meatus, may be decreased 20% from baseline without undue risk.
         (1) Rapid control will require the use of vasodilators such as SNP, NTG, or trimethaphan.
         (2) Less urgent situations may be adequately treated with drugs of slower onset but fewer drawbacks such as the beta blockers, nicardipine, or hydralazine.

    4. Precautions
- **a. Hypovolemia.** Even small doses of vasodilators can cause dramatic hypotension in the presence of hypovolemia.
- **b. Decreased intracranial compliance.** Vasodilators have the potential for cerebral vascular relaxation and thereby increasing cerebral blood volume (CBV). If intracranial compliance is decreased, increases in CBV may act to increase ICP.

D. Lowering HR may be indicated in a number of clinical settings.
1. **Reduce myocardial oxygen consumption.** Tachycardia can increase myocardial oxygen demand and induce ischemia in susceptible patients.
2. **Atrial fibrillation** with a rapid ventricular response might also compromise the heart's ability to deliver an adequate CO.
3. **Hypertension.** Although slowing the HR is not usually sufficient to decrease MAP by a significant degree, less antihypertensive agent is subsequently required due to abatement of reflex tachycardia.
4. **Therapy.** Adenosine and beta blockers such as esmolol, propranolol, and labetalol are often used as first-line drugs due to their rapid onset and relative safety. Some calcium entry blockers such as verapamil and diltiazem are also used to control ventricular rate, particularly for supraventricular tachycardias.
5. **Precautions**
   - a. These drugs have negative inotropic and vasodilatory properties that may result in both low CO and hypotension. Particular caution is necessary when beta blockers and calcium entry blockers are combined.
   - b. Some patients with bronchospastic disease experience exacerbation of their symptoms when receiving a beta blocker.

V. Management of cardiovascular complications of neurologic disorders

A. Cerebral vasospasm
1. **Pathophysiology.** Vasospasm is a misnomer for a potentially devastating complication that occurs after subarachnoid hemorrhage and may be a concern after acute traumatic brain injury. If extensive, vasospasm can decrease CBF to ischemic levels, causing permanent neurologic deficits or death. Although transcranial Doppler is proving to be a useful diagnostic modality, vasospasm is traditionally diagnosed by angiography where beaded narrowing of the cerebral arteries confirms the diagnosis.

2. **Monitoring.** Angiography is the gold standard for vasospasm diagnosis but is impractical for monitoring. Transcranial Doppler (TCD) has the advantage of being portable, noninvasive, and patients may be monitored regularly or even continuously. Transcranial Doppler detects vasospasm by measuring the velocity of blood in a cerebral artery; as vasospasm narrows a vessel, blood velocity through the constriction increases.

3. **Prevention.** A statistical decrease in permanent neurologic deficits in patients at risk has been demonstrated when a cerebral selective calcium entry blocker is used which is not associated with increased diameter in the affected vessels.

4. **Triple-H Therapy.** Hypervolemia, hypertension, hemodilution.

   a. **Rationale.** Triple-H therapy is aimed at increasing blood flow through the narrowed arteries by decreasing the viscosity (hemodilution), increasing the driving pressure (hypertension), and expanding of the blood volume (hypervolemia).

   b. **Invasive monitoring,** usually including pulmonary artery catheterization, is needed as knowledge of intravascular fluid status and the cardiac index are of central importance.

      (1) **Fluids.** Hypervolemia is accomplished by infusion of isotonic fluids or colloids.

      (2) **Vasoactive drugs.** The two hemodynamic goals are increasing MAP and CO. Vasoactive drugs are chosen to increase SVR or contractility, as desired. A selective approach is achieved using phenylephrine for the former and dobutamine for the latter.

   c. **Precautions.** Pulmonary edema is the primary concern even with conscientious management of triple-H therapy. Once detected treatment goals must be adjusted.

5. **Cerebral salt wasting** frequently accompanies SAH and other intracranial pathology. Urinary sodium is elevated in the presence of hyponatremia, an electrolyte picture seen also in syndrome of inappropriate antidiuretic hormone secretion (SIADH). With cerebral salt wasting, unlike SIADH, intravascular volume depletion will develop, which is undesirable when cerebral vasospasm is a risk.

B. **Autonomic hypotension (neurogenic shock)**

1. **Pathophysiology.** Hypotension can occur after a spinal cord injury at a high thoracic or cervical level. Interruption of the sympathetic nervous system causes vasodilatation from loss of sympathetic vascular tone and bradycardia due to involvement of the cardioaccelerator nerves. Young

individuals with high resting vagal tone, normally balanced by sympathetic activity, might experience bradycardia leading to asystole.

2. **Treatment.** Care should be taken in managing low blood pressure in spinal cord injury patients as they do not have intact compensatory mechanisms. They tend to tolerate lower blood pressures without sequelae compared to neurologically intact patients.

   a. Hypotension without bradycardia may be treated with careful administration of fluids if end-organ perfusion is a concern. Urine output in the acute phase of spinal cord injury is typically low regardless of cardiac index or intravascular volume status.

   b. If a vasoactive agent is desired, the clinician should remember that denervation hypersensitivity might produce a much larger response than expected.

   c. Bradycardia might require atropine for the first 72 hours after spinal cord injury. Rarely will bradycardic episodes persist to the point where a pacemaker is needed.

C. **Carotid endarterectomy: postoperative hypotension**

   1. **Pathophysiology.** Patients with atherosclerosis sufficient to require carotid endarterectomy often have underlying cardiovascular disease and are prone to MAP instability in the perioperative period, including bradycardia or dysrhythmias due to abnormal carotid sinus baroreceptor response.

   2. **Treatment** should include administration of fluids to correct any preexisting intravascular volume deficits, atropine if carotid sinus stimulation causes bradycardia, and phenylephrine or dopamine to prevent end-organ compromise if hypotension persists.

D. **Carotid endarterectomy: postoperative hypertension**

   1. **Pathophysiology.** Manipulation of the carotid sinus may contribute to postoperative hypertension. Postoperative hypertension is associated with a higher risk of stroke, death, and postoperative bleeding.

   2. **Treatment.** Hypertension may be effectively managed by intravenous administration of labetalol, nicardipine, hydralazine, or, if severe, SNP.

E. **Acute traumatic brain injury with hypotension**

   1. **Pathophysiology.** In a patient who survives transport to the hospital, hypotension associated with acute traumatic brain injury is most likely due to blood loss. Acute traumatic brain injury sufficient to damage the brain stem vasomotor center is almost always fatal.

2. **Treatment** needs to be prompt as the injured brain is particularly vulnerable to low perfusion pressure, which may already be compromised by increased ICP.

   a. Expand intravascular volume as in any trauma victim suspected of having hypovolemia.

   b. Positive inotropic agents or vasoconstrictors can be used to provide an acceptable MAP rapidly until intravascular volume can be restored.

F. **Acute traumatic brain injury with hypertension**
   1. **Pathophysiology**
      a. Commonly, acute traumatic brain injury (TBI) patients are hypertensive due to excessive secretion of catecholamines. This begins within the first 10 days and may continue for as long as 3 months. Hypertension may be accompanied by tachycardia, tachypnea, restlessness, and diaphoresis limited to the upper body, probably due to disinhibition of central sympathetic reflexes.

      b. **Cushing reflex.** Mean arterial pressure might also be elevated if ICP is approaching systemic values as a protective mechanism to maintain CPP. Original descriptions of the Cushing reflex in animals involved bradycardia, whereas tachycardia is more commonly seen in humans.

   2. **Treatment.** Hypertension in the TBI patient typically is associated with elevated ICP and there are two possible etiologies. First, with impaired autoregulation, increased MAP increases CBF and thus ICP. Second, raised ICP induces arterial hypertension via the Cushing reflex. Treatment must be cautious, monitoring the effect on ICP.

      a. **Sympathetic overactivity.** Hypertension due to posttraumatic brain injury syndrome is responsive to beta blockers, but high doses might be necessary to compete with high levels of endogenous catecholamines. Beta blockers also have the benefit of improving intracranial compliance and do not cause cerebral vascular relaxation. If beta blockade does not adequately decrease MAP, then SNP, NTG, or trimethaphan may be considered. Sodium nitroprusside and NTG can cause cerebral vascular relaxation, increasing CBV and ICP—an effect that may be ameliorated by slow infusion of the drug.

      b. **Cushing reflex.** If hypertension is thought to occur as a result of the Cushing reflex, then attention should be directed to decreasing ICP, as decreasing MAP alone may result in critical CPP reduction.

G. Postoperative hypertension

1. **Pathophysiology.** Patients with no prior history of hypertension will exhibit hypertension after craniotomy. In the absence of raised ICP, postcraniotomy hypertension should be treated to reduce the risk of cerebral swelling and bleeding in the operative site. However, if ICP is elevated, treatment of hypertension may decrease CPP to ischemic levels.

2. **Treatment.** Hypertension after craniotomy may be treated with labetalol or nicardipine with predictable results. If ICH is suspected, then management should follow that outlined above for TBI.

SUGGESTED READINGS

Allen SJ, Parmely CL. Current concepts in treatment of closed head injury. *Curr Opin Anesthesiol* 1998;11:141–145.

Chestnut RM. Avoidance of hypotension: conditro sine qua non of successful head injury management. *J Trauma* 1997;42:54–59.

Harrigan MR. Cerebral salt wasting syndrome: a review. *Neurosurgery* 1996;38:152–159.

Rosner MJ, Rosner SD, Johnson AH. Cerebral perfusion pressure: management protocol and clinical results. J Neurosurg 1995;83:949–962.

Tietkjen CS, Hurn PD, Ulatowcki JA, Kirsch JR. Treatment modalities for hypertensive patients with intracranial pathology: options and risks. *Crit Care Med* 1996;24:311–322.

23

Fluid Management

Concezione Tommasino

Neurosurgical patients often receive diuretics (e.g., mannitol, furosemide) to treat cerebral edema and/or to reduce intracranial hypertension. Conversely, they may also require large amounts of intravenous fluid or blood as part of resuscitation, therapy for vasospasm, correction of preoperative dehydration, or maintenance of intraoperative and postoperative hemodynamic stability.

These two interventions seem to be in conflict: if diuretics are "good" for patients, is it reasonable to argue that fluids (and volume expansion) might be "bad"? In general terms, this is the origin of the belief in fluid restriction and the prohibition against the aggressive administration of fluids. There would be little point in discussing the subject if fluid restriction were benign, if its efficacy were proven, or if the infusion of large amounts of fluid had been conclusively shown to exacerbate cerebral edema or intracranial hypertension. Moreover, fluid restriction, if pursued to excess (hypovolemia), might result in episodes of hypotension, which can increase intracranial pressure (ICP) and reduce cerebral perfusion pressure (CPP). The consequences can be devastating.

It is unfortunate that few substantial human data exist concerning the impact of fluids on the brain that can guide rational fluid management in neurosurgical patients. However, it is possible to examine those factors that influence water movement into the brain and to make some recommendations that we consider reasonable.

I. **Osmolality/osmolarity, colloid oncotic pressure, crystalloids, and colloids.** Before starting our discussion, it is important that the reader be familiar with a number of definitions and distinctions, particularly as they apply to the brain.

A. **Osmotic pressure.** The hydrostatic force acts to equalize the concentration of *water* (H_2O) on both sides of a membrane that is impermeable to substances dissolved in that water. Water will move along its concentration gradient. This means that if a solution containing 10 mM of Na^+ and 10 mM of Cl^- is placed on one side of a semipermeable membrane with H_2O on the other, water will move "toward" the saline solution. The saline solution has a concentration of 20 mosmol/L, and the force driving water will be about 19.3 mm Hg per mosmol, or 386 mm Hg. Note that the driving force is proportional to the *gradient* across the membrane; if two solutions of equal concentration are placed across a membrane, there is no driving force. Similarly, if the membrane is permeable to the solutes (e.g., Na^+ and Cl^-), this will act to reduce the gradient and hence the osmotic forces.

B. **Osmolarity and osmolality.** *Osmolarity* describes the molar number of osmotically active particles per liter of solution. In practice, this value is typically calculated by adding up the milliequivalent (mEq) concentrations of the various ions in the solution. *Osmolality* describes the molar number of osmotically active particles per kilogram of solvent. This value is directly measured by determining either the freezing point or the vapor pressure of the solution (each of which is reduced by dissolved solute). Note that osmotic activity of a solution demands that particles be "independent;" as NaCl dissociates into Na^+ and Cl^-, two osmotically active particles are created. If electrostatic forces act to prevent dissociation of the two charged particles, osmolality will be reduced. For most dilute salt solutions, osmolality is equal to or slightly less than osmolarity. For example, commercial lactated Ringer's solution has a calculated osmolarity of approximately 275 mosmol/L but a measured osmolality of approximately 254 mosmol/kg, indicating incomplete dissociation.

C. **Colloid oncotic pressure.** Osmolarity/osmolality is determined by the total number of dissolved "particles" in a solution, regardless of their size. Colloid oncotic pressure (COP) is that portion of total osmolality that is produced by large molecules, typically plasma proteins. This factor becomes particularly important in biological systems where vascular membranes are often permeable to small ions but not to proteins. In such situations, proteins might be the only osmotically active particles. Normal COP is approximately 20 mm Hg (or equal to about 1 mosmol/kg).

D. **Starling's hypothesis.** In 1898, Starling published his equations describing the forces driving water across vascular membranes. The two major factors that control this movement are (a) the hydrostatic pressure gradient and (b) the osmotic and oncotic gradients. His equation is as follows:

$$FM = k(P_c + \pi_i - P_i - \pi_c)$$

where FM is fluid movement, k is the filtration coefficient of the capillary wall (i.e., how leaky it is), P_c is hydrostatic pressure in the capillaries, P_i is the hydrostatic pressure in the interstitial (extravascular) space, and π_i and π_c are interstitial and capillary osmotic pressures, respectively.

Fluid movement is thus proportional to the hydrostatic pressure gradient minus the osmotic pressure gradient across a vessel wall. The magnitude of the osmotic gradient will depend on the relative permeability of the vessels to solute. In the periphery (muscle, bowel, lung, etc.), the capillary endothelium has a pore size of 65 Å and is freely permeable to small

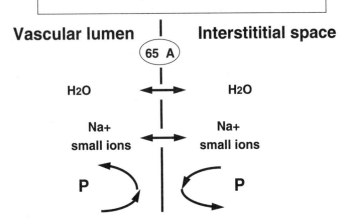

Fig. 23-1. Schematic diagram of a peripheral capillary. The vessel wall is permeable to both water and small ions, but not to proteins.

molecules and ions (Na^+, Cl^-) but not to large molecules, such as proteins (Fig. 23-1). As a result, π is defined only by colloids and the Starling equation can be simplified by saying that **fluid will move into a tissue whenever the hydrostatic gradient increases (either intravascular pressure rises or interstitial pressure falls) or the osmotic gradient decreases.**

In normal situations, the intravascular protein concentration is higher than the interstitial concentration, acting to draw water back into the vascular space. If COP is reduced, e.g., by dilution with large amounts of isotonic crystalloid, fluid will begin to accumulate in the interstitium, producing edema. This fact is familiar to all anesthesiologists who have seen marked peripheral edema in patients given many liters of crystalloid during surgery or resuscitation. By contrast, in the brain where the blood–brain barrier (BBB) is impermeable to both ions and proteins, osmotic pressure is determined by the total osmotic gradient, of which COP contributes only a tiny fraction.

D.   **Interstitial clearance.** In peripheral tissues, there is a net outward movement of fluid (i.e., the value of FM is positive). The reason that edema is not normally present is that this extravasated fluid is cleared by the lymphatics. While many workers agree that there is some lymphatic drainage of the brain, most interstitial fluid is cleared either by bulk fluid flow into the cerebrospinal fluid (CSF) spaces, or via pinocytosis back into the vasculature. This is a slow process and probably does not act as an important buffer to rapid fluid movement.

E. **Hydrostatic forces and interstitial compliance.** In the tissue, the net hydrostatic gradient is determined by (a) intravascular pressure and (b) interstitial tissue compliance. Normally, the direction is outward (capillary to interstitium). There is no question that in the brain (or in any organ) elevated intravascular pressure, such as produced by high jugular venous pressure or a head-down posture, can increase edema formation. However, an often overlooked factor that influences the pressure gradient is the interstitial compliance, i.e., the tendency of tissue to resist fluid influx. The loose interstitial space in most peripheral tissues does little to impede the influx of fluid. This explains the ease with which edema develops around, for example, the face and the eyes even with minor hydrostatic stresses (e.g., a face-down posture).

By contrast, the interstitial space of the brain is extremely noncompliant, resisting fluid movement. As a result, minor changes in driving forces (either hydrostatic or osmotic/oncotic) do not produce measurable edema. However, a vicious cycle can develop, i.e., as edema forms in the brain, the interstitial matrix is disrupted, the compliance increases, and additional edema forms more easily. In addition, the closed cranium and ICP can act to retard fluid influx. This may partially explain the exacerbated edema formation that can occur after rapid decompression of the intracranial space.

F. **Can we explain the influence of certain fluids on the brain?** In contrast to capillaries elsewhere in the body, the endothelial cells in the brain are joined together by continuous tight junctions to form the BBB. There are no intracellular gaps: the membranes are not fenestrated and do not have channels or chains of vesicles that form transendothelial pathways. The effective pore size of the BBB is only 7 Å, making this unique structure normally impermeable to large molecules (plasma proteins and synthetic colloids, such as hetastarch and dextrans) and relatively impermeable to many small polar solutes (Na^+, K^+, Cl^-) (Fig. 23-2). The BBB functions as a semipermeable membrane that allows only water to move freely between the brain's interstitial space and the vasculature. This should serve to make the brain an exquisitely sensitive osmometer (water moves according to osmotic gradients).

We would then predict that **reducing serum osmolality** (e.g., by infusing water or large volumes of nonisotonic crystalloid solution) would increase cerebral edema (or, conversely, increasing osmolality

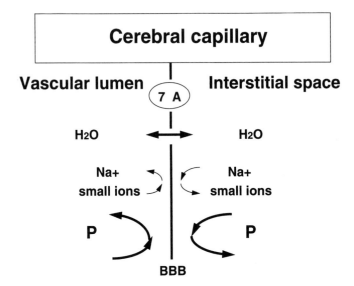

Fig. 23-2. Schematic diagram of a cerebral capillary. The blood–brain barrier is impermeable to small ions and proteins, but not to water.

would reduce brain water content). This experiment was first done in 1919 by Weed and McKibben, who showed a rapid and large increase in brain volume with reduction of serum osmolality. Since that time numerous experiments have shown the exquisite sensitivity of brain water content to changes in serum osmolality. It must be stressed that even small changes in serum osmolality can produce measurable brain water changes; this is not difficult to accept when one realizes that a 5 mosmol/kg gradient is equivalent to an almost 100 mm Hg force driving water (see above). In fact, in experimental animals a reduction in plasma osmolality of as little as 5% under otherwise normal conditions causes brain edema and increases ICP.

G. **What about changes in COP?** As mentioned, colloidally active molecules contribute to only a tiny fraction of total osmolality and when the BBB is intact can be responsible for only a small driving force. Normal plasma COP is approximately 20 mm Hg, whereas that in the brain interstitium is about 0.6 mm Hg. This is equal to the force that could be generated by a change in capillary/tissue osmotic gradient of only 1 mosmol/kg. We would hence predict that changes in COP would have only minimal effect on brain water content. This hypothesis has been tested directly in several animal experiments, which have demonstrated that normal brain water content can be altered by small changes in osmolality, but not by clinically achievable changes in COP. In the normal brain it has not been possible to demonstrate an increase in water content (i.e., brain edema) in any region, even after a very large reduction (around 50%) in COP.

However, **what about more clinically relevant conditions, where the BBB is abnormal**? We can predict that if the BBB is made permeable to both small and large molecules (as is common with several experimental and clinical injuries), it should be impossible to maintain any form of osmotic or oncotic gradient between the blood and brain interstitium. As a result, no changes in brain water content would be expected with a change in either gradient. Indeed, in several animal models resembling human brain injuries (implanted glioma and freezing lesion, which are similar to brain tumor and trauma, respectively), changes induced by reduction in total osmolality were seen only in apparently normal brain regions relatively distant from the injury focus. In keeping with this, several studies have shown that acute hyperosmolality (as with mannitol, urea, hypertonic saline) reduces water content only in relatively normal brain tissue where the BBB is intact.

H. **Summary.** Injury to the brain interferes with the integrity of the BBB to varying degrees, depending on the severity of the damage. In regions in which there is a complete breakdown of the BBB, there will be no osmotic/oncotic gradient; water accumulation (i.e., brain edema) occurs secondarily to the pathologic process and cannot be directly influenced by the osmotic/oncotic gradient. In other regions with moderate injury to the BBB, the barrier might function as in the peripheral tissue (although such areas have not been demonstrated in clinical and experimental studies). Finally, the BBB will be normal in a significant portion of the brain. The presence of a functionally intact BBB is essential if osmotherapy is to be effective.

II. **Fluids for intravenous administration.** Table 23-1 lists a variety of solutions suitable for intravenous use. **Crystalloid** is the term commonly applied to solutions that do not contain any high molecular weight compound and have an oncotic pressure of zero. Crystalloids can be hyposmolar, isoosmolar, or hyperosmolar, and may or may not contain glucose. Crystalloids can be made hyperosmolar by the inclusion of electrolytes (e.g., Na^+ and Cl^-, as in hypertonic saline), low molecular weight solutes such as mannitol (molecular weight 182), or glucose (molecular weight 180). **Colloid** is the term used to denote solutions that have an oncotic pressure similar to that of plasma. Some commonly administered colloids include 5% or 25% albumin, plasma, 6% hetastarch (hydroxyethyl starch,

Table 23-1. Composition of intravenous fluids

Fluid	Dextrose (g/L)	Na+ (mEq/L)	Cl- (mEq/L)	Osmolarity[a] (mosmol/L)[a]	Oncotic P (mm Hg)
5% Dextrose in water	50	—	—	278	—
Crystalloids:					
5% Dextrose in 0.45% saline	50	77	77	405	—
5% Dextrose in Ringer's	50	130	109	525	—
Lactated Ringer's		130	109	275	—
Plasmalyte		140	98	298	—
0.45% Saline		77	77	154	—
0.9% Normal saline (NS)		154	154	308	—
3.0% Saline		513	513	1026	—
5.0% Saline		855	855	1711	—
7.5% Saline		1283	1283	2567	—
20% Mannitol		—	—	1098	—
Colloids:					
Plasma				295	21
Albumin (5%)				290	19
Hetastarch (6%) in NS		154	154	~310	31
Dextran (10%) 40 in NS		154	154	~310	169
Dextran (6%) 70 in NS		154	154	~310	19

[a]Osmolarity = calculated value (osmol/L = mg ÷ molecular weight × 10 × valence).
NS, normal saline; —, no available data; P, pressure.

molecular weight 450), pentastarch (a low molecular weight hydroxyethyl starch, molecular weight 264), and the dextrans (molecular weights 40 and 70). Dextran and hetastarch are dissolved in normal saline, so that the osmolarity of the solution is approximately 290 to 310 mosmol/L with a sodium and chloride content of about 154 mEq/L.

III. **Clinical fluid management of neurosurgical patients**
   A. **Fluid restriction.** Despite a lack of convincing experimental evidence that isoosmolar crystalloids are detrimental, fluid restriction is widely practiced in patients with mass lesions or cerebral edema or at risk for intracranial hypertension. The only directly applicable data indicate that clinically acceptable restriction has little effect on edema formation. However, there is some logic behind modest fluid restriction. One of the few human studies on fluid therapy in neurosurgical patients has demonstrated that patients given standard "maintenance" amounts of intravenous fluid (e.g., 2,000 mL/day of 0.45 N saline in 5% dextrose) in the postoperative period develop a progressive reduction in serum osmolality (Fig. 23-3). On the other hand, patients given half this volume over a period of several days (about a week) show a progressive increase in serum osmolality, which could account for dehydration of the brain (Fig. 23-3). While

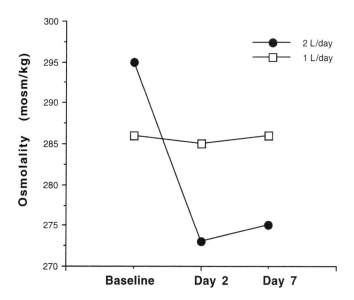

Fig. 23-3. Effect of fluid restriction (1 L/day) on serum osmolality in neurosurgical patients. (Modified by Shenkin et al., 1976).

no central nervous system (CNS)–related parameters were measured, the results suggest that usual maintenance fluids contain excess free water for the typical postoperative craniotomy patient. In this light, fluid restriction can be viewed as "preventing" hyposmotically driven edema. However, this does not imply that even greater degrees of fluid restriction are beneficial or that the administration of a fluid mixture that does not reduce osmolality is detrimental.

B. **Intraoperative volume replacement/resuscitation.** As a general rule, intraoperative fluids should be given at a rate sufficient to replace the urinary output and insensible losses (skin and lung). Table 23-2 illustrates the intravascular volume expansion obtained with different types of fluids. Volume replacement with crystalloid solutions, maintaining the hematocrit around 33%, is calculated approximately on a 3:1 ratio (crystalloid/blood) because of the larger distribution space of the crystalloids.

The available data indicate that volume replacement and expansion will have no effect on cerebral edema as long as normal serum osmolality is maintained, and as long as cerebral hydrostatic pressures are not markedly increased (e.g., due to true volume overload and elevated right heart pressures). Whether this is achieved with crystalloid or colloid seems irrelevant, although the **osmolality of the selected fluid is crucial**. With respect to this issue, it should also be noted that lactated Ringer's solution is not strictly isosmotic (measured osmolality 252 to 255 mosmol/kg), particularly when administered to patients whose baseline osmolality has been increased by either fluid restriction or hyperosmolar fluids (mannitol, hypertonic saline, etc.).

Our recommendation is that serum osmolality be checked repeatedly, with the goal being either to maintain this value or to increase it slightly. Fluid administration that results in a reduction in osmolality should be avoided. Small volumes of lactated Ringer's (1 to 3 L) are unlikely to be detrimental and can be safely used, for example, to compensate for the changes in venous capacitance that typically accompany the induction of anesthesia. If large volumes are needed (due either to blood loss or to compensate for

Table 23-2. Volume replacement

Fluid Infused	Intravascular Volume Increase
1 L isotonic crystalloid	~250 mL
1 L 5% albumin	~500 mL
1 L hetastarch	~750 mL

some other source of volume loss), a change to a more isotonic fluid is probably advisable. This could be normal saline, some other balanced salt solution, or an isotonic colloid (plasma, albumin, hetastarch) (see Table 23-1). Hetastarch should be used with caution due to depletion of factor VIII and possible coagulation difficulties encountered with volumes of more than 1,000 mL. Dextran-40 interferes with normal platelet function and is therefore not advisable for patients with intracranial pathology, other than to improve rheology, such as in ischemic brain diseases.

However, **these recommendations should not be interpreted as "give all the isotonic fluid you like." Volume** *overload* **can have detrimental effects on ICP, by increasing cerebral blood volume (CBV) or by hydrostatically driven edema formation.**

C. **Postoperative period.** In the postoperative period, large fluid requirements should cease. In such cases, the recommendations of Shenkin are probably reasonable (approximately 1,000 mL/day) (Fig. 23-3), although we would again recommend periodic measurements of serum osmolality, particularly if the neurologic status deteriorates. If cerebral edema does develop, further fluid restriction is unlikely to be of value and can cause hypovolemia. Instead, treatment consists of mannitol or furosemide and maintenance of normovolemia with fluids that will sustain the increased osmolality. There is little advantage (and some disadvantage) to inducing hypovolemia such that vasopressors are required to maintain acceptable hemodynamic parameters.

D. **Hypertonic saline solutions.** Hypertonic saline (HS) solutions have been evaluated for use in fluid resuscitation since the 1960s, particularly because hemodynamic improvement can be achieved with very small volumes that can be given very quickly. Because hyperosmolality is known to reduce brain volume, HS has been used in patients who are at risk for increased ICP. In humans, acute resuscitation from hemorrhagic shock with 7.5% HS is associated with improved outcome in multiply traumatized head-injured patients. Clinical studies suggest that HS might be better in hypotensive, brain-injured patients during transport to the hospital.

There is no question that HS can quickly restore intravascular volume while reducing ICP through brain water reduction in uninjured brain. Furthermore, additional benefit may be derived from decreases in CSF production. Unfortunately, what remains unclear is whether this approach is unique—or could the identical CNS benefit be achieved with any resuscitation method that increases osmolality?

The principal disadvantage of HS is the danger of **hypernatremia**. In a recent study in neurosurgical patients during elective supratentorial procedures, we have shown that equal volumes of 20% mannitol and 7.5% HS reduce brain bulk and CSF pressure to the same extent (Fig. 23-3). However, serum sodium increased during the administration of HS and peaked at over 150 mEq/L at the end of the infusion.

Small volumes of hypertonic/hyperoncotic solutions, such as hetastarch and dextran, can restore normovolemia rapidly, without increasing ICP. It is unclear, however, as to whether they offer any advantage over the combination of isotonic fluids and osmotic diuretics. Hetastarch in volumes in excess of 1,500 mL might interfere with hemostasis.

E. **Mannitol and furosemide.** Both mannitol and furosemide (and occasionally other diuretics) are used to control ICP and brain swelling in neurosurgical patients. The mechanism by which **mannitol** acts is by **establishing an osmotic gradient between blood and brain** in the presence of a relatively intact BBB. This promotes removal of water from areas of normal brain. Mannitol might elevate ICP transiently due to the vasodilator effects of hyperosmolality, with a resultant increase in CBV. For both dogs and humans, this phenomenon occurs neither in the presence of intracranial hypertension nor when mannitol is given at moderate rates. Mannitol may, therefore, be given to most neurosurgical patients. The exception might be patients with significant cardiovascular disease in whom the transient volume expansion might precipitate congestive heart failure.

The only other important concern is the repeated use of the drug because excessive hyperosmolality can be deadly. In addition, mannitol does progressively accumulate in the interstitium with repeated doses. If interstitial osmolality rises excessively, it is possible that the normal brain–blood gradient might be reversed, with resultant exacerbation of the edema. Furthermore, if brain osmolality is increased, there is a risk of enhancing edema by subsequent normalization of serum osmolality. The recommended dose is therefore 0.25 to 1.0 g/kg. The smallest possible dose is selected and infused over 10 to 15 minutes.

The exact mechanism of **furosemide's** action remains controversial although it certainly is related to the drug's ability to block Cl^- transport. Furosemide and similar drugs might also act primarily by reducing cellular swelling, rather than by changing the extracellular fluid volume. In several studies it has been demonstrated that furosemide decreases CSF production, and this effect can explain the synergism between mannitol and furosemide on intracranial compliance. However, **furosemide's maximal effect is delayed compared with that of mannitol**. For this reason, mannitol probably remains the agent of choice for rapid ICP control.

F. Glucose-containing solutions. Intravenous salt-free solutions containing glucose are avoided in patients with brain pathology. Free water reduces serum osmolality and increases brain water content. Furthermore, there is solid evidence in animals and humans that **excessive glucose exacerbates neurologic damage** and can worsen outcome from both focal and global ischemia. This is because glucose metabolism enhances tissue acidosis in ischemic areas. Alternatively, the reduction of adenosine levels with hyperglycemia could be detrimental. Adenosine inhibits the release of excitatory amino acids, which play a major role in ischemic cell damage.

Although clinical studies have indicated a negative relationship between plasma glucose on admission and outcome in patients after stroke, cardiac arrest, and head injury, more recent studies suggest that this correlation is not necessarily one of cause and effect (i.e., perhaps the high glucose reflects worse primarily CNS damage), nor has it been possible to demonstrate that the administration of glucose to humans is detrimental. Nevertheless, since withholding glucose from adult neurosurgical patients is not associated with hypoglycemia, it is prudent to withhold glucose-containing fluids from acutely injured and elective surgical patients. This caveat does not apply to the use of hyperalimentation in such patients, perhaps because such hyperglycemic solutions are typically started several days after the primary insult.

G. Should insulin be administered to correct hyperglycemia in patients with brain pathology? While there is laboratory evidence that preischemic correction of hyperglycemia with insulin improves outcome, this has not been studied in humans.

H. Summary. In neurosurgical patients blood sugar should be controlled carefully, the goal being to avoid both hypo- and hyperglycemia, and to maintain glucose between 100 and 150 mg/dL. Glucose-containing solutions should be withheld, except in the case of neonates and patients with diabetes, in whom hypoglycemia can occur very rapidly and be detrimental.

IV. Hemodilution. One common accompaniment of fluid administration is a reduction in hemoglobin/hematocrit. In the face of active blood loss, the use of asanguineous fluids can cause marked anemia. This hemodilution is typically accompanied by an increase in cerebral blood flow (CBF), and physicians have long argued as to whether the hemodilution is beneficial, benign, or detrimental. The answer probably depends on the degree of hemodilution and on the disease state.

From a theoretical vantage, a hematocrit of 30% to 33% gives the optimal combination of viscosity and oxygen-carrying capacity. In the normal brain, the increase in CBF produced by hemodilution is almost certainly an active compensatory response to a decrease in arterial oxygen content, and this response is essentially identical to that seen with hypoxia. In the face of brain injury, however, the normal CBF response to hypoxia and hemodilution is attenuated, and both conditions can contribute to secondary tissue damage.

The one situation in which hemodilution might be beneficial is the period during and immediately after a focal cerebral ischemic event. Several animal studies have shown that regional oxygen delivery may be increased (or at least better maintained) in the face of modest hemodilution (hematocrit approximately 30%) with improvement in CBF and reduction in infarction volume. In spite of this, several clinical trials have failed to demonstrate any benefit from hemodilution in stroke patients, except in those who were polycythemic to begin with. The lack of success, however, may reflect delayed institution of therapy or inadequate hematocrit reduction.

A. **What clinical lesson can be learned from the work on hemodilution?** It is our opinion that in elective neurosurgical patients and patients suffering from head injuries, hemodilution to a hematocrit below 30% to 35% is unlikely to be any more "beneficial" than hypoxia. Hemodilution to 30% to 35% might be better tolerated in patients at risk for focal ischemia. Nevertheless, active attempts to lower hematocrit are probably not advisable at the present time.

B. **Water and electrolyte disturbances.** Table 23-3 summarizes the principal differences among the commonest water and electrolytes disturbances in patients with brain pathology.

C. **Diabetes insipidus.** Diabetes insipidus (DI) is a common sequela of pituitary and hypothalamic lesions, but it can also occur with other cerebral pathology, such as head trauma, bacterial meningitis, intracranial surgery, phenytoin use, and alcohol intoxication. Patients with markedly elevated ICP and brain death also commonly develop DI.

Diabetes insipidus is a metabolic disorder caused by the decreased secretion of antidiuretic hormone (ADH). This results in failure of tubular reabsorption of water. Polyuria (more than 30 mL/kg/hour or, in an adult, more than 200 mL/hour), progressive dehydration, and hypernatremia occur subsequently. Diabetes insipidus is present when the urine output is excessive, the urine osmolality is inappropriately low relative to serum osmolality (which is above normal because of water loss), and the urine specific gravity is less than 1.002.

1. **Management.** The management of DI requires restoration of normal serum sodium, along with careful balancing of intake and output to avoid fluid overload. The patient should receive hourly maintenance fluids plus either three fourths of the previous hour's urine output or the previous

Table 23-3. Principal water-electrolyte disorders

Factor	DI	SIADH	CSWS
Etiology	Reduced secretion of ADH	Excessive release of ADH	Release of brain natriuretic factor
Urine:			
Output	>30 mL/kg/h		
Sp. gr.	<1.002		
Sodium	<15 mEq/L	>20 mEq/L	>50 mEq/L
Osmolality vs. serum osmolality	Lower	Higher	Higher
Serum:			
Sodium	Hypernatremia	Hyponatremia	Hyponatremia
Osmolality	Hyperosmolality	Hypoosmolality	
Intravascular volume	Reduced	Normal or increased	Reduced

DI, diabetes insipidus; SIADH, syndrome of inappropriate antidiuretic hormone secretion; CSWS, cerebral salt wasting syndrome.

Table 23-4.   Management of diabetes insipidus

Hourly monitoring of UO

Maintenance fluids +75% of the previous hour's UO *or*

Maintenance fluids + the previous hour's UO minus 50 mL.

If UO > 300 mL/h: vasopressin or desmopressin

UO, urinary output.

hour's urine output minus 50 mL (Table 23-4). Half-normal saline and free water are commonly used as replacement fluids, with appropriate potassium supplementation. Serum sodium, potassium, and glucose are checked frequently.

If the urine output is greater than 300 mL/hour for 2 hours, it is now standard practice to administer aqueous vasopressin (5 to 10 IU, i.m. or s.c., q6h) or the synthetic analog of ADH, desmopressin acetate (0.5 to 2 μg i.v., q8h; or by nasal inhalation, 10 to 20 μg).

D. **Syndrome of inappropriate antidiuretic hormone secretion.** Various cerebral pathologic processes (mostly head trauma) can cause excessive release of ADH, which leads to the continued renal excretion of sodium (more than 20 mEq/L), despite hyponatremia and associated hypoosmolality. Urine osmolality is therefore high, relative to serum osmolality. Syndrome of inappropriate antidiuretic hormone secretion (SIADH) can also result from over administration of free water in patients who cannot excrete free water because of excess ADH.

1. **Management.** The mainstay of treatment of SIADH is fluid restriction to 1,000 mL/24 hours of isoosmolar solution. If hyponatremia is severe (less than 110 to 115 mEq/L), administration of hypertonic (3% to 5%) saline and furosemide might be appropriate. Since rapid correction of hyponatremia has been associated with the occurrence of central pontine myelinolysis, it is advisable to restore serum sodium at a rate of about 2 mEq/L/hour.

E. **Cerebral salt wasting syndrome.** Cerebral salt wasting syndrome (CSWS) is characterized by hyponatremia, volume contraction, and high urine sodium concentration (more than 50 mEq/L). This syndrome is frequently seen in patients after subarachnoid hemorrhage (SAH) and the causative factor seems to be an increased release of a natriuretic factor from the brain.

1. **Management.** The therapy is to reestablish normovolemia with the administration of sodium-containing solutions.

The **distinction between SIADH and CSWS is very important** because treatment of these two syndromes is quite different: fluid restriction versus fluid infusion. It should be stressed that in patients with SAH, in whom normo- to hypervolemia is advocated, fluid restriction (i.e., further volume contraction) might be especially deleterious.

V. **Conclusion.** As neuroanesthesiologists/intensivists we should always remember that we treat patients and not only brains. Thus, with the exception of patients with SIADH, we should abandon the old dogma that patients with intracranial pathology must be "run dry" and replace it with "run them isovolemic, isotonic, and isooncotic."

VI. **Key points**
- *Movement of water* between the normal brain and the intravascular space is dependent on osmotic gradients.
- Reducing *serum osmolality* by administration of free water or hypotonic crystalloid solutions (0.45% NaCl) results in edema formation in all tissues, including normal brain tissue.
- Reduction of *colloid oncotic pressure* (COP) with maintenance of serum osmolality is associated with increased water content in many tissues, but not in the normal brain. Colloid solutions exert little influence on brain water content and ICP.
- In the setting of *brain injury*, reducing serum osmolality increases edema and ICP. Therefore, the objective of fluid management in neurosurgery is to avoid reduction of serum osmolality. Reduction of COP, with careful maintenance of osmolality, does not increase edema in the injured brain.
- *Hypertonic solutions*: Mannitol decreases brain water content in normal brain and is commonly used to reduce ICP. Hypertonic saline decreases brain water content and ICP, but can cause hypernatremia.
- *Glucose*-containing solutions should not be used in patients with brain pathology and are avoided in patients at risk for brain ischemia.
- *Fluid restriction* minimally affects cerebral edema and, if overzealously pursued, can lead to hemodynamic instability, which is detrimental in neurosurgical patients.
- *Isotonic crystalloid solutions* are widely used to maintain and/or restore intravascular volume.

SUGGESTED READINGS

Gemma M, Cozzi S, Tommasino C, et al. 7.5% hypertonic saline versus 20% mannitol during elective neurosurgical supratentorial procedures. *J Neurosur Anesthesiol* 1997;9:329–334.

Rudehill A, Gordon E, Ohman G, Lindqvist C, Andersson P. Pharmacokinetics and effects of mannitol on hemodynamics, blood and cerebrospinal fluid electrolytes, and osmolality during intracranial surgery. *J Neurosurg Anesthesiol* 1993;5:4–12.

Shenkin HA, Benzier HO, Bouzarth W. Restricted fluid intake: rational management of the neurosurgical patient. *J Neurosurg* 1976;45:432–436.

Tommasino C, Todd MM. Fluid management in neurosurgical patients. In: Van Aken H, ed. *Neuroanaesthetic practice.* London: BMJ, 1995:133–149.

Zornow MH, Scheller MS, Todd MM, Moore SS. Acute cerebral effects of isotonic crystalloid and colloid solutions following cryogenic brain injury in the rabbit. *Anesthesiology* 1988;69:180–184.

Nutritional Support

Linda L. Liu

The goal of nutritional support is to design a regimen that is tailored to the needs of the individual patient. Since the early 1980s, the importance of nutritional support in the patient with severe neurologic injury has been appreciated. Delays in the initiation of nutritional support can cause muscle atrophy, weaning failure, gastrointestinal (GI) atrophy, and possibly heart failure. Most of the studies on nutrition and neurologic injury have focused on head trauma but recent studies are also reporting the same nutritional and metabolic requirement in patients with acute ischemic injury and other critical neurologic illnesses.

I. **Pathophysiology.** The effects of elective operations, trauma, and critical illness activate the neural and endocrine systems. The increase in sympathetic outflow leads to lipolysis, proteolysis, and decreased glucose uptake due to the antagonism of insulin by growth hormone and epinephrine. Because of this sympathetic surge, energy expenditure, tissue catabolism, and mobilization of protein, fat, and carbohydrate are increased. Other effects include hyperglycemia, poor wound healing, decreased serum proteins, and depressed immune function.

After the neurologic injury this hyperdynamic state leads to increased oxygen consumption and calorie requirements. Recent studies using indirect calorimetry demonstrate that severely head-injured patients are hypermetabolic and hypercatabolic. This has been shown in patients treated both with and without steroids. In addition, there is also delayed gastric emptying, bacterial translocation, and altered vascular permeability leading to intestinal edema and malabsorption.

II. **Nutritional assessment.** Delivery of appropriate metabolic support begins with the assessment of nutritional status. It is important to identify patients who present with subtle signs of deficiencies in caloric, protein, vitamin, or trace metal intake. These patients should be considered for earlier and more aggressive support.

   A. **History.** In most cases, a history of recent unintentional weight loss raises the possibility of malnutrition. Other diseases such as renal failure might suggest loss of amino acids, vitamins, and trace metals during dialysis. Patients with cancer may have deficiencies due either to the underlying disease or to chemotherapy (e.g., methotrexate).

   B. **Physical examination.** Caloric intake can be assessed by the amount of fat in the extremities, buttocks, and buccal fat pad. Protein can be evaluated from the bulk and strength of extremity muscles and the temporal muscle. Vitamin deficiencies may be manifested as changes in skin texture, cheilosis, glossitis, change in quality and texture of hair, or loss of vibration and position sense.

C. **Anthropometrics.** Measurements are used to estimate the stores of body fat and protein. Body fat is approximated by the thickness of the triceps skin fold (TSF) and protein is estimated by the midarm muscle circumference (MAMC).

$$MAMC = midarm\ circumference - fat$$
$$= midarm\ circumference - (0.314 \times TSF)$$

These data are then compared with normal values to determine nutritional status. Two assumptions that are made but might not be correct are that body fat is uniformly distributed and that population standards apply to the critically ill. In fact, anthropometric measurements are generally invalid in the critically ill patient due to anasarca.

D. **Biochemical measurements.** A variety of biochemical and metabolic measurements have been studied as potential indices of nutritional status. Although many of these tests are of significant value in assessing stable patients scheduled for elective surgery or patients well on the way to recovery, their applicability to critically ill patients is questionable. Trends between the same patient's measurements on different days can be used if other factors are relatively stable.

1. **Plasma proteins.** Plasma protein levels are a reflection of nutritional status because levels are dependent on rates of hepatic synthesis, which is dependent on substrate levels. Unfortunately, a decrease in level is not specific, since biological half-life, the catabolic rate, and a variety of nonnutritional factors can alter plasma protein levels. For example, expansion of the extracellular fluid compartment will result in a reduction in albumin concentration. In addition, some serum protein levels decrease promptly in response to trauma, sepsis, or severe illness as a result of fluid shifts, alterations in capillary permeability, and changes in rates of synthesis and degradation. Liver disease, nephrotic syndrome, eclampsia, and protein-losing enteropathies are additional causes of hypoproteinemia.

   a. **Albumin** has a half-life of approximately 18 days. It is the most common test used for the diagnosis of protein calorie undernutrition, but depending on albumin values alone it can lead to delays in treating nutritional deficits. Plasma levels can be maintained for a long time due to the long half-life. In critical illness, albumin levels may also remain low until the inflammatory response remits despite adequate nutritional intake.

b. Transferrin has a half-life of approximately 8 days and therefore levels more accurately reflect changing nutritional status. Iron deficiency, pregnancy, and hypoxia stimulate transferrin synthesis whereas chronic infection, sepsis, and iron overload decrease transferrin levels.

c. Thyroxine-binding prealbumin and retinol-binding protein have a half-life of 2 to 3 days and 8 to 12 hours, respectively. These are much more sensitive to short-term alterations in protein and total calorie intake, and low levels can return to normal after only 3 days of adequate nutritional support. Unfortunately, many nonnutritional factors can influence these levels as well. Infection and trauma depress prealbumin levels. Stress and vitamin A deficiency lead to low retinol-binding protein concentration and renal failure can lead to an erroneously elevated level of retinol-binding protein.

2. Immunologic functions. Total lymphocyte count (TLC) and reactivity to skin test antigens are immunologic functions that can be used to assess nutritional status, but they are not routinely used in critically ill patients. Any stressful situation and especially any disease process that requires a stay in the intensive care unit (ICU) can depress cellular immunity, leading to a nonspecific test result.

III. Estimation of energy requirements. Since all the prior tests measure nutritional status indirectly, other more sensitive and specific techniques have been developed.

A. Predictive equations

1. Harris-Benedict equation. The resting energy expenditure (REE) is the energy requirement at rest and can be estimated using the Harris-Benedict equation.

Women: REE (kcal/day) = $65 + 9.6W + 1.8H - 4.7A$

Men: REE (kcal/day) = $66 + 13.7W + 5H - 6.8A$

where W = actual body weight (ABW) in kilograms or ideal body weight (IBW) in kilograms if the patient is edematous, H is height in centimeters, and A is age in years. If the patient is obese, then an adjusted IBW should be used:

Adjusted IBW = IBW + 0.25 (ABW − IBW)

2. Adjustments to resting energy expenditure. Energy expenditure (EE) can vary greatly from daily resting energy requirement in active sub-

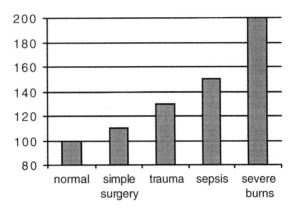

Fig. 24-1.   Energy expenditure as a percentage above normal in several disease states.

jects. Brain injury induces a hyperdynamic state; and elevated energy expenditure levels are usually associated with total body surface area burns of 20% to 40%. Figure 24-1 shows the energy expenditure as percent above normal in several disease states. A common practice is to adjust the estimated REE for the hypermetabolism that characterizes critically ill patients. Usual correction factors are:

Fever: REE × 1.1 (for each degree Celsius above normal)

Mild stress: REE × 1.2–1.3

Moderate stress: REE × 1.4–1.5

Severe stress: REE × 1.6–1.8

B. **Indirect calorimetry.** Indirect calorimetry relies on measurement of oxygen consumption (VO_2) and the production of carbon dioxide (VCO_2). The oxygen consumed in a given period of time is the amount required for oxidation of carbohydrate, fat, and protein. Simultaneously, carbon dioxide is produced from the oxidation of carbohydrate, fat, and protein. If the patient inspires a known concentration of oxygen and carbon dioxide, measurement of VO_2 and VCO_2 can be used to calculate the REE. Usually measurements taken over a minimum period of 20 to 30 minutes generate better baseline values. To account for sedation, ICU activity, dietary-induced thermogenesis, anabolism, and work of breathing, an extra percentage is added to the measured EE. Examples of usual correction factors are:
Thermogenesis: 5% to 10%
ICU activity: 10%

Anabolism: 5% to 10%
Sedation: 0 to 30%

IV. **Estimation of protein requirements.** The daily protein requirements are usually estimated first and measured later.

A. **Predictive equations.** The goal of protein supplementation is to decrease the degree of loss of lean body mass, since there are no protein stores in the body. Approximate protein requirements can be estimated based on patient weight, degree of illness, and organ system failure. High-dose steroids, which are often given to the patients in a neurologic ICU, will also increase protein requirements.

Normal protein requirement: 0.8 to 1.0 g protein/kg/day

Mild stress requirements: 1.0 to 1.2 g protein/kg/day

Moderate stress requirements: 1.2 to 1.4 g protein/kg/day

Severe stress requirements: 1.4 to 1.6 g protein/kg/day

Patients with renal failure on hemodialysis: 1.2 g protein/kg/day

Patients with encephalopathy: 0.8 g protein/kg/day

For the head injury patient, studies of patients receiving 1 to 1.5 g protein/kg/day have still reported negative nitrogen balances. Current recommendations are to provide 2 g protein/kg/day if renal function is normal and reassess the nitrogen balance in a few days.

B. **Nitrogen balance.** Nitrogen balance is used to assess the adequacy of caloric and/or protein intake and whether the anabolic state has been achieved in response to nutritional therapy.

Nitrogen balance equals nitrogen intake minus nitrogen output. Total nitrogen output equals urine urea nitrogen from a 24-hour urine collection and 2 to 4 g/day of nonurinary losses. In the critically ill, this may be up to 6 g/day due to increased fecal nitrogen loss from diarrhea, blood loss, or increased mucosal sloughing. Because protein is 16% nitrogen, each gram of urinary nitrogen (UN) represents 6.25 g of degraded protein.

$$\text{Nitrogen balance} = \text{nitrogen intake} - \text{nitrogen output}$$

$$\text{Nitrogen balance} = (\text{protein intake}/6.25) - (\text{urine urea nitrogen} + 2 \text{ or } 4)$$

Nitrogen balance measurements might not be reliable in patients with renal and hepatic failure due to altered protein synthesis and clearance. For renal failure, the creatinine clearance must be greater than 50 mL/minute for a valid result.

V. Specific nutrients

A. **Carbohydrates.** As long as adequate energy and protein are provided in the diet there is no specific requirement for dietary carbohydrate, but current recommendations are to provide 50% to 60% of total calories as carbohydrates. Much of this is used by the central nervous system, which relies on glucose as its primary fuel source.

B. **Fat.** The goals of lipid supplementation include providing for essential fatty acids, promoting nitrogen sparing, and offering a balanced approach to fulfilling energy requirements. Increased fat decreases the incidence of hepatic steatosis and the production of carbon dioxide from a high-carbohydrate diet. Lipid oxidation as an energy source is increased in the critically ill patient, so recommendations suggest that 30% to 40% of the total calories be provided as lipid.

C. **Protein.** The goal of protein supplementation is to provide substrate for cellular protein synthesis and the maintenance of lean body mass. Protein requirements increase if there are excessive losses from the GI tract, skin, or draining wounds. It is often difficult to achieve positive balance in critically ill patients, but effort should be made to minimize negative nitrogen balance.

D. **Vitamins.** Vitamins are involved in metabolism, wound healing, and immune function. They are essential and cannot be synthesized by the body. There are 12 essential vitamins that should be supplied daily and they are divided into fat- and water-soluble. Recommended dietary allowances of vitamins are listed in Table 24-1.

E. **Trace elements.** There are nine essential trace elements. Deficiencies in these can lead to problems in several organ systems such as insulin resistance, myopathy, increased susceptibility to infections, or pancytopenia. Recommended dietary allowances of trace elements are listed in Table 24-2.

In patients with renal failure, zinc and chromium

Table 24-1.   Recommended dietary allowance of vitamins for a healthy 25- to 50-year-old man

Vitamin	Amount	Vitamin	Amount
Vitamin A	1000 μg	Vitamin D	5 μg
Vitamin E	10 mg	Vitamin K	80 μg
Vitamin C	60 mg	Thiamine	1.5 mg
Riboflavin	1.7 mg	Niacin	19 mg
Vitamin B_6	2 mg	Folate	200 μg
Vitamin B_{12}	2 μg		

Table 24-2. Recommended dietary allowance of trace elements for a healthy 25- to 50-year-old man

Element	Oral	Intravenous
Zinc	10–15 mg	2.5–4.0 mg
Chromium	50–290 μg	10–15 μg
Copper	1.2–3 mg	0.5–1.5 mg
Manganese	0.7–5 mg	0.15–0.8 mg
Selenium	50–200 μg	40–120 μg
Molybdenum		200 μg

should be reduced or omitted because they are excreted in the urine. Similarly, when biliary tract obstruction is present, intake of copper and manganese should be reduced or omitted because they are excreted primarily in the bile.

Decreased serum zinc levels and increased urinary zinc losses have been reported after head injury, although the mechanism and clinical significance are unknown. No other specific changes in vitamin and mineral metabolism after neurologic injury have been identified.

VI. **Timing and route of feeding.** Although some patients can safely handle protein and calorie deprivation for several days, nutritional support should not be delayed in critically ill patients who are not expected to tolerate oral intake for a prolonged period. Nutritional support should also not be delayed in patients who will have massive calorie requirements from burns, sepsis, trauma, or head injury. The decision as to which route (enteral or parenteral) should be used involves an assessment of the functional capacity of the gut. It is important to remember that enteral and parenteral feeding are not mutually exclusive and combinations are often appropriate. Each has specific advantages and complications.

A. **Enteral feeding.** If the GI tract is functional, then enteral feeding is preferred because it is easier, safer, and less expensive. Auscultation of the abdomen for bowel sounds can lead to false signs of bowel function. The absence of bowel sounds does not mean the absence of bowel function. If there is no air present there will be no bowel sounds but the small bowel will likely still have peristalsis and absorptive function. Contraindications for the use of tube feedings include ileus or obstruction, or the need for total bowel rest. Studies in animals have shown that villus atrophy and increased intestinal permeability and bacterial translocation occur after parental nutrition and gut disuse. Although this has yet to be shown in humans, it has been extrapolated from clinical cases where bacteria of the gut region have been found in critically ill patients with no clear focus of abdominal infection.

1. **Types of formulas.** Selection of an enteral formula should be based on the patient's digestive capacity and specific nutritional needs. Table 24-3 lists some enteral formulas and their nutritional components.

   a. **Polymeric** contains intact nutrients and requires normal digestion and absorption.

   b. **Fiber-enriched** is frequently used in patients experiencing diarrhea or constipation.

   c. **Calorically dense** is used in patients with cardiac, renal, or hepatic failure and when fluid restriction is required.

   d. **Elemental** contains one or more partially digested macronutrients and is used in patients with compromised GI function.

   e. **Modular** is composed of individual nutrient modules to produce a formula customized to meet a patient's specific needs. They can also be used to modify a preexisting commercial formula to add caloric and/or protein density.

2. **Routes of enteral feeding**

   a. **Gastric.** Gastric feeding can be established via a feeding tube from the nose or can be surgically obtained from a gastrostomy tube. The method takes advantage of the reservoir capacity of the stomach but many patients, especially those with elevated intracranial pressure, might not tolerate this due to decreased gag reflex, delayed gastric emptying, and/or gastric atony.

   b. **Duodenal.** The proposed advantage is that there is reduced risk for reflux and aspiration, but unfortunately there is no evidence to support this hypothesis. Patients can still aspirate even with jejunal feeds. Feedings given via this route must be as continuous infusions since large boluses are not tolerated.

3. **Initiation and advancement.** Isotonic solutions can be started slowly at full strength and then the rate advanced every 8 hours as tolerated until the goal rate is achieved. Hypertonic solutions should be diluted to isotonicity and concentration should be advanced to full strength before the infusion rate is increased.

4. **Complications**

   a. **Mechanical.** Misplaced nasal feeding tubes might end up in the bronchus or in the brain in patients with cribriform plate fractures. There is also a higher incidence of epistaxis and sinusitis because the tube passes through the nares.

Table 24-3. Enteral formulas and their components

Product	Formula type	kcal/mL	mosmol	Composition per liter (g) Protein	Fat	CHO
Osmolite	Polymeric	1.06	300	37	38	145
Osmolite HN Plus		1.2	360	56	39	158
Jevity	Fiber-enriched	1.06	300	44	36	151
Jevity Plus		1.2	450	56	39	175
Glucerna		1	375	42	56	94
Two Cal HN	Calorically dense	2	690	84	91	217
Peptamen	Peptide-based (semielemental)	1	270	40	39	127
Peptamen VHP		1	300	62	39	104
Crucial		1.5	490	94	68	135
Vivonex Plus	Elemental	1	650	45	6.7	189

CHO, carbohydrate.

      b. **Gastrointestinal.** Nausea and vomiting might occur due to postinjury ileus and gastric atony. Diarrhea might be a problem due to volume of administration, concentration, and osmolarity of tube feeds; presence of lactose, fat, or gluten; low residue; or bacterial contamination.

      c. **Pulmonary.** Pulmonary aspiration is probably the most common serious, potentially fatal complication of enteral nutrition. Reported incidence is highly variable (0 to 95%) depending on the population of patients studied and the definition of aspiration, since chemical evidence of aspiration is more common than clinically diagnosed aspiration pneumonia. The presence of tube feeds in the pulmonary secretions can be detected by checking for glucose or adding food coloring to the feeds and checking the secretions for a color change.

      d. **Metabolic.** Hyperosmolarity or volume overload must be carefully monitored. Electrolyte imbalance, e.g., hyponatremia, is common, especially in head injury patients who are at risk for syndrome of inappropriate antidiuretic hormone secretion or diabetes insipidus. Hypophosphatemia, hypokalemia, and hypomagnesemia can be common during refeeding.

B. **Parenteral feeding.** Total parenteral nutrition (TPN) should be initiated when gut failure is demonstrated.

    1. **Parenteral solutions.** There are three elemental nutrients in parenteral nutrition:

      a. **Dextrose** is available in concentrations ranging from 10% to 70%. The higher the dextrose percentage, the higher the osmolarity and the greater the need for central access.

      b. **Amino acids** provide for protein requirement.

      c. **Fat emulsions** are rich in linoleic acid. The infusions are given over several hours. Infusion rates should be adjusted for patients receiving propofol for sedation. Propofol is in a fat emulsion and provides the equivalent of 1.1 kcal/mL of fat calories.

      d. **Additives** such as electrolytes, vitamins, and trace elements are added directly to the dextrose and amino acid infusion.

    2. **Routes of parenteral feeding.** Intravenous calories can be given peripherally or centrally.

      a. **Peripheral access** should be used only for short-term nutritional support. The hyperosmolarity and low pH of TPN predispose small veins to thrombophlebitis. It is also difficult to provide the necessary caloric requirements via this route due to the limitations imposed by dextrose and amino acid concentrations. Long peripheral lines that extend into a central vein can be used as a central line and do not have the same limitations from dextrose and amino acid concentrations.

b. **Central access** should be used when longer periods of parenteral feeding are necessary or the patient is seriously ill.

3. **Initiation and advancement.** Parenteral nutrition is usually started at a slow rate and then the infusion rate is advanced every 12 to 24 hours until the goal rate is achieved. When discontinuing the infusion, the rate should be tapered so that hypoglycemia does not result from the increase in insulin production stimulated by the parenteral nutrition.

4. **Complications**

a. **Mechanical.** Significant venous thrombosis requires removal of the catheter and heparinization. This can usually be diagnosed by ultrasound or injection of radiopaque contrast. Catheter infections must always be suspected, and meticulous catheter care and a high index of suspicion are necessary.

b. **Gastrointestinal.** Elevated transaminases are common while starting TPN but they should not persist for long. Fatty liver might develop due to excess carbohydrates or total calories in the diet. Cholelithiasis or gallbladder sludge might be secondary to changes in bile composition as well as decreased frequency of gallbladder contractions. These usually resolve once enteral alimentation is initiated.

c. **Metabolic.** Elevations in glucose can occur early on from relative insulin resistance and might require an insulin infusion. Hypercapnia can result from refeeding a malnourished patient who cannot adequately increase minute ventilation. Carbon dioxide production may be reduced by decreasing the daily calories or replacing dextrose with fat. Any electrolyte abnormality can occur, so daily adjustments must be made in conjunction with the laboratory results. Suggested laboratory monitoring guidelines are listed in Table 24-4. The most common vitamin deficiency is that of vitamin K, which is not contained in the multivitamin preparations.

VII. **Future directions.** Because the response to injury is characterized by greatly increased energy demands and

Table 24-4. Suggested monitoring guidelines for enteral and parental nutrition

Schedule	Enteral	Parenteral
Baseline	Electrolytes, BUN, Cr, Ca, Mg, PO$_4$, glucose, albumin	Electrolytes, BUN, Cr, Ca, Mg, PO$_4$, glucose, liver function tests, triglycerides, cholesterol, albumin
Daily	Intake and output, weight	Intake and output, weight
Daily until stable; then 2–3 times/ week	Electrolytes, BUN, Cr, glucose	Electrolytes, BUN, Cr, glucose
Every other day until stable; then 1–2 times/ week	Ca, Mg, PO$_4$	Ca, Mg, PO$_4$
Every 10–14 days	Albumin	Liver function tests, albumin, triglycerides
Weekly	PT, prealbumin	PT, prealbumin

BUN, blood urea nitrogen; PT, prothrombin time.

clinical malnutrition, appropriate nutritional support might prevent the multisystem organ failure that often occurs in the critically ill. The gut is now being seen as an important metabolic organ, with a critical need for certain substrates. Clinical trials are being conducted to evaluate diets enriched with immunomodulatory components. Although use of these components has been advocated, their benefits remain controversial for now.

  A. **Glutamine.** The primary fuel for the intestine, glutamine is important in maintaining intestinal structure and function, preventing mucosal atrophy during starvation, decreasing bacterial translocation, and stimulating the intestinal immune system in sepsis and stress. Glutamine might also decrease intestinal injury during ischemia by preserving gut glutathione levels.

  B. **Arginine.** Arginine improves wound healing, stimulates immune function by increasing production of natural killer and helper T cells, and enhances intestinal absorption and proliferation. Arginine is also responsible for the synthesis of nitric oxide, which maintains the integrity of microvascular structure in the gut after injury.

  C. **Omega 3 Fatty acids.** The omega 6 fatty acids have been shown to decrease immune response by generating degradation products that suppress T-cell and macrophage activity. Replacement of dietary omega

6 fatty acids with omega 3 fatty acids might down-regulate several aspects of the inflammatory response and thereby improve immune function. There have been a few reports that omega 3 fatty acids may impair wound healing and so balance should be obtained between the two fatty acids.

D. Dietary nucleotides. Dietary nucleotides are important for intestinal structure and function. In animals, supplementation of dietary nucleotides in TPN diminishes the intestinal mucosal atrophy. Ribonucleic acid (RNA) nucleotides have also been shown to stimulate the immune system by promoting the development of T lymphocytes.

E. Growth hormone. In the critically ill, growth hormone has beneficial anabolic effects. It mobilizes fat stores as an energy source and enhances whole-body protein stores in trauma patients. It has been shown to increase total lymphocyte count and serum albumin and transferrin levels. It also enhances intestinal function directly by binding to growth hormone receptors in the gut, and indirectly by stimulation of insulin-like growth factor.

F. Anabolic steroids. Anabolic steroids are sometimes used as a replacement for growth hormone because of their beneficial effect on the deposition of lean tissue. They lead to less hyperglycemia than growth hormone and also cost substantially less.

ACKNOWLEDGMENT

The author acknowledges the assistance of Annette Stralovich, RD, CNSD in the preparation of this manuscript.

SUGGESTED READINGS

Baudowin S, Evans T. Nutrition in the critically ill. In: Hall J, Schmidt G, Wod L, eds. *Principles of critical care,* 2nd ed. New York: McGraw-Hill, 1998:205–220.

Souba W. Nutritional support. *N Engl J Med* 1997;336(1):41.

Thompson J. The intestinal response to critical illness. *Am J Gastroenterol* 1995;90(2):190.

Twyman D. Nutritional management of the critically ill neurologic patient. *Crit Care Clin* 1997;13(1):39.

Weekes E, Elia M. Observations on the patterns of 24-hour energy expenditure changes in body composition and gastric emptying in head-injured patients receiving nasogastric tube feeding (comments). *J Parent Ent Nutr* 1996;20(1):31.

25

Head Injury

Audrée A. Bendo

Head injuries are a significant cause of morbidity and mortality. An estimated 500,000 persons in the United States sustain severe head injuries each year. Both nonoperative and postoperative head-injured patients will require critical care management. In the critical care unit (CCU), the main objectives are to optimize recovery from primary brain injury and to prevent secondary injury. This requires the provision of optimal systemic support for cerebral energy metabolism and cerebral perfusion pressure (CPP) and normalization of intracranial pressure (ICP) for injured brain.

Secondary brain injury represents complicating processes initiated by the primary injury, such as ischemia, brain swelling and edema, intracranial hemorrhage, intracranial hypertension, and herniation. Prompt recognition and treatment of systemic complications (Table 25-1) that aggravate the initial injury and contribute to secondary injury are essential to the successful management of head injury. An outcome study using data from the Traumatic Coma Data Bank (Table 25-2) revealed that hypotension after head injury is associated with greater than 70% morbidity and mortality. The combination of hypoxia and hypotension is significantly more detrimental than hypotension alone; more than 90% of these patients die or are severely disabled.

I. **Initial presentation and neurologic assessment**
   A. **Admission evaluation**
      1. The following conditions require evaluation and treatment as necessary:
         a. Adequacy of gas exchange.
         b. Associated injuries and hemodynamic status.
         c. Presence of intracranial problems, e.g., increased ICP, hematoma, hydrocephalus, massive edema.
         d. Metabolic abnormalities.
         e. Concurrent medical problems and chronic medications.
      2. Initial diagnostic procedures include:
         a. Computed tomography (CT) scan and cervical spine radiographs.
         b. Examination of airway and chest, arterial blood gases, chest radiograph, and electrocardiogram.
         c. Other studies as indicated by history and examination to diagnose concurrent injuries, e.g., peritoneal lavage, long bone radiographs.
         d. Measurement of electrolytes, hematocrit, hemoglobin, prothrombin time (PT), partial thromboplastin time (PTT), and platelets.

Table 25-1. Systemic complications contributing to secondary injury

Minutes to hours after initial impact:
    Hypoxia   Anemia
    Hypercarbia   Hyperglycemia
    Hypotension
Hours to days after initial impact:
    Seizures   Electrolyte disturbances
    Infection/sepsis   Coagulation abnormalities
    Hyperthermia

B. **Neurologic assessment** forms the basis for determining the severity of injury, the need for immediate therapeutic interventions, and the selection of diagnostic studies. The examination includes determination of the Glasgow Coma Scale (GCS) score, and complete neurologic assessment and evaluation of CT scan and cervical spine radiographs. Baseline neurologic examination must be followed by repetitive exams at regular intervals to determine neurologic stability, improvement, or deterioration.

  1. The GCS provides a quantitative measure of neurologic injury with good interevaluator agreement and an estimate of progress and prognosis. It defines neurologic impairment in terms of eye open-

Table 25-2. Impact of hypoxia and/or hypotension[a] on outcome after severe head injury (GCS $\leq$ 8)

Secondary Insults	Number of Patients	Outcome Percentage		
		Good or Moderate	Severe or Vegetative	Dead
Total	699	43	21	37
Neither	456	51	22	27
Hypoxia	78	45	22	33
Hypotension	113	26	14	60
Both	52	6	19	75

GCS, Glasgow Coma Scale; SBP, Systolic blood pressure.
Hypoxia = PaO_2 < 60 mm Hg; hypotension = SBP < 90 mm Hg.
[a] At time of hospital arrival.
Data adapted from the Traumatic Coma Data Bank. Chesnut RM, Marshall LF, et al. *J. Trauma* 1993; 34:216–222.

Table 25-3.   Glasgow Coma Scale

Eye opening:	Spontaneous	4
	To verbal command	3
	To pain	2
	None	1
Best verbal response:	Oriented, conversing	5
	Disoriented, conversing	4
	Inappropriate words	3
	Incomprehensible sounds	2
	None	1
Best motor response:	Obeys verbal commands	6
	Localizes pain	5
	Flexion/withdrawal	4
	Flexion/abnormal (decorticate)	3
	Extension (decerebrate)	2
	None	1
	Total:	3–15

ing and verbal and motor responses (Table 25-3). The total score is 15 with severe head injury defined as less than or equal to 8, persisting for 6 or more hours; moderate injury, 9 to 12; and mild injury, 13 to 15.

2. General neurologic evaluation should include:
   a. Level of consciousness (awake, lethargic, stuporous, comatose);
   b. Mental status examination (orientation, insight, memory, general information, behavior, capacity);
   c. Pupillary assessment (size, equality, light reactivity);
   d. Eye movements [eye position, oculocephalic (doll's eyes) reflex];
   e. Observation for motor symmetry;
   f. Corneal and gag responses, response to noxious stimulus, and Babinski reflex, when indicated.

3. **Signs and symptoms of increased ICP (Table 25-4). Syndrome of transtentorial herniation**–altered mental status, unilateral pupillary dilatation, contralateral hemiparesis, hemiplegia—is considered diagnostic of hemispheric mass lesion requiring immediate therapy.

II. **Routine critical care management.** Primary considerations include the following: control of gas exchange, ICP, CPP [mean arterial pressure (MAP) minus ICP], temperature, glucose, and electrolytes.
   A. **Airway management/control of gas exchange**
      1. **Airway management.** Important neurosurgical considerations are concurrent airway and cervical spine injury, hemodynamic status, level of con-

**Table 25-4.   Signs and symptoms
of increased intracranial pressure**

Headache
Nausea, vomiting
Papilledema
Unilateral pupillary dilatation
Oculomotor or abducens palsy
Depressed level of consciousness
Irregular breathing
Midline shift (0.5 cm) or encroachment of expanding brain on
  cerebral ventricles (CT or MRI)

CT, computed tomography; MRI, magnetic resonance imaging.

sciousness, increased ICP, presumed full stomach, and adequacy of gas exchange. Endotracheal intubation is required according to routine indications for respiratory failure (pulmonary complications, thoracoabdominal injury, shock) and for neurosurgical considerations (impaired gag reflex, increased ICP, respiratory dysrhythmias). For a GCS score of 8 or less, patients need intubation with respiratory support for neurosurgical considerations.

2. **Gas exchange**
   a. **Oxygenation** is continuously monitored with pulse oximetry and intermittent blood gas analysis, when indicated. Causes of **hypoxia** include aspiration, atelectasis, decreased cardiac output, pneumothorax, neurogenic pulmonary edema, lung contusion, fluid overload, embolism, and mechanical problems with the endotracheal tube. Initial treatment is to increase the fraction of inspired oxygen (FiO_2). If adequate oxygenation is not achieved with controlled ventilation and FiO_2 0.55 or less, PEEP (positive end-expiratory pressure) is added. The PEEP at 5 to 10 cm H_2O does not adversely affect ICP. A PEEP of greater than 10 cm H_2O might increase ICP and decrease MAP and CPP. Therefore, the effect of PEEP on ICP, MAP, and CPP must be monitored.
   b. During controlled ventilation, arterial CO_2 is maintained in the lower range of normal ($PaCO_2$ 30 to 35 mm Hg) to avoid inducing or exacerbating cerebral ischemia. Temporary hyperventilation ($PaCO_2$ 25 to 30 mm Hg) is instituted for control of intracranial hypertension and/or herniation syndrome. The duration of effectiveness of hyperventilation for lowering ICP may be as short as 4 to 6 hours.

Once established, the degree of hyperventilation should be intermittently confirmed using blood gas analysis.

B. Intracranial hypertension

1. There are two types of intracranial hypertension categorized according to cerebral blood flow (CBF) as **hyperemic** or **oligemic.**

2. Untreated intracranial hypertension (ICP more than 20 mm Hg) can lead to global cerebral ischemia (CPP = MAP − ICP) and brain herniation.

3. **ICP monitoring**

   a. After CT imaging and any necessary surgical procedures, an **ICP monitor** is inserted. Treatment is directed to controlling ICP and maintaining CPP more than or equal to 70 mm Hg (Table 25-5).

   b. Techniques used to monitor ICP include ventricular catheters, subdural-subarachnoid bolts or catheters, epidural transducers, and intraparenchymal fiberoptic devices.

   c. **An external ventricular drain** (EVD, ventriculostomy) measures ICP reliably and allows therapeutic cerebrospinal fluid (CSF) drainage. Such drains require meticulous attention to sterility and to their position relative to the patient. The EVD is the standard method for monitoring ICP.

4. **Treatment (Table 25-5)**

   a. First **normalize physiologic variables**—adequate oxygenation and ventilation ($PaCO_2$ 30 to 35 mm Hg), euvolemia, cardiovascular stability.

   b. Elevate the head of the bed 15° to 30°. Head elevation lowers ICP by 3 to 5 mm Hg when the patient is euvolemic.

   c. Sedation and pharmacologic paralysis. Sedation is effective in reducing intracranial hypertension. The choice of agents is left to the practitioner. Any agent with potential hypotensive side effects must be administered carefully.

   Neuromuscular blockade is administered to patients exhibiting motor activity not adequately controlled by sedation. Patients who are confused, agitated, or exhibiting motor posturing and who require complete absence of motor activity or who are "bucking" the ventilator are candidates for these drugs.

   d. When a ventriculostomy has been employed, **CSF drainage** should be the first ICP-specific reducing maneuver. When the catheter is open for drainage, ICP measurement is unreliable. Therefore, drainage should be intermittent and treatment based on pressures

**Table 25-5.   Severe head injury—
treatment of intracranial hypertension**

- Insert ICP monitor
- Maintain CPP > 70 mm Hg
- Intracranial hypertension

First-tier therapy:
Ventricular drainage (if available)
Mannitol 0.25 to 1 g/kg i.v. (may repeat if serum osmolarity
    <320 mosmol/L and patient euvolemic)
Hyperventilation to $PaCO_2$ 30 to 35 mm Hg

Second-tier therapy:
Hyperventilation to $PaCO_2$ < 30 mm Hg (SjO_2, $AVDO_2$ and/or
    CBF monitoring recommended)
High-dose barbiturate therapy
Consider hypothermia
Consider hypertensive therapy
Consider decompressive craniectomy

ICP, intracranial pressure; CPP, cerebral perfusion pressure; SjO_2, jugular bulb oxyhemoglobin saturation; $AVDO_2$, arteriovenous difference in oxygen content; CBF, cerebral blood flow.
Adapted from 1995 Brain Trauma Foundation. Guidelines for the management of severe head injury. *J Neurotrauma* 1996;13:641.

measured when the system is closed. Major complications of CSF drainage are infection, hemorrhage, and iatrogenic damage from errant catheter.

e. **Diuresis.** Rapid brain dehydration and decrease in ICP can be produced by administering an **osmotic diuretic** (mannitol, 0.25 to 1 g/kg i.v., begins to work within 10 to 15 minutes and lasts about 2 hours) or a **loop diuretic** (furosemide, 0.5 to 1 mg/kg i.v. alone or 0.15 to 0.3 mg/kg i.v. in combination with mannitol).

   (1) Because mannitol might initially increase ICP (mannitol-induced vasodilatation), it should be administered slowly (over 10 minutes or longer). A mannitol-induced increase in intravascular volume might precipitate left ventricular failure in patients with preexisting cardiovascular disease. Furosemide may be a better agent for ICP reduction in patients with impaired cardiac reserve.

   (2) Prolonged use of mannitol might produce dehydration, electrolyte disturbances, hyperosmolarity, and impaired renal function. During diuresis, the patient must remain euvolemic, with serum osmolarity less than 320 mosmol/L,

and normal serum electrolyte concentrations. Then mannitol administration may be repeated as necessary for ICP control.

(3) Combined mannitol and furosemide diuresis is more effective than mannitol alone but can produce more severe dehydration and electrolyte imbalance.

(4) For control of intracranial hypertension, diuresis is recommended before hyperventilation.

f. **Hyperventilation** of the patient's lungs to maintain a PaCO$_2$ of 25 to 30 mm Hg (every mm Hg decrease below 40 mm Hg decreases CBF by 1 to 2 mL/100 g/minute, but this effect might last for only 4 to 6 hours depending on the pH of the CSF) is initiated when intracranial hypertension is refractory to "conventional therapy" (see above).

To detect cerebral ischemia during hyperventilation, monitoring of jugular bulb oxygen saturation, CSF lactate, CBF, or cerebral oxygen consumption is recommended (Table 25-6).

g. **High-dose barbiturate therapy** can be effective in treating refractory intracranial hypertension.

(1) The most significant complication is cardiac depression and instability. Therefore intensive hemodynamic monitoring is required. Hypovolemia and hypotension must be avoided.

(2) Barbiturate treatment is begun with a slow intravenous infusion of pentobarbital, 5 to 10 mg/kg over 10 to 30 minutes.

(3) The limits of therapy are determined by the occurrence of burst suppression on **electroencephalographic (EEG) monitoring.** Once burst suppression is achieved, a constant infusion is maintained.

Table 25-6. Measurement of jugular bulb oxyhemoglobin saturation and cerebrospinal fluid lactate

SjO$_2$	CSF Lactate	CBF	Hyperventilation
>75	Normal	↑	Indicated
<50	Normal	↓	Not indicated
Variable	↑	↓	Not indicated

SjO$_2$, jugular bulb oxyhemoglobin saturation; CSF, cerebrospinal fluid; CBF, cerebral blood flow; ↑ increased; ↓ decreased.

(4) Serum barbiturate levels should range between 30 and 50 mg/dL.

   h. Surgical decompressive craniectomy is another treatment option for patients with refractory intracranial hypertension. The most common procedure used for cranial decompression is hemicraniectomy or large unilateral cranial flaps with dural patching.

C. Cerebral perfusion pressure. The therapeutic goal is to maintain CPP (MAP − ICP) at or above 70 mm Hg. If ICP increases to a greater extent than MAP, CPP is reduced and the brain becomes ischemic. Careful maintenance of circulating volume (euvolemia to mild hypervolemia) and the use of pressors and/or inotropes may be required to meet the desired CPP (70 to 110 mm Hg).

1. Measurement of central cardiac filling pressures is required for resuscitation and management of fluid shifts resulting from trauma and/or the use of diuretics.

2. When vasopressors and inotropes are administered, insertion of a pulmonary artery catheter is recommended to optimize cardiac output in parallel with the CPP level, and to measure systemic vascular resistance (SVR) and pulmonary capillary wedge pressures (PCWP). The PCWP should be maintained between 14 and 16 mm Hg with a cardiac index of greater than 3.0 L/minute/m^2 and SVR (systemic vascular resistance) in the normal range.

3. Fluid balance should be tightly controlled to avoid hypovolemia from repeated doses of diuretics. An hourly 1:1 replacement of urine volume and electrolytes is an effective method of avoiding a negative fluid balance.

D. Temperature regulation

1. **Hypothermia** induced to 32°C to 34°C might improve outcome after head injury and has been demonstrated to reduce ICP by decreasing brain metabolism, CBF, CBV, and CSF production. Hypothermia can be induced in the ventilated patient through application of external cooling (hypothermia blankets, ice packs). A centrally measured temperature, e.g., esophageal, tympanic membrane, or nasopharyngeal sensor, must be used to guide temperature management.

2. **Hyperthermia** must be avoided because of potential adverse effects on the injured brain. Antipyretic therapy (acetaminophen, external cooling) should be administered for any temperature elevation. The cause of fever should be sought (cultures obtained, vascular catheters changed) and treated.

E. Glucose and electrolytes

1. **Glucose.** In head-injured patients, hyperglycemia is associated with a poor outcome. The stress

response to head injury increases glucose levels. Hyperglycemia augments ischemic damage by promoting neuronal lactate production, which worsens cellular injury. Blood glucose levels should be monitored and maintained at around 200 mg/dL in hyperglycemic head-injured patients.

2. **Electrolytes** can become abnormal with head injury. The stress response which includes elevated catecholamines, corticotropin, and antidiuretic hormone can cause fluid retention with an excessive retention of water over sodium, causing **hyponatremia.**

   a. **Cerebral salt wasting** may occur with the release of a natriuretic factor that produces loss of sodium in the urine.

   b. The **syndrome of inappropriate antidiuretic hormone secretion** is associated with hyponatremia, serum and extracellular fluid hyposmolality, renal excretion of sodium, urine osmolality greater than serum osmolality, and normal renal and adrenal function.

      (1) The patient develops signs and symptoms of water intoxication (anorexia, nausea, vomiting, irritability, personality changes, and neurologic abnormalities).

      (2) Syndrome of inappropriate antidiuretic hormone secretion usually begins 3 to 15 days after trauma and lasts for no longer than 10 to 15 days with appropriate therapy.

      (3) Treatment includes water restriction with or without hypertonic saline.

   c. **Diabetes insipidus** (DI) can occur after craniofacial trauma and basal skull fracture.

      (1) The clinical presentation includes polyuria, polydipsia, hypernatremia, high serum osmolality, and dilute urine.

      (2) If DI is transient, treatment is based on water replacement. If the patient cannot maintain fluid balance, replacement therapy with either aqueous vasopressin (5 to 10 U i.v. or i.m.) or desmopressin (1 to 4 mg subcutaneously every 6 to 12 hours) is administered.

   d. **Nonketotic hyperosmolar hyperglycemic coma** can occur in these patients because of steroids, prolonged mannitol therapy, hyperosmolar tube feedings, phenytoin, and limited water replacement.

      (1) Diagnostic findings are hyperglycemia, glucosuria, absence of ketosis, plasma

osmolality of greater than 330 mosmol/ L, dehydration, and CNS dysfunction.

(2) Hypovolemia and hypertonicity are the immediate threats to life.

(3) Serum sodium might be high, normal, or low, depending on the state of hydration. Serum potassium is low.

(4) Serial laboratory tests are essential. Once sodium deficits are replaced and blood pressure and urine output are stable, water deficits are replaced with 0.45% saline.

(5) Hyperglycemia responds to small doses of insulin.

III. **Systemic sequelae of head injury.** Systemic effects of head injury are diverse and can complicate its management (Table 25-7). These systemic complications must be diagnosed quickly and treated aggressively to reduce morbidity and mortality.

IV. **Seizure prophylaxis.** Seizures after head injury are categorized as (a) immediate—occurring within 24 hours after injury; (b) delayed early—occurring during the remainder of the first week; and (c) late—occurring more than 1 week after trauma.

   A. Risk factors include a GCS score of less than 10, hematoma, contusion, penetrating injury, early seizures, and depressed skull fracture.

Table 25-7. Systemic sequelae of head injury

Cardiopulmonary:
   Hypotension/shock
   Aspiration
   Pneumonia
   Adult respiratory distress syndrome
   Neurogenic pulmonary edema
   ECG changes
Hematologic:
   Disseminated intravascular coagulation
Endocrinologic:
   Diabetes insipidus
   SIADH
   Cerebral salt wasting
Metabolic:
   NHHC
Gastrointestinal:
   Stress ulcers
   Hemorrhage

ECG, electrocardiogram; SIADH, syndrome of inappropriate antidiuretic hormone secretion; NHHC, nonketotic hyperosmolar hyperglycemic coma.

B.   The administration of prophylactic anticonvulsants is controversial. However, phenytoin is generally administered to patients who are at risk.

SUGGESTED READINGS

Chesnut RM, Marshall LF, Klauber MR, et al. The role of secondary brain injury in determining outcome from severe head injury. *J Trauma* 1993;34:216.

Guidelines for the Management of Severe Head Injury. Brain Trauma Foundation, American Association of Neurological Surgeons, Joint Section on Neurotrauma and Critical Care. *J Neurotrauma* 1996;13:641.

Obrist WD, Langfitt TW, Jaggi JL, et al. Cerebral blood flow and metabolism in comatose patients with acute head injury. Relationship to intracranial hypertension. *J Neurosurg* 1984;61:241.

Muizelaar JP, Marmarou A, Ward JD, et al. Adverse effects of prolonged hyperventilation in patients with severe head injury: a randomized clinical trial. *J Neurosurg* 1991;75:731.

Shiozaki T, Sugimoto H, Taneda M, et al. Effect of mild hypothermia on uncontrollable intracranial hypertension after severe head injury. *J Neurosurg* 1993;79:363.

Marion DW, Penrod LE, Kelsey SF, et al. Treatment of traumatic brain injury with moderate hypothermia. *N Engl J Med* 1997; 336:540.

Subject Index

Subject Index

Page numbers followed by 't' indicate tables; page numbers in *italics* indicate figures.